Complementary and Alternativ
for Child and Adolescent Care

D1761300

*This book is dedicated to my father, Christopher Mantle,
whose translation skills were so sorely
missed during the writing of this book.*

Commissioning Editor: Susan Young
Project Development Editor: Catherine Jackson
Project Manager: Samantha Ross
Designer: George Ajayi

Complementary and Alternative Medicine for Child and Adolescent Care

Fiona Mantle BSc(Hons) RN RHV CertEd RNT
Staff Nurse, The Emergency Department,
John Radcliffe Hospital, Oxford, UK

Foreword by

Anne Casey FRCN RSCN RGN MSc
Editor, Paediatric Nursing,
RCN Publishing Company, Harrow, UK

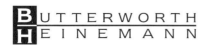
BUTTERWORTH
HEINEMANN

EDINBURGH   LONDON   NEW YORK   OXFORD   PHILADELPHIA   ST LOUIS   SYDNEY   TORONTO   2004

BUTTERWORTH-HEINEMANN
An imprint of Elsevier Science Limited

First published 2004

ISBN 07506 5175 X

British Library Cataloguing in Publication Data
A catalogue record for this book is available from the British Library

Library of Congress Cataloging in Publication Data
A catalog record for this book is available from the Library of Congress

Notice
Medical knowledge is constantly changing. Standard safety precautions must be followed, but as new research and clinical experience broaden our knowledge, changes in treatment and drug therapy may become necessary or appropriate. Readers are advised to check the most current product information provided by the manufacturer of each drug to be administered to verify the recommended dose, the method and duration of administration, and contraindications. It is the responsibility of the practitioner, relying on experience and knowledge of the patient, to determine dosages and the best treatment for each individual patient. Neither the Publisher nor the author assumes any liability for any injury and/or damage to persons or property arising from this publication.

The Publisher

The URLs quoted were correct at the time of going to press, however, information on the internet, including URLs, is subject to constant change.

ELSEVIER SCIENCE your source for books, journals and multimedia in the health sciences
www.elsevierhealth.com

Printed in China

Contents

Foreword   vii

Preface   ix

Acknowledgements   xiii

Section 1   Professional issues   1

Chapter 1   Complementary and alternative medicine   3
Chapter 2   Clinical effectiveness, clinical supervision and legal and professional issues   33

Section 2   0–11 years   47

Chapter 3   Problems related to breathing   49
Chapter 4   Problems related to rest and sleep   70
Chapter 5   Problems related to pain   79
Chapter 6   Problems related to eating and drinking   94
Chapter 7   Problems related to elimination   109
Chapter 8   Problems related to mobility   118
Chapter 9   Problems related to washing and dressing   134

Section 3   11–18 years   147

Chapter 10   Problems with communication   151
Chapter 11   Problems related to sleep   162
Chapter 12   Problems related to expressing sexuality   167
Chapter 13   Problems related to washing and dressing   177
Chapter 14   Problems with eating and drinking   185
Chapter 15   Problems with elimination   192
Chapter 16   Problems related to working and playing   196

Recommended reading   207
Appendix 1   CAM usage client assessment tool   209
Appendix 2   Useful addresses   210
Appendix 3   Useful web sites   214

Index   215

Foreword

In the early 1970s when I trained as a nurse – and I use the word 'trained' intentionally – complementary therapies were known as 'alternative medicine' and were frowned upon in the medically dominated world of nursing. Over the years my feelings about such therapies have been mixed, swinging positively with reports of benefit and negatively with the inevitable stories of bizarre and damaging practices.

Until recently, my attitude reflected that of many professionals: even if a therapy has no real effect on the underlying problem, the patient will feel better for the extra time and attention and therefore it is worthwhile. Provided the therapy is safe and does not interfere with any conventional treatment, it is acceptable. However, there is now a critical mass of evidence in paediatric nursing and other literature that demonstrates the real and lasting benefits of therapies such as reflexology, massage and hypnosis. I suspect I am now at a similar stage in my understanding of complementary and alternative therapies as most nurses: convinced that they have something to offer but with very little understanding of the detail of different therapies and their application in the care of children and young people with specific health problems. This is exactly the gap that this books fills. It clearly locates complementary and alternative therapies in relation to the discipline of nursing and brings together the scattered evidence to inform practitioners, at least to the level where they will feel competent in discussing options with a family and with other professionals. The classification of therapies on the first page of the introduction may be well known to some but for me it was an immediate aid to understanding, giving an early insight into the professional responsibilities so well presented in Chapter 2. For the first time in many years I have read a nursing text that introduces completely new perspectives. For example, the idea that the writer (and the nurse in practice) understands and adopts the 'language of the patient's medical belief system' should be picked up as a challenge for education and practice.

Many of you reading this book will be inspired to learn more and to become competent in the delivery of different forms of therapy. Expansion of the scope of nursing practice into areas that build on philosophies of holism, patient choice and patient experience is eminently desirable. We can, however, learn from our experience of expansion into traditional medical roles and ensure that the same principles are applied: clarity of purpose; consideration of additional resources, education and development needs, accountability, authority and responsibility; evaluation and audit.

The core focus of nursing is human responses to and experience of health problems and health care. Children and young people and their families respond in different ways to illness and injury but many of them will continue to have negative experiences of traditional health care. In the coming years many more will make their preferences known and will choose to explore complementary and alternative therapies, particularly for chronic conditions. Supporting patient decision-making by providing balanced, evidence-based information is a core nursing intervention: this book gives nurses caring for children and young people the basis for exploring options with them and the basis for deciding where complementary and alternative therapies fit into their own practice.

2004   Anne Casey

Preface

There are a number of excellent books on the market addressing the role of complementary and alternative medicine (CAM) in nursing, midwifery and physiotherapy (Rankin-Box 2001, Tiran 2000, Charman, 2000) which review, in general, a range of themes relevant to the discipline. As far as possible I have tried to avoid going over the same ground in this book, however, there will be inevitably some overlap. In addition I have assumed that the reader has a prior level of knowledge covering paediatric, professional and legal issues in nursing. I, therefore, aim to focus this book on the specific issues relating to the use of CAM therapies and in particular to their use in paediatric care. The review is not, and probably could never be, comprehensive, since the diversity of the world of CAM means that any text is unlikely to be comprehensive. I apologise if some readers are disappointed that their particular interests have not been included. However, in an attempt to ensure that the text includes a diversity of approaches I have included not only those CAM therapies for which there is a high standard of scientific evidence and which are supported by the House of Lords Select Committee on Science and Technology (2000), but also other readily available over-the-counter remedies, which parents and children may be using as part of their healthcare options. These have been included because nurses will need to have a working knowledge of the mode of action, safety levels and potential interactions of these interventions when discussing their use in the care of a child. This decision was based on my experience as a health visitor during which time I frequently visited families who routinely used CAM as part of their health care.

The layout of this book is also slightly different from other publications in that most books or articles on CAM for healthcare professionals are therapy-based (Tiran 2000, Rankin-Box 2001). In this text, instead of taking a therapy-centred focus, I have taken a developmental, problem-solving approach and for this reason I have adopted the format of Roper et al's (1985) model of nursing. This format has been chosen because its framework is familiar to British nurses. However, I have to confess that the categories developed by Roper et al have been used, in this instance, as a convenient descriptive and organisational tool and not, in the strictest sense, as a nursing model since I have included the CAM treatment of contributing medical conditions. In addition, not all of Roper's categories have been included since I have subsumed some of them into other sections. For example, in the context of this book, maintaining a safe environment is enshrined in evidence-based practice as well as in the indicators for safety levels within the therapies. Communication is inherent in all nursing interactions, therefore, a separate section has not been used, since a number of therapies involve touch, the most basic form of communication. Similarly, those interventions dealing with problems such as constipation, eating and drinking, and pain can be applied in a wide range of clinical situations including the care of the dying.

The aim of the book is not to turn nurses into CAM experts nor to suggest that they use the therapies or techniques without training, but to highlight the contribution of CAM to the field of paediatric health care so that, if practitioners felt that the therapy or therapies could make a significant difference to the children they are caring for, they may decide either to train in the therapy themselves or be in a position to discuss the potential use of the therapy with patients and carers. They will also be able to indicate if the therapy is safe to use alongside conventional treatments and to guide the parents towards selecting a suitably qualified practitioner. Where possible, research to support the therapy is offered and critically evaluated. However, since research into many of the therapies is limited, other levels of evidence, as discussed by Muir Gray (1997), will be offered.

The book is divided into three sections. Section 1 covers the history of CAM: its re-emergence over the last 50 years, its philosophy and culture and the fusion of nursing and CAM as a holistic, and caring intervention. The role of evidence-based practice is discussed and within this, the particular issues related to CAM research are highlighted. Although this book is not a 'how to' but more of an 'about', advice is offered on the issues relating to implementing CAM into nursing care whether in an advisory capacity or as a hands on intervention.

Section 2 covers 0-11 years and addresses early childhood problems based on the activities of living. It also examines when CAM interventions may be used advantageously. In each chapter there is a description of the problem in general, the conventional approach and then how CAM can help with the main problem or contributing factors. One condition is then used as an example to illustrate the point. For example, in the chapter on problems related to sleeping, general measures using CAM to promote restful sleep are suggested and then a prime cause of insomnia, in this instance pain, is addressed. As an example of where CAM is effective in treating a specific painful condition, headaches and migraine are examined in some depth.

In Section 3 the categories discussed in Section 2 are developed, and, where appropriate, more age-related treatments are described. In addition, problems specific to adolescence, such as acne, are discussed.

Therapies to be included, when age appropriate, are music therapy, reflexology, massage and aromatherapy, homeopathy, hypnosis, herbalism, Alexander technique, Ayurvedic medicine, Traditional Chinese Medicine (TCM) and Anthroposophical medicine. These have been chosen for a number of reasons: they are the therapies most commonly used (by the general public) alongside conventional medicine in nursing care, as an over-the-counter remedy, are accessed by visiting a therapist, or they reflect an approach to health care which is different from standard Western medicine but which may be used by many members of our multicultural society. Increasingly, some of those patients who would normally adhere to the Western medical tradition are turning to these alternative belief systems to seek solutions to problems for which Western medicine has little to offer. The population of Great Britain is 56.3 million of which 3.4 million is made up of ethnic minorities who have brought with them a variety of different cultural patterns. In her review, Boi (2000) emphasises the need for nurses to be aware of their patients' cultural and spiritual beliefs in order to provide effective care. However, little has been written on the need for nurses to understand patients' health belief systems in relation to what is referred to as alternative medicine as opposed to 'lay' health beliefs. Moreover, many of these traditional medical interventions are being practised alongside Western medicine and offer patients a more familiar way of expressing their signs and symptoms. In fact, the charity MIND (1993) has advocated that, when caring for patients from another culture, we should digress from the standard Western diagnosis and adopt the language of the patient's medical belief system. It is for this reason that I have included some of these diverse languages into the text. An understanding of, and a sympathy for, these medical traditions and health belief systems will enhance a nurse's ability to work collaboratively with patients and their families. Of particular importance is the understanding that not only may the description of an illness differ between cultures but that other cultures actually suffer from different conditions, either because a condition is not recognised as a separate pathology or because cultural differences, such as diet and lifestyle, do not provide an appropriate aetiology for the condition to occur. For example, TCM does not recognise diabetes since genetically the Chinese very rarely develop diabetes as their diet and lifestyle mitigate against the development of the condition. When diabetes does develop it is treated under the general rubric of weakness. This will be obvious in the text when it becomes difficult to align Western conditions with other cultural interpretations. The interventions discussed are not intended to replace medical treatment but to indicate where it might have been shown to be of value and could be used by parents or relatives both in hospital and in the community.

Whilst examples of the use of CAM will inevitably be related to one area of child health care, much of what is in the book will be of relevance to all areas of paediatric nursing and I envisage that practitioners will select the relevant information applicable to their particular clinical area as a basis for providing clients and their families with the information to make an informed choice in relation to their health belief system. Cole and Shanley (1998) suggest that CAM offers nurses the opportunity to enhance their nursing care and that it is an area that may offer the best opportunity for developing their scope in professional practice. Although the book is aimed at all practitioners dealing with children, including physiotherapists, occupational therapists, school nurses, health visitors, paediatric nurses in hospitals or the community and nursery nurses, for clarity, the term nurse has been used throughout the book.

Information was obtained by searching the databases MEDLINE, CINAHL, Psycinfo and AMED as well as a manual follow-up of reference lists and biographical sources.

Oxford, 2004   Fiona Mantle

REFERENCES

Boi S 2000 Nurses' experiences in caring for patients from different cultural backgrounds. Nursing Times Research 5(5): 382–389

Charman R 2000 Complementary therapies for physical therapists. Butterworth Heinemann, Oxford

Cole A, Shanley E 1998 Complementary therapies as a means of developing the scope of professional nursing practice. Journal of Advanced Nursing 27: 1171–1176

House of Lords Select Committee on Science and Technology November (2000) Sixth report on complementary and alternative medicine. HMSO, London

MIND 1993 MIND's policy on black and minority ethnic people and mental health. MIND, London

Muir Gray J 1997 Evidence based health care: how to make policy and management decisions. Churchill Livingstone, Edinburgh

Rankin-Box D 2001 The nurse's handbook of complementary therapies: a guide for nurses and the caring professions. Baillière Tindall, London

Roper N, Logan W, Tierney A 1985 The elements of nursing. Churchill Livingstone, Edinburgh

Tiran D 2000 Complementary therapies for pregnancy and childbirth, 2nd edn. Baillière Tindall, Edinburgh

Acknowledgements

Authors are only as good as the libraries they use and my heartfelt thanks go to the excellent and ever helpful staff of the Cairns library at the John Radcliffe Hospital in Oxford for their patient help both with reference searches and obtaining some quite obscure inter-library loans. I am indebted to a number of people who have kindly given their time and expertise, either in person, via telephone conversations, emails or meetings: Denise Tiran for her continual encouragement and support; Jo Code, Head of Studies at Norland College; Vivian Dawson for her help with Traditional Chinese Medicine; and many friends and colleagues at the John Radcliffe Hospital, including: Elizabeth Bowran for her help with Anthroposophical medicine; Karen Webb, infection control nurse; and Sandy Clayton, Senior Nurse Manager Infection Control; Leone Willis, oncology staff nurse, ward 4b. I would also like to thank Anne Taylor, Senior Lecturer, Oxford Brookes University and Annette Dearmun, Principal Lecturer/Specialist Nurse Paediatrics, for their valued comments on the text. My particular thanks go to my sister Andrea Kachellek, staff nurse in the Adolescent Unit of the John Radcliffe Hospital, for her expertise in adolescent care and for patiently re-reading the text as it evolved, but most of all, thanks to my mother, Lilian Mantle, for her continuing support, both domestic and literary, and for endlessly re-reading the text for sense, grammar and punctuation.

Section

1

Professional issues

SECTION CONTENTS

Chapter 1 Complementary and alternative medicine 3

Chapter 2 Clinical effectiveness, clinical supervision and legal and professional issues 33

INTRODUCTION

In a thoughtful article Hodes (2000), following an epiphany with a faith healer in Africa, has suggested that 'there are many rooms in our mansion of medicine and many ways to the truth and that no system of medicine should be denied'.

Chapter 1 of this section establishes just what is meant by complementary and alternative medicine (CAM), the reasons for its popularity and the philosophy behind it. The use of CAM in paediatrics and the nurse's role in this are discussed, focusing on issues of safety. The chapter then goes on to describe the main therapies in use, briefly covering the history, background and mode of action of each one.

In Chapter 2 the theoretical basis for the use of CAM is examined, and a critical appraisal is offered of the evidence base for the clinical effectiveness of CAM therapies. The chapter goes on to highlight the importance of clinical supervision and legal and professional issues.

REFERENCE

Hodes M 2000 Folk medicine deserves our respect. Medical Economics (March 6) 119–123

1 Complementary and alternative medicine

CHAPTER CONTENTS

- **What is complementary and alternative medicine (CAM)?** 3
- **Who uses CAM?** 4
- **Philosophy of CAM** 5
  - *Vitalism* 5
  - *Holism* 6
- **The use of CAM in paediatrics** 8
  - *Role of the nurse* 9
- **Safety issues** 10
- **CAM interventions** 12

Traditional Chinese Medicine (TCM) 12
Anthroposophical medicine 15
Ayurveda 17
Hypnosis 19
Homeopathy 20
Bach flower remedies 22
Aromatherapy 24
Massage 25
Reflexology 26
Herbalism 27
Music therapy 28
- **References** 29

WHAT IS COMPLEMENTARY AND ALTERNATIVE MEDICINE (CAM)?

Practices which fall under the general description of CAM comprise a wide diversity of interventions, from the officially regulated to the totally unsubstantiated, and it is almost impossible to gauge how many different CAM therapies are currently practised in the UK, although an early estimate by the BMA (1993) was a conservative 160.

The latest classification is the one proposed by the House of Lords Select Committee on Science and Technology (2000).

- *Group 1* Professionally organised alternative therapies, including acupuncture, chiropractic, herbal medicine, homeopathy and osteopathy.
- *Group 2* Complementary therapies, i.e. Alexander technique, aromatherapy, Bach flower remedies, massage, hypnotherapy, meditation, reflexology, shiatsu, nutritional medicine and yoga.
- *Group 3a* Alternative disciplines, including long established and traditional systems of health care, such as Anthroposophical medicine, Ayurvedic medicine, Chinese herbal medicine, Traditional Chinese Medicine and naturopathy.
- *Group 3b* Other alternative disciplines, including crystal therapy, dowsing, iridology, kinesiology and radionics.

In addition, a number of therapies are now available as over-the-counter (OTC) remedies, having migrated from their original home in health-food shops to the high street chemist chains and supermarkets where they are available as own-brand therapy products. Sales of books on CAM have also proliferated over the years.

WHO USES CAM?

A number of attempts have been made to determine the extent to which members of the public are using complementary and alternative medicine as part of their healthcare system. Recent surveys have indicated that the rise in the use of CAM continues amongst all social classes, though classes one and two predominate. Simpson and Roman (2001) noted that whilst CAM use was not related to income, cost was an issue.

In their survey Boutin et al (2000) reported that it was only a lack of information about CAM that precluded a greater use not only by the general public, but also by doctors. They also highlighted the issue of availability, reporting that even more patients would use CAM therapies if they were more readily available.

In a review of the literature on the use of CAM by the public, Harris and Rees (2000) identified the difficulty of getting an accurate picture of the phenomenon because of the diversity of the therapies, the lack of differentiation between visiting a practitioner and using an over-the-counter remedy, and the fact that many practitioners use more than one therapy to address the presenting problem.

In the main, users of complementary therapies are sufferers of long-term chronic or painful conditions for which orthodox medicine has little to offer, such as musculoskeletal conditions, asthma, eczema, hypertension, fatigue, sleep disorders and stress-related conditions. Grenfell et al (1998) noted the differences in CAM use between different ethnic groups. In a survey of CAM users attending outpatient clinics at a London hospital, 68% had used some form of CAM intervention in the previous year. Of these, the figures were highest for black people at 78%, and Asians at 77%. For Caucasians, acupuncture was the most popular treatment, at 38%, whilst for black people and Asian patients herbal remedies were preferred, at 65% and 44% respectively. Of the last two groups, half obtained their remedies from their country of origin.

Although to many people CAM therapies represent a new way of tackling disease, to many millions of people worldwide they represent mainstream medical care and, far from being new, many have been used successfully for thousands of years. What we now refer to as CAM stretches back to the dawn of medicine when the use of oils and herbs and taking the waters were the main sources of medical aid. Sometimes these practices were promoted, whilst at other times they were undermined by suspicion and prejudice. Within all medical systems there have always been alternatives to the mainstream medical provision, usually stemming from an economic imperative, often informal and involving folk remedies or other nursing or medical interventions.

The pervasiveness of injury, disease and general ill health has meant that, from earliest times, every human society has developed ways to heal, mend and maintain health. Before the advent of antibiotics, people relied on their own natural ability to throw off illness or injury. In spite of the high death rate, some patients did survive, relying on what a naturopath would prescribe today: diet, sunlight, fresh air and herbal medicines. The advent of biomedicine, the introduction of more sophisticated surgical techniques (vouchsafed by better and safer anaesthetics), and the discovery of antibiotics resulted in traditional medicine falling into disuse and being replaced by a more mechanistic, interventionist, reductionist paradigm.

However, along with technological advances in medicine, there has been not only an increase in patient survival rate, but also a concomitant rise in morbidity in place of previously fatal conditions, sometimes resulting in a lifetime of disability and pain. In addition, changes in lifestyle relating to faulty diet, increased leisure and more sedentary working conditions have resulted in an escalation in the incidence of chronic and degenerative diseases in adults and, increasingly, in children. An example is obesity leading to a growth in the incidence of type 2 diabetes in a progressively younger population. Conventional medicine, preoccupied as it is with disease, assumes that treatment rather than health care and prevention is the basis of health. Therefore, in the main, the therapies fell into abeyance until the 1960s when a groundswell of interest challenged medical orthodoxy, partly as a result of the thalidomide disaster (1962–1963) when public confidence in orthodox medicine was severely shaken, but also as a result of people's higher expectations of health care and a general disenchantment with the delivery of modern health care.

As Micozzi (2001) points out, the philosophy of Western medicine has been the deconstruction of health into its smallest component parts. He then adds: 'However, the resulting biomedical system is not always able to account for and use many observations in the realms of clinical and personal experience, natural law and human spirituality.'

PHILOSOPHY OF CAM

The philosophy behind CAM interventions differs from the biomedical model in a number of important ways. First, the emphasis is on wellbeing rather than disease, and on the encouragement of self-healing, which is attained by focusing on the patient as an individual rather than as a diseased entity to be cured. This involves collaboration in care, with patients being responsible for much of their own treatment, the aim of the intervention being to mobilise the body's own resources to effect a return to health. A second important concept is that of vitalism (or vital force) and a third is holism. Each of these will be discussed in turn and related to nursing care.

Vitalism

Ancient medical systems such as Traditional Chinese Medicine (TCM), Ayurvedic medicine, herbal medicine and, more recently, homeopathy, all aim to augment the natural healing process, restoring and maintaining health by ensuring the balance and flow of the body's vital energy. Vitalism is a key concept behind the healing power of CAM. This idea of a vital force is not unique to CAM but was originally a tenet of Western medicine. Prior to the development of reductionism, the medieval concept of humanity was that mind and body were indivisible, neither being able to exist without the other. The idea of anything being totally inert and passively dependent on external influences was inconceivable. As developments in medical science progressed, human beings began to be regarded as machines which from time to time break down and need to be repaired. However, there was a backlash against this new philosophy, which was seen as being too simplistic. It was felt that there was more to human beings than a collection of biological systems and that some sort of life force was responsible for differentiating humans from inorganic matter. However, by the 19th century the rational deconstructive school of science had prevailed and the concept of a 'vital force' was discredited. The idea left mainstream medicine, but it has always been and remains an integral part of alternative forms of healing (Kaptchuk 2001). The balance and flow of this energy is seen as vital for restoring and maintaining health. This concept of 'energy' can be problematic to Western medicine, though Western medicine does measure a number of energy systems within the body, for example by using the electrocardiogram or electroencephalogram. Certainly patients have a concept of energy, frequently complaining of a lack of it, although this is usually attributed to a medical cause which is subsequently diagnosed and treated.

Holism

Definition

Germane to the philosophies of both CAM and nursing is the concept of holism, which again involves an emphasis on self-determination and collaboration, patients having a responsibility for their own health, and being partners in treatment. The concept of holism is quite old. The word comes from the Greek *holos* meaning whole, and holism looks beyond patients' immediate, obvious symptoms to encompass the social and psychological contexts of their condition. It emanates from the view that a person is a complex and integrated being involving mind, body and spirit and includes the concept of the vital force, mentioned above, called prana in Ayurvedic medicine and Qi in Traditional Chinese Medicine (TCM). These ancient systems of health care have long taken into account the patient's lifestyle, social circumstances and spiritual health when diagnosing and treating a condition.

In a more modern context, the word holism was first used by Jan Smuts the South African statesman who coined the word in 1926. However, it is not always appreciated that his application of the term was meant to apply not only to the anti-mechanistic approach, but also to the anti-vitalistic concept germane to most CAM. He argued that the 'entirety of an organism necessarily implied a teleologic purpose which could not be explained by the laws governing component parts' (Kaptchuk 2001). In spite of this, the word holism has entered the medical domain where it has been seized upon almost as a mantra of care (whether holistic or not) and over-used to the point of trivialisation. The author noted an illustration of this which occurred in an article in a magazine devoted to complementary therapies. The article described the work of a woman who was offering 'holistic' riding lessons. This innovative procedure involved the pupils cleansing their own and their horses' auras with a candle (in a sawdust strewn riding school) and choosing two aphorisms to use during the lesson, one for the pupil and one for the horse. Sadly, this type of misuse of the term holistic for commercial reasons devalues the concept as a powerful therapeutic force.

Holism and nursing

The philosophy of holism within nursing has been addressed by a number of authors and a number of definitions have been considered. Boschma (1994) points out that for nurses, holism includes a major emphasis on self-help and self-awareness, with individuals accepting responsibility for their own health and well-being which, as we have seen, is in concordance with CAM philosophy. The ethos involves the promotion of healthier habits to increase wellbeing, and illness is seen as a potential for growth with the gaining of self-knowledge. Of particular importance is the development of the therapeutic relationship between client and practitioner to facilitate healing. Watson (1985) sees the nurse as a catalyst assisting clients to grow and change.

Ham-Ying (1993) found that the term holism had two common usages in the context of nursing: first, when a person is seen as a holistic being and, secondly, when holism is seen as a specific approach to nursing care. She also highlighted a number of variations in definition, but suggested that the key concept was the idea that people are more than the sum of their parts and are not just a collection of sub-systems, i.e. the bio-, psycho- and social beings reflected in a number of nursing models (e.g. Rogers 1970, Levine 1983, Orem 1985 and Roper et al 1985). These have been challenged by Mantle (2001), who proposed that the use of a personal construct approach would provide a truly integrated pathway, enabling CAM to blend seamlessly into nursing care.

However, other definitions of holism have advocated a different approach. Newbeck and Rowe (1986), in their essay on holism in nursing, suggest that 'holistic nursing means offering an extended range of interventions to the clients, such as: massage, relaxation therapy, meditation, reflexology and acupuncture'. Todd (1990) suggests that many people now tend to define holism as a treatment modality, focusing on the complementary therapies themselves, rather than on the philosophy, but she suggests that true holism is 'the feelings and perspectives of holism, rather than the tools of practice, that define the approach'. She also suggests, as do Vincent and Furnham (1997), that complementary therapies are not intrinsically holistic, although as Buckle (1993) points out, modern discourse tends to suggest that 'holism is rapidly becoming a pseudonym for complementary'. Stevensen (2001) defined holistic nursing as 'meeting the most appropriate needs of the patient whatever they may be'. This approach is reflected in an attempt to capture the essence of holism by Long et al (2000). These authors have developed a tool with which to measure holistic practice, and suggest that it offers a missing dimension and outcome measure in CAM research.

It can be seen that, as far as the traditions and philosophies are concerned, a comparison of nursing and most complementary therapies reveals a certain synergy. Both aim to treat the patient holistically. Both complementary therapies and nursing work in partnership with patients, who retain control over their illness. In the light of Florence Nightingale's statement that the goal of nursing was to 'put the patient into the best condition for nature to act upon him [*sic*]' (Nightingale 1859, republished 1980) nursing and CAM could be said to share the same philosophies and values.

Given the synergy between nursing and CAM, it is not surprising that nurses have embraced the use of CAM in their practice. In her survey of members of the Royal College of Nursing Complementary Therapy Forum, Rankin-Box (1997) found that, at the time of the survey, therapies were being used more frequently in the private sector than in the National Health Service (NHS), but when they were used in the NHS the most common areas of practice were community palliative care and oncology. The most frequently used therapies were aromatherapy and massage, reflexology, relaxation, visualisation and acupuncture, which are the therapies that can be introduced most easily into nursing care. Chadwick (1999) sought nurses' views as to why they used CAM and was interested to discover that they enjoyed the extended role that it offered and felt it provided a vehicle for enhancing care.

THE USE OF CAM IN PAEDIATRICS

Since there is a growing demand for the use of CAM amongst adults, it would seem safe to assume that children also use the therapies. As Vessey and Rechkemmer (2001) have pointed out, our ancestors relied heavily on herbs and other natural remedies for treating their children and today, parents and children are increasingly turning to CAM for their health needs, not only for treating existing conditions but also in terms of health promotion.

In his review Ernst (1999) found that there was a high and growing use of CAM by children and that generally it was perceived as being helpful, whilst Verhoef et al (1994) noted (unsurprisingly) that children seemed to be influenced by their parents regarding the usefulness of CAM. In particular, surveys have shown that children suffering from chronic conditions for which there is no known cure were amongst the highest users (Pendergrass & Davis 1981, Sawyer et al 1994). Grootenhuis et al (1998) have reviewed the use of CAM amongst paediatric oncology patients in Holland and found that about one third of the families consulted had used or were using some form of CAM. In Simpson and Roman's (2001) survey, the reasons given by parents for using CAM for their children included:

- Word of mouth recommendation 59.7%
- Dissatisfaction with conventional medicines 37%
- Fear of side effects from conventional medicines 31.8%
- More personal attention 13.2%
- Having a child with a chronic condition 8.4%.

CAM was also used very commonly for acute, self-limiting conditions. These figures suffer from the common problem of CAM survey research in that the types of CAM and length of usage are not congruent across studies and may well reflect only a fraction of the use of CAM by paediatric patients. Of particular concern is the discovery that not all patients tell their doctors of their use of CAM. Sawyer et al (1994) noted that less than 50% of the patients using CAM had discussed its use with their doctor.

Spigelblatt (1997) raises the issue of whether children should be using CAM at all. She specifically highlights the 'lay' aspect of practitioners' claims and the fact that their health philosophy may be in direct conflict with children's health needs, in particular citing the fact that a number of CAM philosophies are antipathetical to immunisation. It is a fact that many CAM practitioners are not medically qualified and certainly not qualified paediatricians, and thus may have little experience of paediatric problems. Of particular concern is the plethora of lay advice available to parents about CAM in many popular over-the-counter magazines.

The issue of medical advice being given via the media has been raised by Goodman (2001) who, in a strong attack on CAM in general, usefully high-lighted the problem of press control of the industry. It would seem that, provided an article is clearly titled and does not intend to mislead the reader, the Press Complaints Council are unable to do anything about its content. Goodman also points out that book shops are crammed with books that he refers to as 'health fiction'. Schmidt (2002) highlights the fact that 93% of people who use the inter-net for health purposes in France and the USA believe that the information is trustworthy and of good quality. However, not only is some of the information highly suspect, it may also offer false hope in the treatment of serious illnesses such as cancer, when prescriptions for so called cures are offered over the inter-net. Reputable web sites are listed in Appendix 3 for readers to access.

Role of the nurse

It has been shown that patients approach CAM practitioners as a result of rec-ommendations from family and friends as well as the media, therefore it is extremely important that informal advice is tempered with professional guid-ance and that nurses are able to give advice as to the suitability of the CAM ther-apy to the problem being addressed.

Chez et al (1999) have delineated the role of the physician (which can just as well apply to nurses) in advising patients about the use of CAM as follows:

■ Protect patients against dangerous practices
■ Permit [sic] practices which are harmless and may assist with comfort and palliation
■ Promote and use those which are proven safe and effective
■ Partnership with patients by communicating with them about the use of specific CAM therapies and products.

The role of nurses as gatekeepers of medical information has long been recog-nised and, increasingly, specialist nurses (particularly in the community) are becoming the first point of contact for patients seeking medical care. Irish (1989) has suggested that the nurse's role in CAM integration is as 'a critical link between the individual and the health care complex for optimum communica-tion, comfort and care in the pursuit of health'. Zagorsky (1993) has suggested that there is an inherent challenge for nurses to accommodate patients and fam-ilies who adopt CAM by acting as a liaison, enabling them to reap the benefits from both CAM and orthodox systems. She goes on to demonstrate the potential that CAM offers for health promotion. In particular she emphasises that to keep patients within the orthodox system and reduce non-compliance with essential treatment, attention must be paid to the personal reasons for the family turning to CAM in the first place. Of value at this stage is the Ullrich–Hodge Alternative Therapy Assessment Model (Ullrich & Hodge 1999), an adapted version of which is in Appendix 1. The full version of the model is a conceptualised process useful for identifying patients who use CAM and for evaluating the degree of risk involved and the patient's motivation in using CAM. This may be of value to nurses if used routinely in their patient assessment process to indicate the nurses' acceptance of the use of CAM and to give patients the chance to discuss any therapies they may be using. This is extremely important if a child is having any procedure done under anaesthetic. Murphy (1999), Norred et al (2000) and Tsen et al (2000) discuss the potential effect of herbal remedies in surgery.

SAFETY ISSUES

The safety of CAM has been an issue which has been debated for some time. One perennial problem is the lay perception that CAM therapies are intrinsically safe because they are 'natural', with the implication that they have no side effects. This perception can be wrong but may prove difficult to dislodge.

A potential risk can be assessed in two ways, as relative risk or as absolute risk. The risk associated with an intervention is the 'probability' that an adverse effect will occur. Probability is something which is likely to happen and implies a higher potential than 'possible'. Therapies are not, of course, viewed in isolation and in each case, a risk benefit assessment needs to be made. Key issues around the topic of safety in CAM include:

- Qualifications and competence of the practitioner
- Standardisation of products
- Safety of products, especially herbal medicines, which can be made unsafe either by adulteration or by mislabelling of the contents, leading to a more toxic effect than anticipated.

Examples of these problems are highlighted here.

Some therapies, such as the Bach flower remedies and homeopathic medicines, are generally considered to be safe, although Jonas (1998) discusses the misdiagnosis, misclassification and misinterpretation of the function and clinical methodology of homeopathy. Other therapies, however, have the potential for harm in unskilled hands. For example, following acupuncture there have been reported cases of pneumothorax (Gray et al 1991), cardiac-tamponade and haemothorax (Hasegawa et al 1991) and spinal epidural haematoma and subarachnoid haemorrhage (Keane et al 1993). In a review of the reported side effects of acupuncture by Rampes and James (1995), a total of 395 incidences are listed. However, these were collated world wide over 20 years and included such minor reactions as syncope (53 incidences), bruising (2), and pain (2). The largest categories were hepatitis (126 incidences, which can be eliminated by the use of disposable needles), drowsiness (79), syncope (53) and pneumothorax (32). A further report of adverse reactions from a Norwegian study again indicated that pneumothorax and fainting during treatment were the most predominant adverse reactions.

Of particular concern are the safety standards for imported Indian or Chinese herbs, for which there are a number of adverse reports either because the herb itself is toxic (Dickens et al 1994) or has been mixed with other toxic substances (Treleaven et al 1993), or because it has been adulterated with a conventional drug, in one case mefenamic acid (Abt et al 1995).

A number of serious consequences have been reported following chiropractic manoeuvres (Horn 1983, Sinel & Smith 1993). Coe and Rykan (1979) and

Judd et al (1985) have reviewed the potential dangers of hypnosis and, whilst the role of hypnosis in the treatment of psychopathology is debated, they conclude that hypnosis per se is a safe therapy if used following proper training. Clearly, each therapy is only as safe as the practitioners who use it and, even when there is a regulating framework and register of practitioners, problems can still occur.

Indirect risks include the appropriateness of the intervention for the condition presented and the dangers of misdiagnosis by the practitioner, who may or may not be medically qualified or qualified in any of the professions allied to medicine (PAMs). As Rankin-Box (2001) points out, non-medically qualified practitioners of CAM are free to practise under common law irrespective of their levels of training or clinical competence. Problems that can arise include an existing condition not being recognised or a condition which is not present being wrongly identified. I was recently talking to a friend who, following a visit to a reflexologist (not medically qualified), was taking kelp tablets. When I asked why, she replied that the reflexologist had diagnosed something wrong with her thyroid. The reflexologist did not know whether the thyroid was under- or overactive, so my friend decided to take kelp as she had heard that the iodine in it was good for the thyroid!

Another risk is the possibility of a delay in seeking or a refusal to undergo orthodox treatment, even when that treatment would be more appropriate. In addition, some therapies advocate practices which are potentially dangerous, particularly to children. For example, naturopathy advocates dietary manipulation, which can involve cutting out key food groups, commonly wheat and dairy products; it also occasionally advocates fasting, which would be unsuitable for children.

Some herbal medicines may interfere adversely with orthodox medication, which is of particular concern to cardiology, diabetes, haematology and oncology nurses, whilst reflexology has the effect of reducing blood sugar in diabetics (see Ch. 6 on eating and drinking).

Ernst and Barnes (1998) discuss methods for ensuring the safety of CAM interventions and list the classification of adverse effects used in conventional medicine, in which there are four different categories:

■ Type A, pharmacologically predictable; usually dose dependent; can often be predicted.
■ Type B, idiosyncratic reactions, not predictable on the basis of pharmacological properties; not dose dependent; usually rare; often serious and potentially fatal.
■ Type C, develop during long-term therapy; usually predictable.
■ Type D, delayed effects, such as carcinogenicity and teratogenicity.

They suggest that herbal remedies, aromatherapy and homeopathic medicines can be classified using the same system, but that the more physical therapies such as acupuncture, manipulation and massage are not so easily classified. In these, harm can generally be attributed to the practitioner rather than the therapy itself, so they suggest that a further category of adverse effects, relating to the practitioner's insufficient medical competence, would be pertinent in CAM (although why, in the light of recent medical scandals, this category should be confined to complementary therapists is not at all clear).

Of particular concern for nurses is the confusion surrounding the therapeutic values, methods of dispensing and safety of aromatherapy oils and, in particular, the issue of what constitutes toxicity (Mantle 1996a, Vickers 1996). Fowler and

Wall (1997, 1998) attempt to address this by relating aromatherapy to the Control of Substances Hazardous to Health (COSHH) and Chemical Hazard Information and Packaging (CHIP) regulations. Unfortunately, even with this initiative, confusion and conflicts arise. For example, the authors refer to an alleged incident of hypersensitivity to citrus oils and point out that an occupational dermatitis has been identified among workers who are regularly in contact with lemon and orange peel, which rather begs the question as to the relationship between workers who are in contact with the substance all day and practitioners who use one drop of essential oil diluted in 10 mL of carrier oil. They also point out that some essential oils contain phenols which are harmful to health. Again, the small quantities involved in aromatherapy and the amount of neat phenol that would be harmful to health are not comparable. Inappropriate examples like this do not add anything to the debate.

One of the key problems in therapies of all forms is those adverse reactions that fall into the B category described above, i.e. idiosyncratic, not predictable on the basis of pharmacological properties, not dose dependent, usually rare, with serious and sometimes fatal results. The literature abounds with reports of this type of adverse reaction, from mild skin reactions to the more serious manifestations. However, it would be a pity if therapies were to be banned because of these occurrences when we bear in mind that allergies to everyday substances such as eggs, milk and feathers can provoke equally strong reactions, but none of these have been designated as dangerous to health or banned from public use.

One particular difficulty in policing the effects of CAM is the absence of a reporting system for adverse reactions, similar to the medical yellow card system which has been in place since 1964. However, common sense tells us that there may be other legitimate ways of highlighting adverse reactions to substances. For example, aromatherapists are exposed to oils on a daily basis and it would seem reasonable, given the length of time aromatherapy has been practised, that serious adverse reactions would have come to light. This is supported by Buckle (1997) who suggests that, although aromatherapy has been used for thousands of years, there appear to be very few cases of sensitivity, allergy or fatality when oils are used within established guidelines. Tisserand and Balacs (1995) indicate the safety margins of a wide range of essential oils, and should be consulted in connection with the use or recommendation of any essential oils.

CAM INTERVENTIONS

The following pages describe the main therapies referred to in this book and provide a brief outline of each therapy's origins, history, mode of action and application. Reference sources for the use of the therapies are found in Chapters 3–16 in Sections 2 and 3, but some relevant sources are also included here.

Traditional Chinese Medicine (TCM)

The first recorded medical text for Traditional Chinese Medicine is *The Yellow Emperor's Inner Classic* (Huang Di Nei Jing), ostensibly written by Huang Di between 2698 and 2598 BC (although it may have been written by a number of writers some centuries later). This text is the originator of the traditional medicine of China. Since then, several key figures have contributed to the development of TCM. Zhang Zhongjing established the principles of treatment, including the importance of a differential diagnosis. The first Chinese herbal, called *The Divine Husbandman's Classic of Materia Medica,* was written between 25 and 220 AD, whilst Qigong has a verbal history going back 10 000 years and a written history of about 4000 years.

In this text I have followed Maciocia's (2000) style in using initial capitals for the terms specific to TCM to distinguish them from their Western interpretations.

Enshrined within the philosophy of TCM (in common with many other medical systems) is the concept of internal harmony and balance, exemplified by the ideal balance between Yin and Yang energy which are present simultaneously within the person. Yin element reflects the dark, cold, female, slow, down, inside aspects of the person whilst conversely, Yang represents the light, warm, male, quick, up, outside aspects of the person. The terms Yin and Yang are used to describe normal physiology and pathology. The vital force, discussed earlier, is represented in TCM by the idea that the body is pervaded by a subtle material which enables physiological function to occur to restore and maintain the health and welfare of the person. In TCM this vital force is called Qi. The body comprises more than one Qi, according to its organ, location and function. Since every movement and activity of the body is a manifestation of Qi flowing, entering and leaving the body, any disharmony in Qi, i.e. any interruption or deviation of this flow or any reduction in the level of Qi, will interrupt the body's normal functions and result in poor health and illness. Qi emanates from the organs of the body such as the liver (Liver-Qi), spleen (Spleen-Qi), or lungs (Lung-Qi). Allowing Qi to travel around the body is a system of meridians or channels, punctuated at intervals by points which are stimulated during acupuncture and acupressure to enhance the flow of Qi if it becomes blocked. There are 12 main meridians either side of the body and each meridian is related to specific organs, i.e. meridians relating to the Lung, Large Intestine, Stomach, Spleen, Heart, Small Intestine, Bladder, Kidney, Pericardium, Triple Energiser, Gallbladder and Liver, and two special meridians known as Vessels, i.e. the Governor Vessel and the Conception Vessel. Some of these meridians are of relevance in the section on reflexology.

Another element is Blood, not the type circulating through the veins but, in TCM terms, a substance which nourishes the body, moistening it and aiding the mind (Shen), leading to clear and stable thought processes. Qi, together with Essence and Shen, make up the three treasures. Essence, or Jing, in contrast to Qi which is responsible for everyday health and energy, is the slow burning underpinning of Qi and is responsible for the body's organic development through life, whilst Shen is the mind or spirit of the person and is responsible for human consciousness. Deficiencies of Shen will result in slow and muddled thinking, anxiety or insomnia. Deficiency of Jing will lead to developmental disorders such as learning difficulties or physical disabilities.

TCM also includes the Five Element theory in which the human body is seen as a microcosm of the universe. This theory is found in other medical systems such as Ayurveda. The Five Elements are:

1 Water: wet, cooling, descending, flowing, yielding
2 Fire: dry, hot, ascending, moving
3 Wood: growing, flexible, rooted

4 Metal: cutting, hard, conducting

5 Earth: productive, fertile, potential for growth.

Each Element has a number of affiliations with the material world and the human body and, because they are the processes of the body, they support and interact with each other. TCM recognises that body disharmonies can be caused by internal and external factors such as the Seven Emotions, i.e. anger, joy, sadness, grief, pensiveness, fear and fright, and external forces i.e. Wind, Cold, Damp, Fire and Heat.

The principle of treatment in TCM involves the rebalancing of the disharmonies and includes those arising:

- When a deficiency exists and the energy needs to be tonified
- When an excess of energy exists and it must be reduced
- When too much Heat is present and it is expelled or cooled
- When too much Cold is present and it is expelled or warmed
- When Damp is present and it needs to be resolved
- When Phlegm is present and it needs to be resolved.

The TCM system accepts the interaction of these factors and sees mind and body as indivisible. Treatments include the use of herbs, massage, acupuncture, diet, t'ai chi and Qigong to restore the body's balance and regain harmony. Qigong is a mind/body approach to health widely used in China. Its aim is to:

- Calm the mind
- Promote good health
- Prolong a healthy life
- Cure disease
- Develop strength and prowess.

If the basis of TCM seems hard to grasp, it is interesting to note what Helman (2000) records concerning the reactions and observations of patients in his general practice in north London. When asked how they viewed the causes of their ill health, they commonly described their symptoms using terms such as hot, cold, chill, wet and dry, and saw these symptoms as products of external forces such as damp, heat, cold and wind. It is interesting to note that two such diverse cultures both attribute ill health to an imbalance between the person and the forces of nature. It is less surprising that Ayurvedic medicine and TCM share such similarities, since these two cultures are geographically adjacent and share the ancient philosophy of the human being as a microcosm of the universe.

The diagnostic process in TCM includes a number of observations very seldom used in Western diagnostic techniques, if at all. Specifically, in addition to routine examinations common to both systems, observation of the tongue is part of the diagnostic process, the tongue being seen to represent the internal organs; the appearance of the tongue, its colour and the location of striations are noted and analysed for diagnosis. Of prime importance is the examination of the pulses. In TCM this is taken at three main sites on both arms, with each point corresponding to a different internal organ and used to determine the organ's energy level. Note is taken of the pulse rate, width, strength, quality, rhythm and depth.

Herbal prescriptions in TCM follow a hierarchy of effectiveness. First is the chief (principal) ingredient which treats the principal disease; next comes the deputy (associate), which assists the chief ingredient; then comes the adjutant ingredient, which enhances the chief ingredient; and this is followed by the envoy (guide) ingredient, which focuses the formula on the specific parts of the body. Other interventions will be described in the chapters of the book in which they have specific application.

Although Western paediatrics is a comparatively recent discipline, paediatrics in TCM has a much longer history. Texts began appearing in the first century BC when paediatric massage (Tui Na) was first mentioned in the *Nei Jing*, the classic acupuncture text book. By 200 AD childhood was recognised as a separate state from adulthood and in the 12th century the paediatrician Qian Yi wrote the first paediatric text book. In TCM children are seen as having a different physiology, not just being smaller but having different predominant life forces. Children are mostly Yang with small amounts of Yin. This makes sense, since Yang is associated with growth, development and upward movement. A newborn baby has maximum Kidney-Yang and Pre-Heaven Essence, both of which deteriorate with age. Since the child is Yin deficient, Blood and therefore fluid are insufficient and delicately balanced. In Western terms this means that the child will dehydrate very easily and even minimal blood loss can be critical.

TCM divides childhood into five developmental stages, although there is no abrupt transition from one to the other at any set time. In this theory the children are strengthened as they move from one stage to another. For example, children in the Water phase of development are vulnerable to Kidney imbalances and would benefit from regular prophylactic stimulation of the Kidney meridians; as they pass into the next stage, the Liver stage, they become susceptible to Liver-Qi imbalances which can be addressed prophylactically. TCM lays great stress on the value of diet in health and this is addressed in greater detail in Chapter 6.

Great emphasis is placed on health promotion in TCM and it follows the ancient wisdom of 'winter disease, summer cure'; for example, seasonal conditions such as asthma are treated during the summer before the winter symptoms begin. Although the Chinese were amongst the first to vaccinate, starting with the smallpox vaccine, their approach to mass vaccination of small babies is more cautious. As with Anthroposophical and Ayurvedic medicine, it is felt that too many vaccinations given at one time will seriously weaken the child's constitution and it is advocated that vaccinations should be given singly. TCM promotes the concept that children should achieve levels of immunity naturally by having the disease. There is evidence that acupuncture can tonify the immune system and this is done routinely in children from birth. Although it may seem an unusual treatment for small children, they can tolerate needle acupuncture and techniques, and needle types are adapted to suit children of different ages including babies. Children are also taught meditation, t'ai chi and Qigong to strengthen themselves physically and mentally.

The study of TCM is fascinating and this section can only provide a glimpse of its variety and richness. In Sections 2 and 3 the specific application of TCM to childhood conditions will provide further insight into its effectiveness and show where it can be incorporated into nursing care. Evidence for the efficacy of TCM is predominantly through empirical observations made and recorded over many centuries; more recently, however, aspects of TCM (particularly acupuncture) have been subjected to clinical trials. (Source material Loo 2002, Maciocia 2000.)

Anthroposophical medicine

This is an approach to healing inspired by the work of Rudolph Steiner (1861–1925), who understood the nature of humankind as being not just body but soul and spirit. In common with some other medical approaches, Anthroposophical medicine looks to the cause of the problem rather than suppressing the symptoms, aiming to treat the patient not the disease. The Anthroposophical approach embraces a range of interventions including conventional medicine as well as homeopathic and herbal remedies. These remedies would be prescribed in conjunction with diet, massage, hydrotherapy, eurhythmy, art therapy or music therapy as an integrated package of care tailored to suit each patient. However, where Anthroposophical remedies differ is in the preparation of the medication, which takes into account cosmic influences such as the seasons and solar, lunar and planetary influences, in accordance with ancient tradition. The choice of remedy would depend on the patient and system affected. The efficacy of the medication is not confined to its chemical effect; it also acts as a catalyst to stimulate changes in the patient's life energy. Anthroposophical medicine is part of Steiner's wider philosophy, which includes special and mainstream education, architecture and painting. Steiner was not a medical doctor but worked alongside conventional doctors to develop Anthroposophic medicine. The name is derived from the Greek *anthropos* (human) and *sophia* (wisdom). Steiner saw the human condition as comprising the life forces which make up the physical body. The physical body is perfused by the non-physical formative forces, called the etheric body, which have a particular role to play in growth and nutrition. Humans also have a third body called the astral body or soul, which acts with and through the nervous system. In addition, there is what Steiner described as the spiritual core or ego, which expresses itself through the musculature and blood.

Anthroposophical medicine tries to understand and treat the presenting illness on the basis of how the four bodies interrelate. Again, a key concept of the system is maintaining equilibrium. The four different bodies are each more active during different stages of life. They interact with each other and form the whole person. The etheric body is predominant during the embryonic stage. The astral body is the seat of consciousness, thoughts and feelings, whilst the etheric body is concerned with development and growth. The astral body is engaged in the breaking down of the body and tends towards illness. The ego aids the work of the astral body to break down (catabolism) and the etheric body to build up (anabolism). The ego is concerned with thinking and the will and enables people to think for themselves. Each human element is related to a natural element: for example, the ego relates to fire, the astral body to air, the etheric body to water and the physical body to earth. This alignment of the human body with cosmic elements is also common to Ayurvedic medicine and Traditional Chinese Medicine.

In Anthroposophical medicine there are three main systems: the nervous sense system, i.e. the spinal column, the brain and the nerves; the metabolic limb system, which is responsible for the assimilation of nourishment, metabolism and activity of the limbs; and the rhythmic system, which includes breathing and the pulse. Each of the four bodies has particular affinities to these systems. Of the three systems, two are polar opposites and the third, the rhythmic system, is in the middle mediating between the others.

Human growth and development in Anthroposophical medicine is seen as occurring in 7-year cycles, the end of the first cycle at 7 years of age coinciding with the completion of the second dentition, and the end of the second cycle coinciding with puberty (i.e. around the age of 14 years).

Up until the age of 7 years, children are considered to be at particular risk of illness. However, paediatric nurses need to be aware that the Anthroposophical approach to illness and immunisation involves the idea that suffering from a particular illness is part of the child's destiny and has a special meaning for that child, and that removing the opportunity for the child to have the disease will result in the child's growth and spiritual development being retarded. Some illnesses, depending on how they present themselves, are regarded as a way of bringing about changes in people, and the way the illness manifests itself in an individual can reveal something of that person's being. As a result of this, the general feeling within anthroposophy is to avoid immunisation of children. For a full account of this stance see Kummer (1995). A more considered approach is offered by Glöckler and Goebel (1990) who, working in partnership with parents, encourage parental choice in this area. However, they do express concern about the number and timing of immunisations in small babies affecting the child's immune system, and suggest confining immunisation to tetanus and polio in the first year and rubella at adolescence, discouraging immunisation against whooping cough and measles. They feel that to repress the illness by immunisation is to interfere with the physical and spiritual connection. If the illness is artificially prevented, the body is reinforced at the cost of the soul in its development. It is considered that, whilst the body might be fit, the soul will become shallow and less active. When a child is ill, Glöckler and Goebel believe that the role of the doctor and nurse is to guide the patient through the illness which destiny has decreed the child should have.

Anthroposophical medicine is the most integrated of all CAM interventions since Anthroposophical doctors and nurses are conventionally trained but use Anthroposophical medicine alongside orthodox medical care. There are a number of such doctors and nurses practising in the UK, both in private practice and in the NHS. There is also an Anthroposophical hospital, Park Attwood Clinic, in Worcestershire. (Source material Glöckler and Goebel (1990), Bott (1996), Evans and Rodger (2000).)

Ayurveda

One system of medicine that is now becoming popular in this country is the traditional medical system of India called Ayurveda, which is rooted in the culture of the subcontinent. The term comes from the words *ayur* (life) and *veda* (knowledge). The first recorded medical text is the *Rig Veda*, dating from 1500 BC, which is a poem detailing medical information. This medical system, which started as an oral tradition some 5000 years ago, with the first written texts dating from around 1000 BC, is a dynamic one and texts have incorporated traditions and techniques from other migrating cultures. More recently Maharishi Ayurveda (MAV), a new development of the traditional Ayurveda, has evolved, which has the aim of researching into Ayurveda and publishing the results. For convenience, both the traditional evidence and more recent clinical trials are included in this text.

Central to the philosophy of Ayurvedic medicine is the concept of primordial energy, which can only exist in pure awareness and is central to the maintenance of health. Ayurveda holds that everything in the universe is composed of five elements: air, fire, earth, ether (or space) and water. These elements are in a state of perpetual motion, each element affecting the others, and are proportionally different in varying situations. In combination they form the three vital energies or doshas, which encapsulate the physical and psychological aspects of the human being, and particular combinations of doshas form particular constitutional types. The three doshas are:

- Pitta, which is a combination of fire and water with fire predominating
- Vata, which is air and ether with air predominating
- Kapha, which is water and earth with water predominating.

Each energy or dosha has a specific role. Vata is the energy of movement, pitta is the energy of digestion and metabolism and kapha is the energy that deals with the body's structure and holds the body together. In human development terms the period between birth and 16 years is a kapha period. In a healthy individual the doshas work together in harmony, resulting in physical and emotional stability and creating a unique individual. The dominance of a particular dosha will result in a tendency to specific conditions. For example, vata dominant people tend towards emotional illnesses such as anxiety and depression, low back ache, painful joints, dry skin and hair and respiratory conditions; pitta individuals tend to suffer from migraine, skin rashes, fevers, inflammations and sore throats; while kapha dominance leads to catarrhal conditions, diabetes and water retention. Imbalances of the three doshas affect the body's natural resistance or agni, which leaves the body vulnerable to infection. Each dosha has a range of functions and an affinity with specific areas of the body. When the ratio of the doshas differs from that of the constitutional type, Ayurvedic medicine seeks to restore the balance.

Ayurvedic medicine describes the disease process as following five stages:

- Accumulation: at this stage the aggravated dosha begins to build up in its location in the body, i.e. kapha in the stomach, pitta in the small intestine and vata in the colon.
- Provocation: the dosha continues to accumulate but now begins to affect the respective organ.
- Spread: at this stage the dosha leaves the primary location and starts to spread around the body and may move in any direction. The direction of the dosha and the type of dosha will determine the symptoms experienced by the patient.
- Deposition: the dosha settles into a weak spot in the body and begins to accumulate again. It is at this stage that the condition's prodromal symptoms begin.
- Manifestation and differentiation: cardinal signs appear and the disease is diagnosed.

Treatment is aimed at rebalancing the dosha and is accomplished by the use of the herbal compound triphala, consisting of amalaki, a regulator for pitta energy, bibhitaki, a regulator for kapha energy, and haritaki, a regulator for vata energy. In addition, other specific herbs might be prescribed depending on the presenting symptoms. Other treatments include panchakarma, meaning five actions, which is a deep cleansing process to remove any excess dosha. Preparation for the procedure includes a massage with oil, which may be facilitated by a steam treatment.

Yoga is an integral part of Ayurvedic medicine and positions (or asanas) are prescribed according to the presenting condition. Treatment is individualised for each patient. In addition, dietary adjustment may be advised. Other therapeutic interventions in Ayurvedic medicine include therapeutic vomiting, enemas and massage.

Evidence for the efficacy of Ayurvedic medicine is predominantly based on tradition and empirical observation but also, more recently, on clinical trials. There is an Ayurvedic charitable hospital in London. (Source material Lad (1985), Morrison (1994), Warrier (2002).)

Hypnosis

Inducing an altered state of consciousness by using drugs, dance, rhythmic music or chanting has been part of religious ceremonies throughout the ages, but it was Anton Mesmer (1734–1815) who identified this altered state as being of therapeutic value. Not fully understanding the nature of the phenomenon, he called it animal magnetism. Using a variety of ingenious contraptions he induced a state of trance in his subjects and as a result he noticed that certain conditions (usually physiological) got better. A number of other people took up the practice of animal magnetism and it became a common feature of Parisian salons. Although hypnosis became discredited following an investigation into Mesmer's work, other physicians were aware of the potential for its use in medicine, particularly in surgery, and a number of other investigators have increased our knowledge of how it can be used. Mesmer's student, the Marquis de Chastenet de Puységur, adapted Mesmer's methods and developed his own approach, which involved a more relaxed, quiet state of mind that he referred to as 'artificial somnambulism'.

The Abbe de Faria called hypnosis lucid sleep and induced the state by verbal suggestion. James Braid used hypnosis for surgical procedures and promoted the term hypnotism. Later, the French psychologist Pierre Janet (1859–1947) suggested that the hypnotic state was a form of disassociation. With the advent of psychoanalysis, hypnosis fell into a decline until the 1950s, when there was a resurgence of interest in it as a valuable therapeutic technique.

Understanding exactly what hypnosis is has engaged the minds of psychologists for many years, with the debate focusing on whether this phenomenon is a separate state of consciousness or the extension of an everyday experience. Whatever the case, it is generally felt that hypnosis is not a therapy in itself but an additional therapeutic modality employed to enhance the effect of an established treatment. It is probably best described as the therapeutic utilisation of daydreaming, in which a state of trance is induced. The concept of trance includes three elements:

- Focused attention
- Disattention to extraneous sounds
- Absorption in some activity, image, thought or feeling.

This state does not have to be induced by someone else, but can be entered quite easily by anyone who is bored, or perhaps carrying out some repetitive or familiar task.

Key to this state of trance is a heightened susceptibility to suggestion. We are all, to some extent or other, open to suggestion but the use of hypnosis enhances this tendency, allowing suggestions to be accepted and acted upon much more readily than in a non-hypnotic state.

Hypnosis and children

There are age-related differences in hypnotic susceptibility, with young children between the ages of 7 and 12 being the most receptive. It has been suggested that this is due to the fact that many of the features of the hypnotic state are akin to a child's normal waking state. For example, the narrowed focus of attention and heightened concentration achieved in hypnosis are normal in children, since their cognitive skills are not fully developed. Children tend to focus their attention more on the immediate present and are usually completely absorbed in whatever activity is in progress, to the exclusion of everything else. In addition, they think in concrete, literal terms, which facilitates the acceptance of appropriately worded hypnotic suggestions. Because of their limited experience on which to base reality testing, and their enjoyment of story telling and fantasy, the barrier between fantasy and reality is more permeable. Children are by nature more open to new experiences and, once their confidence has been gained, will enter into the spirit of hypnosis very easily. One of the most valuable effects of hypnosis in children and adults is their capacity to gain mastery of their condition through learning a new skill. Since children are particularly motivated to learn new skills they are often very enthusiastic about the method. This particularly relates to learning self-hypnosis and the compliance with practice is high.

The first goal in undertaking therapy with children is to gain their confidence and this is achieved by giving an explanation of hypnosis which is appropriate to their age. For very small children, hypnosis can be described as playing a game, whilst older children may be invited to use their imagination to solve problems. Of particular importance is the need to address and dispel any reservations and misconceptions that the child's parents may have. Often these revolve around perceptions of hypnotism gained as a result of the entertainment media. Further concerns include issues of inherent risk, unregulated practice, religious objections or perceived lack of control. However, if parents can be reassured as to the safety and value of the procedure, many children will accept their parents' assurance and enter into the spirit of the exercise. Evidence for the efficacy of hypnosis as an intervention includes empirical observations, expert opinion and controlled trials.

Homeopathy

Homeopathy is a system of vibrational or energy medicine (medicine that works on the patient's vital force), based on the concept of 'like treating like', i.e. the symptoms presented by the patient are matched with the toxic effects of the remedy. Two patients with the same condition might present with different symptoms (think of how variously the symptoms of the common cold may present), in which case the remedy would be selected to match the particular symptoms rather than the specific condition, and the patients would have different remedies. If two people presented with different conditions but with the same symptoms, the remedy would again be selected to match symptoms, and so the patients would have the same remedy.

This philosophy of medication and treatment was noted in Hindu writings over 3000 years ago. It was mentioned in the writings of Hippocrates (460–377 BC), and Galen confirmed its therapeutic value in Rome in 200 AD. However, the German physician Samuel Hahnemann (1755–1843) was credited with developing homeopathy as we know it today, when he initiated the concept of the minimum dose. Hahnemann discovered, during a series of experiments, that remedies were still effective in dilutions which were too small to be detected chemically. This idea that a minimal amount of a substance can have as dramatic effect on a condition as a larger dose is perhaps one of the most difficult ideas in homeopathy for people to accept.

Substances used in homeopathy can include whole plants, animal products, mineral and ores. These substances are extracted through four stages of preparation: maceration, in which the substance is ground down in various alcohol strengths and filtered; extraction, in which the macerated material is treated with ethanol and distilled water; ageing, when the solution is stored to allow it to mature; and filtration, when further filtering is done to refine the final mother tincture. The solution is then serially diluted and succussed, i.e. shaken very vigorously between dilutions until none of the original substance remains in the solution. Dilutions may be in the ratio of 1:10 (the decimal potencies), 1:100 (the centennial potencies) and 1:1000 (the millemisimal potencies).

There is no generally accepted explanation as to how homeopathy works, but it is thought that when the remedy is being succussed the memory of the remedy is somehow imprinted onto the water. Homeopathic medicine works at different levels and can be used by anyone for minor or short-lived health problems. In addition, it can have a profound healing effect when dispensed by a homeopathic doctor or nurse following an in-depth assessment of the patient and the condition.

The homeopathic interview elicits a long and detailed account of the patient's illness or condition, past and present, given by the patient in their own words, and is acknowledged to be a therapeutic and healing experience in its own right. The history covers not only the signs and symptoms of the condition and when it first started, but also what else was going on in the patient's life at that time. It addresses the current psychology of the patient, referred to in some texts as the *mentals*, as well as the *modalities* of the condition, identifying the external influences which affect its presentation, such as temperature, whether better or worse for being outdoors or indoors, whether worse for standing up or lying down, or better or worse at different times of the day or seasons of the year. Food preferences are discussed as well as fears and anxieties. One other area of enquiry unique to homeopathy is the section of the assessment which covers 'strange, rare and peculiar symptoms'. Thus, a complete and comprehensive picture is built up not only of the condition but of the person.

Dosage and prescription methods in homeopathy are not laid down but depend on the presenting symptoms and their severity, doses being given frequently initially, sometimes as often as every 5 minutes, and reducing in frequency as the condition improves. This differs from orthodox practice, where a prescribed regime is set out; however, readers may note a similarity between the homeopathic regime and their own approach to treating headaches, in which dosage and frequency of medication will depend on how severe the headache is, the day's demands and how well the first dose of analgesia works. Practitioners may note differences between suggested prescribing regimes in various publications, but the principle of prescribing remains the same. In general, the potency is less important than matching the patient's symptoms with the symptom picture of the remedy.

Remedies are normally prescribed singly and tailored to address the patient's presenting symptoms, but there are a number of composite over-the-counter remedies that are dispensed to address a range of presenting symptoms within one condition. This form of prescribing is common in Germany, 80% of remedies being prescribed in this way, normally for chronic conditions. The style of prescribing described in this text is known as specific, i.e. a single remedy is prescribed for a specific symptom. This is in contrast to the constitutional remedy style, which takes into account not only the symptoms but also the personality and physical characteristics of the patient. However, these factors may not always be relevant in addressing the presenting problem, and in any case, given the variability of humankind, it is not always possible to identify a constitutional remedy for a client. However, Herscu's (1991) classic homeopathy text, which gives a classification of eight paediatric constitutional types, is referred to in this book as appropriate. It is important to realise that there are many ways of selecting a remedy, depending on time, prescribing style and experience.

Homeopathic remedies are now freely available over the counter and in this country are dispensed at the 6c or 30c potency. In general, the 30c potency can be used for both chronic and acute conditions. As a general guide, the 30c potencies are used when the condition has a marked emotional overtone and the 6c for more physical conditions. The remedies are dispensed for children in a number of formats: pilules are dissolved on the tongue (for babies and small children they can be crushed first between two clean spoons); tablets can be chewed or sucked; and tinctures, which are the most suitable for babies, can be dispensed by droplet or granules. The remedies are completely safe for babies and children and do not interfere with orthodox medicine.

The healing process in homeopathy follows the path laid down in what is known as Hering's (1800–1880) law, which states that:

- Symptoms resolve in the reverse order of their onset
- Symptoms resolve from above downwards
- Symptoms resolve from inside outwards
- The most important organs resolve first.

Along with other CAM interventions, homeopathy does not seek to suppress symptoms and as part of the healing process, there may be an exacerbation of the original condition following the onset of treatment. This is normal and will resolve as the remedy takes effect. Homeopathic remedies can be used alongside orthodox medication without adverse interaction. Evidence for the efficacy of homeopathy includes randomised controlled trials, expert opinion and empirical observations. (Source material Boyd (1989), Lockie (1990), Downey (1997), Gemmell (1997), Swayne (1998a, b.)

Bach flower remedies

Nurses may well come across these remedies being used by patients both in and out of hospital, and they are readily available in many high street chemists and health food shops. The therapeutic effect of the remedies is aimed at rebalancing negative emotional states rather than at treating a physical condition. The Bach flower remedies were identified and developed (some say rediscovered) by Dr Edward Bach, a physician and homeopath born in 1886 in Warwickshire, who trained and qualified at University College London. On starting his medical career he became more interested in the effect of an illness on his patients than in the illness itself. In particular, he noted that patients often reacted differently to the same condition and that prescribing the same treatment did not always result in an improvement in the patient's condition. He was a great observer of people and quickly deduced that a person's mood and personality were important considerations in the planning of their treatment, since they appeared to have a significant effect on the course of the illness.

For a while he practised at the Royal London Homeopathic Hospital and was greatly influenced by the work of Hahnemann, whom he admired. However, he eventually rejected the practice of homeopathy on the grounds that many homeopathic remedies were made from bacteria. Surprisingly for his generation, Bach did not feel that medical interventions should be the sole province of the doctor. He thought that ordinary people should have the wherewithal to treat themselves, a philosophy of patient empowerment well ahead of its time. His avowed aim was to establish a system of emotional healing which would be available to everyone. To this end he spent the next few years discovering and developing the 38 flower remedies which bear his name. These 38 remedies correspond with the 38 negative emotions he identified in his patients.

The remedies are divided into two groups, one group comprising the type remedies (similar to homeopathy's concept of constitution) and the other group consisting of mood remedies, which address the presenting emotional state of the patient. Bach recognised that the presenting mood of the patient might not be a permanent or normal part of their personality but might represent a reaction to current circumstances. Hahnemann's influence can be detected in the flexibility of the flower remedy prescriptions, which are adjusted over time to accommodate the patient's changing emotional state. In fact, the two groups of remedies can be used interchangeably since one person's predominant personality may be markedly altered by a changing situation. This idea of plasticity of personality was out of step with the prevailing theories of the time.

There are two ways of distilling the flower essences used in the remedies. The first is the sun method. Fresh flowers are picked, put into a glass bowl of spring water and left in the sun for several hours so that the sun's rays can energise the water. This is similar to the homeopathic concept of imprinting energy onto water. The flower essence is then preserved in brandy and becomes the mother tincture. The second method, known as the boiling method, involves boiling the flowers in water for half an hour, the resulting essence being preserved in brandy. Up to six remedies can be prescribed at one time and are dispensed by adding 2 drops of the tincture to 30 mL of spring water; then 4 drops are taken, either directly onto the tongue or in fluid four times a day. The most well-known remedy is Rescue Remedy, a composite remedy including Star of Bethlehem (for loss, bereavement or trauma), Rock Rose (for terror and panic, often following an accident), Impatiens (for irritation and impatience), Cherry Plum (for fear of losing control, uncontrollable rage) and Clematis (for inattention and the slightly disorientated feeling following shock). Rescue Remedy is also available as a cream, which has honey as one of the ingredients and does not contain any animal fats.

The process of diagnosis lies in the ability of the patient or Bach practitioner to uncover the emotional layers and ascertain which underlying condition needs to be treated. The remedies are safe for children of all ages (in common with homeopathy, the dosages being the same for children as for adults) and do not interfere with orthodox medication.

At present, evidence for the efficacy of the flower remedies remains anecdotal with some support through empirical observations, but the remedies do appear to offer a measure of comfort and support to many people. (Source material Howard (1994), Mantle (1997).)

Aromatherapy

The term *aromatherapie* was coined by the French chemist Rene-Maurice Gattefosse in 1928 following his successful work using essential oils as a treatment for burns, gangrene and other war wounds during the First World War. The dictionary defines it as the use of essential plant oils to treat human ailments. A number of authors have reviewed the history of essential oils, tracing their use from ancient times until their recent resurgence as a modern therapeutic intervention. Records show that the antibacterial properties of essential oils were known to the Egyptians, who used them in the mummification of their dead, and the use of aromatic oils is mentioned repeatedly in the Bible.

The therapeutic use of plants was widespread in the ancient world, but an Arab healer called Ibn Sina, also known as Avicenna, was thought to be the first person to distil the essential oil from the mother plant, although earlier artefacts have been found in the Indus valley which suggest that the distillation of the oils was achieved 5000 years ago. The recent resurgence of the use of essential oils was led by Madame Maury, who brought the discipline to the UK from France. Her success in promoting the use of these oils, particularly combined with massage, has led to an explosion of interest in the therapy which nurses have identified as being of particular value in nursing care.

The oils are highly concentrated, volatile substances and are usually obtained by distillation (though other methods might be used) from all or specific parts of the plant, and it is the chemical constituents which give them their therapeutic action. The oils can consist of between 100 and 300 components, which include hydrocarbons such as monoterpenes, diterpenes and sesquiterpenes. Monoterpenes are found in nearly all essential oils in varying amounts and have antibacterial, antiviral and mildly analgesic properties. Sesquiterpenes are anti-inflammatory, antispasmodic and anti-infective, whilst diterpenes are mildly anti-infective and expectorant. Some oils exhibit a differential antiseptic effect on specific systems of the body. Other constituents of essential oils include esters and aldehydes, which are sedative and antiseptic, phenols, which are stimulant and antibacterial, and ketones, alcohols and oxides. Since some of the constituents of essential oils are skin irritants, the oils must be properly diluted in a carrier oil before use. However, with the potential for an allergic reaction, the use of nut-based carrier oils should be avoided.

Oils may be administered in a number of ways including inhalation, massage, compresses and by being added to a bath. As indicated above in the section on safety, there is considerable concern about the lack of consensus amongst aromatherapists regarding the therapeutic properties, dispensation and toxicity of essential oils. In addition, a number of academics have critically evaluated some of the assumptions underlying aromatherapy. Lis-Balchin (1997) suggests that much of aromatherapy folklore about the effects of essential oils has been extrapolated erroneously from the works of Culpeper and other English herbalists. She points out that the pharmaceutical action of herbs and essential oils is fundamentally different and suggests that aromatherapy can help some illnesses sometimes, but that there is scant evidence that massaging with highly diluted oils will have any effect on internal organs (Lis-Balchin 1995).

Buchbauer (1992) suggests that it is a waste of time applying essential oils by massage because of the evaporation time, and that the preferred route should be by inhalation. Evidence for the efficacy of the use of essential oils includes randomised controlled trials, expert opinion and empirical observations. Evidence for the efficacy of the use of aromatherapy with children and the value of aromatherapy as an intervention in a range of conditions is given in subsequent chapters as appropriate. (Source material Davis (1996), Tiran (2000).)

Massage

Massage is an instinctive, probably innate, behaviour used by humans and animals as a form of therapy, communication and comfort. Massage has been used therapeutically for centuries and is mentioned in ancient medical texts within the Greek, Egyptian, Indian and Chinese medical systems. Hippocrates made extensive use of it for the treatment and prevention of disease. In Egypt it was considered a sacred art and the Romans used it to prepare gladiators for the arena.

Child massage (Tui Na) is an integral part of TCM and is incorporated into the daily home regime for parents, who are taught basic massage and acupressure skills to use on both babies and older children. Each massage takes about 3–4 minutes for general application, but parents are taught to massage the relevant acupressure points if the child has a particular condition. Abdominal massage is considered to be particularly beneficial in TCM because it is believed that the Five Elements are situated in a circle round the abdomen with the umbilicus, the seat of the Middle Energiser (see previous section on TCM meridians), in the centre, and it is by massaging the abdomen that the Five Elements are harmonised. Child care also includes a regular back massage and the stimulation of acupressure points to harmonise the flow of Qi to all the organs, particularly the Yin organs (remembering that children are predominantly Yang, so promoting Yin will effect a balance). In order to stimulate the flow of Qi, parents can massage the major meridians, encouraging the flow of Qi around the body.

Ayurvedic medicine also advocates the use of massage for children, again starting in infancy. An abhyanga (oil massage) is used, which takes a maximum of half an hour. Recommended oils include sesame, coconut and ghee, although the same caution in the use of nut oils which was highlighted for aromatherapy should be used.

In Anthroposophical medicine the astral body experiences the massage in three ways, depending on the vigour of the massage. A light pressure will have only a limited effect on the astral body, but the effect will be enhanced with a more strongly applied technique. Muscles are closely related to the astral body since both work in polarities, one movement counterbalancing the other, and it is believed that different massage movements relate to the different polarities. For example, finger pressure will obtain its effect from the nervous sense pole, use of the thumb will energise the metabolic pole, whilst the palm of the hand will benefit the rhythmical system. The massage intervention will be determined by the physician, depending on the clinical diagnosis and the need to balance the underlying imbalance of the system that is causing the disease.

Massage is not a single therapy but a group of interventions and techniques that can range from the gentle, soothing movements of baby massage and aromatherapy massage, through Swedish massage and sports massage, to the deep massage technique known as Rolfing, which seeks to make structural alterations in the musculature and to liberate tensions. Other massage systems include stimulating shiatsu or reflexology points. Massage is used to promote wellbeing, improve circulation and enhance the movement of the musculo-skeletal system.

Massage has been an integral part of nursing care since the development of modern nursing. An article in the first edition of the *Nursing Times* encourages nurses (particularly private nurses) to train in massage or they may find that, without this skill, they do not get many referrals. Evidence for the efficacy of massage as a therapeutic intervention includes anecdotal reports, empirical observations and controlled trials. (Source material Morrison (1994), Field (2000), Tiran (2000), Loo (2002).)

Reflexology

In common with a number of other therapies which have developed over many centuries, reflexology has evolved into a number of styles and formats, such as traditional reflexology (Ingham 1984), holistic multidimensional reflexology (Ashkenazi 1993), reflex zone therapy (Goodwin 1992) and vacureflexology (Griffiths 2001); however, for convenience and continuity, the general term reflexology will be used throughout.

Reflexology is a form of massage or touch in which the organs of the body are mapped, primarily on the foot but also on the hands, face and back. However, reflexology is more than just a massage. It is a holistic therapy dedicated to the generation and maintenance of health and wellbeing, producing harmony and balance within the patient as well as addressing specific health problems. A lively ongoing debate concerns whether reflexology can be used as a diagnostic tool, some therapists claiming that, by being able to feel minute gritty areas or granules under the skin at explicit points, they can detect an underlying condition. However, the use of feel and touch on the skin over the reflex points is usually seen as only one aspect of a general assessment of the patient rather than an exact tool for diagnosis.

The use of foot massage as a therapy would appear to be part of many long established medical systems. Archaeologists have found evidence suggesting that a form of reflexology was practised in such diverse cultures as those found in India, Assyria and Egypt. It is also thought that the Chinese used it as long ago as 4000 BC, although its use died out as the art of acupuncture became more refined and entered mainstream Traditional Chinese Medicine. There are two main theories as to how reflexology works. The first is the zone theory, which postulates that the body is divided into 10 vertical zones, 5 on each side of the body; the respective organs within that longitudinal division are reflected in the corresponding area of the foot. The other key theory is that the link between the soles of the feet and the organs is via the six main Chinese meridians (discussed under TCM). The six main meridians running through the feet are the Liver, Spleen, Pancreas, Stomach, Gall Bladder and Kidney meridians. In the West, evidence that a form of reflexology was known and practised as far back as the

14th century is to be found in a book by Adamus and A'tatis published in 1582 on the subject of zone therapy.

More modern developments in reflexology have their roots in neurological studies in Russia and Germany, but it was the Americans who brought reflexology to the attention of the general public. Dr William Fitzgerald of Connecticut, who practised in Vienna and London, recognised the role of reflex zones in effecting a local anaesthesia, allowing him to perform minor operations. Following this discovery he attempted to map the various zones of the foot and their corresponding internal organs. The theory was further developed and refined by a number of practitioners, many of whom have developed their own schools and techniques.

Reflexology is a safe, non-invasive therapy which is easy to incorporate into nursing care, and applicable to babies and children as well as adults. The length of treatment and amount of pressure used is adjusted according to the child's age and physical condition. Relevant reflex points will be indicated as appropriate for particular conditions discussed in subsequent chapters. Research evidence for reflexology includes randomised controlled trials, expert testimony and anecdotal reports. (Source material Dougans (1996), Lett (2000), Mackereth and Tiran (2002).)

Herbalism

Herbalism has a long and honourable tradition of providing health care to the poor and rich alike, long before the advent of the NHS, and is thought to be the oldest form of therapy practised by humankind. Our ancestors observed the behaviour of sick animals and noted which plants they ate to heal themselves. Since plants tend to vary from one region to another, local formularies were developed; however, where the same herb has been identified in different parts of the world there is very often a high level of concordance between quite isolated populations about its therapeutic use. This knowledge was probably passed on by word of mouth from one healer to the next, although early written records have been discovered in Sumeria listing botanical remedies. The ancient Egyptians listed 850 plant medicines on a papyrus scroll dating from 1500 BC.

It is suggested that the first Western herbal was written by Theophrastus (371–287 BC) in the 3rd century BC, and its instructions about the collection and preparation of plant remedies were used for 2000 years. With the marching Roman legions came the march of medical knowledge across Europe. Unfortunately, a great deal of the accumulated medical knowledge was lost when the Christians burnt the medical library at Alexandria in the 4th century AD. In England, a number of herbals were published during the Renaissance, for example, by John Gerard (1545–1612) and Nicholas Culpeper (1616–1654). In 1621 the first physic garden was cultivated at Magdalen College, Oxford, whilst the Worshipful Society of Apothecaries founded the physic garden in Chelsea in 1674.

With the growth of orthodox medicine, herbal medicine lost ground, largely because the folklore surrounding the cultivation and gathering of plants was considered to be the result of ignorance and superstition. For example, it was held that gathering certain plants should be done at certain times of the day or month according to the lunar cycle. However, these early observations have now been shown to be correct since plants do vary in their therapeutic potential at different times of the day or year.

Diagnosis by modern herbalists follows a similar pattern to orthodox medicine; in fact the diagnosis is often already made since many people approach herbal medicine as a last resort. However, treatment will encompass a number of approaches including addressing the main complaint, but also will include supportive treatments to aid the body's own healing capacity. This might include a tonic or relaxant, a diuretic to enhance elimination, or an aid to digestion. Herbal remedies are prepared as teas, tinctures, pills, juices, creams or lotions. The whole of the herb is used in preparing the prescription, the ingredients working synergistically rather than an 'active ingredient' being extracted and isolated. By using the whole of the plant many of the side effects that result from isolation of the active ingredient can be avoided. For example, by using the whole of the dandelion plant (*Taraxacum officinale*) as a diuretic, the loss of potassium is avoided since potassium is found in the dandelion leaves, rendering additional supplementation unnecessary.

Remedies are classified according to their actions, which are described slightly differently from those of orthodox medication:

- Warming remedies, such as vasodilators and circulatory stimulants
- Cooling remedies, such as relaxants and bitters (for allergies, inflammatory conditions, migraines and fevers)
- Diuretics
- Expectorants, including stimulating and warming expectorants, relaxing expectorants and antitussives
- Alteratives, for detoxification and cleansing, e.g. for chronic inflammatory conditions of the skin and connective tissues
- Tonic and hormonal remedies
- Healing remedies.

There are a number of over-the-counter herbal remedies that parents may be interested in using. Some of these remedies are not suitable, in their commercial form, for use on children under a certain age (variable), so nurses should encourage parents to seek the advice of a medical herbalist before administering anything other than simple teas for colic or relaxation. Herbal remedies described in this text are simply examples of what a herbalist might prescribe and the evidence for their efficacy is given. Much of the research falls into the empirical domain but is more commonly now backed up by clinical trials. If children are being given herbal remedies it is important that this is brought to the attention of the anaesthetist if the child is to undergo an operation, since some herbs may affect the amount or type of anaesthetic given (Murphy 1999, Tsen et al 2000). See also Chapter 4 on sleep in Section 2. (Source material Mills (1989), Mills and Bone (2000), Sumner (2000).)

Music therapy

Biley (2001) makes the distinction between music as therapy and music therapy, the former being an intervention that can be used informally by healthcare professionals, whilst the latter can only be performed by a qualified music therapist. Since there is evidence for the efficacy of both approaches, both have been included in the text. Music as a therapeutic intervention has been recorded for many thousands of years. Our earliest ancestors would appear to have fashioned and used musical instruments, possibly in the first instance to frighten away wild animals or evil spirits. In ancient Egypt, music was called the physic of the soul and the effect of music on the mind is recorded in a wide range of ancient texts, for example the Biblical accounts of David playing the lyre to King Saul. Both Homer and Plato believed that music promoted physical and mental health, dispelling negative emotions and thoughts, and many ancient healers were also musicians.

Although music therapy is not indicated as a therapeutic component in TCM, the Chinese recognised the value of music and believed that it could convey essential truth. Confucius believed that a society's music reflected the state of that society, a feeling no doubt harboured by many who deplore modern musical trends.

Anthroposophical medicine, on the other hand, uses music therapy as an integral part of the diagnostic and healing process. The therapist works with the doctor and therapy is aimed at dealing with a specific diagnosis and tailored to suit individual patients. Central to treatment is attentive listening and the alternation of making and listening to music. Physical changes have been identified as a result of music therapy, including changes in metabolism, heart rate, blood pressure and energy levels.

Music has been shown to enhance paediatric care in neonatal units, in pain relief and as distraction. For young children who are in hospital, in a world that is completely different from their home, playgroup or school, the comfort of a familiar tune or song can be very beneficial. Music can enable these children to express their feelings, and techniques used by the music therapist may include encouraging children to write songs, sing or play an instrument.

REFERENCES

Abt A, Oh J, Huntington R, Burkhart K 1995 Chinese herbal medicine induced acute renal failure. Archives of Internal Medicine 155(2): 211–212

Ashkenazi R 1993 Multidimensional reflexology. International Journal of Alternative and Complementary Medicine 11(6): 8–12

Biley F 2001 Music as therapy. In: Rankin-Box R (ed) The nurse's handbook of complementary therapies. Baillière Tindall, London

Boschma G 1994 The meaning of holism in nursing: historical shifts in holistic nursing ideas. Public Health Nursing 11(5): 324–330

Bott V 1996 Spiritual science and the art of healing: Rudolf Steiner's anthroposophical medicine. Healing Arts Press, Vermont

Boutin P, Buchwald D, Robinson L, Collier A 2000 Use and attitudes about alternative and complementary therapies among outpatients and physicians at a municipal hospital. The Journal of Alternative and Complementary Medicine 6(4): 335–343

Boyd H 1997 Introduction to homeopathic medicine, 2nd edn. Beaconsfield Publishers, Beaconsfield

British Medical Association 1993 Complementary medicine: new approaches to good practice. Oxford University Press, Oxford

Buchbauer G 1992 Biological effects of fragrances and essential oils. 12th International Congress of Flavours, Fragrances and Essential Oils. Vienna, Austria, Oct 4–8, 1992. Available from the British Library

Buckle J 1993 When is holism not complementary? British Journal of Nursing 2(15): 744–745

Buckle J 1997 Clinical aromatherapy in nursing. Arnold, London

Chadwick D 1999 What are the reasons for nurses using complementary therapy in practice? Complementary Therapies in Nursing and Midwifery 5(5): 144–148

Chez R, Jonas W, Eisenberg D 1999 The physician and complementary and alternative medicine. In: Jonas W, Levin J (eds) Essentials of complementary and alternative medicine. Lippincott, Williams & Wilkins, Philadelphia

Coe W, Rykan K 1979 Hypnosis and risk to human subjects. American Psychologist 34(8): 673–681

Davis P 1996 Aromatherapy: an A–Z. CW Daniel, Saffron Walden

Dickens P, Tai Y, But P 1994 Fatal accidental aconite poisoning following ingestion of Chinese herbal medicine: a report of two cases. Forensic Science International 67(1): 55–58

Dougans I 1996 Complete reflexology: therapeutic foot massage for health and well-being. Element Books, Shaftesbury, Dorset

Downey P 1997 Homeopathy for the primary health care team. Butterworth-Heinemann, Oxford

Ernst E 1999 Prevalence of complementary/ alternative medicine for children: a systematic review. European Journal of Pediatrics 158: 7–11

Ernst E, Barnes J 1998 Methodological approaches to investigate the safety of complementary therapy. Complementary Therapies in Medicine 6: 115–121

Evans M, Rodger I 2000 Healing for body, soul and spirit. Floris Books, Edinburgh

Field T 2000 Touch therapy. Churchill Livingstone, Edinburgh

Fowler R, Wall M 1997 COSHH and CHIPS: ensuring the safety of aromatherapy. Complementary Therapies in Medicine 5(2): 112–115

Fowler P, Wall M 1998 Aromatherapy: control of substances hazardous to health (COSHH) and assessment of the chemical risk. Complementary Therapies in Medicine 6(2): 86–93

Gemmell D 1997 Everyday homoeopathy. Beaconsfield Publishers, Beaconsfield, UK

Glöckler M, Goebel W 1990 A guide to child health. Anthroposophical Press, Floris Books, Edinburgh

Goodman N 2001 The Observer's barefoot doctor: explanations for the credulous. The British Journal of General Practice (November) 952–953

Goodwin H 1992 Reflex zone therapy. In: Rankin-Box D (ed) Complementary health therapies: a guide for nurses and the caring professions. Chapman & Hall, London

Gray R, Maharajh G, Hyland R 1991 Pneumothorax resulting from acupuncture. Canadian Association of Radiologists Journal 42(2): 139–140

Grenfell A, Patel N, Robinson N 1998 Complementary therapy: general practitioners' referral and patients' use in an urban multi-ethnic area. Complementary Therapies in Medicine 6(3): 127–132

Griffiths P 2001 Reflexology. In: Rankin-Box D (ed) The nurse's handbook of complementary therapies. Churchill Livingstone, Edinburgh

Grootenhuis M, Last B, de Graaf-Nijkerk JH, van de Wel M 1998 Use of alternative treatment in pediatric oncology. Cancer Nursing 21(4): 282–288

Ham-Ying S 1993 Analysis of the concept of holism within the context of nursing. British Journal of Nursing 2(15): 771–775

Harris P, Rees R 2000 The prevalence of complementary and alternative medicine use among the general population: a systematic review of the literature. Complementary Therapies in Medicine 8: 88–96

Hasegawa J, Noguchi N, Yamasaki J et al 1991 Delayed cardiac tamponade and hemothorax induced by an acupuncture needle. Cardiology 78: 58–63

Helman C 2000 Feed a cold, starve a fever. In: Davey B, Gray A, Seale C (eds) Health and disease: a reader. Open University Press, Bucks

Herscu P 1991 The homeopathic treatment of children. North Atlantic Books, Berkeley, California

Horn S 1983 The 'locked in' syndrome following chiropractic manipulation of the cervical spine. Annals of Emergency Medicine 12(10): 648–650

House of Lords Select Committee on Science and Technology 2000 Sixth report on complementary and alternative medicine. HMSO, London

Howard J 1994 Growing up with the Bach flower remedies. CW Daniel, Saffron Walden

Ingham E 1984 Stories feet have told. Ingham, Florida

Irish A 1989 Maintaining health in persons with HIV infection. Seminars in Oncology Nursing 5(4): 302–307

Jonas W 1998 Safety in homeopathy. In: Ernst E, Hahn E (eds) Homeopathy: a critical appraisal. Butterworth-Heinemann, Oxford

Judd F, Burrows G, Dennerstein L 1985 The dangers of hypnosis: a review. Australian Journal of Clinical and Experimental Hypnosis 13: 1–15

Kaptchuck T 2001 The history of vitalism. In: Micozzi M (ed) Fundamentals of complementary and alternative medicine, Churchill Livingstone, Edinburgh

Keane J, Ahmadi J, Gruen P 1993 Spinal epidural haematoma with subarachnoid haemorrhage caused by acupuncture. American Journal of Neuroradiology 14(2): 365–366

Kummer K-R 1995 Childhood immunisation programs: questions from the anthroposophical point of view, part I. Journal of Anthroposophical Medicine 12(4): 34–45

Lad V 1985 Ayurveda the science of self healing: a practical guide. Lotus Press, Wisconsin

Lett A 2000 Reflex zone therapy for health professionals. Churchill Livingstone, Edinburgh

Lis-Balchin M 1997 Essential oils and 'aromatherapy': their role in modern healing. Journal of the Royal Society of Health 117(5): 324–329

Lockie A 1990 The family guide to homeopathy. Penguin Books, Middlesex, UK

Long A, Mercer G, Hughes K 2000 Developing a tool to measure holistic practice: a missing dimension in outcomes measurement within complementary therapies. Complementary Therapies in Medicine 8(1): 26–31

Loo M 2002 Pediatric acupuncture. Churchill Livingstone, Edinburgh

Maciocia G 2000 The practice of Chinese medicine. Churchill Livingstone, Edinburgh

Mackereth P, Tiran D 2002 (eds) Clinical reflexology: a guide for health professionals. Churchill Livingstone, Edinburgh

Mantle F 1996 Safe practices. Nursing Times 92(6): 36–39

Mantle F 1997 Bach flower remedies. Complementary Therapies in Nursing and Midwifery 3(5): 121–148

Mantle F 2001 Complementary therapies and nursing models. In: Rankin-Box D (ed) The nurse's handbook of complementary therapies, 2nd edn. Baillière Tindall, Edinburgh

Micozzi M 2001 Characteristics of complementary and alternative medicine. In: Micozzi M (ed) Fundamentals of complementary and alternative medicine. Churchill Livingstone, Edinburgh

Mills S 1989 The complete guide to modern herbalism. Thorsons, London

Mills S, Bone K 2000 Principles and practice of phytotherapy: modern herbal medicine. Churchill Livingstone, Edinburgh

Morrison J 1994 The book of Ayurveda: a guide to personal well being. Gaia Books, London

Murphy J 1999 Preoperative considerations with herbal medicine. AORN Journal 69(1): 173–175

Newbeck I, Rowe D 1986 Going the whole way. Nursing Times (February) 19: 24–25

Nightingale F 1980 Skeet M (ed) Notes on nursing: what it is and what it is not. Churchill Livingstone, Edinburgh

Orem D 1985 Nursing: concepts of practice. McGraw-Hill, New York

Pendergrass T, Davis S 1981 Knowledge and use of alternative cancer therapies in children. American Journal of Pediatric Haematological Oncology 3: 339–345

Rampes H, James R 1995 Complications of acupuncture. Acupuncture Medicine 13: 26–33

Rankin-Box D 1997 Therapies in practice: a survey assessing nurses' use of complementary therapies. Complementary Therapies in Nursing and Midwifery 3(4): 91–120

Rogers M 1970 The theoretical basis of nursing. Davis, Philadelphia

Roper N, Logan W, Tierney A 1985 The elements of nursing. Churchill Livingstone, Edinburgh

Sawyer M, Gannoni A, Toogood I 1994 The use of alternative therapies by children with cancer. Medical Journal of Australia 160: 320–322

Schmidt K 2002 CAM and the desperate call for cancer cures and alleviation. What can websites offer cancer patients? Complementary Therapies in Medicine 10(3): 179–180

Simpson H, Roman K 2001 Complementary medicine use in children: extent and reasons. A population-based study. British Journal of General Practice (November) 914–916

Sinel M, Smith D 1993 Thalamic infarction secondary to cervical manipulation. Archives of Physical Medicine and Rehabilitation 74(5): 543–546

Spigelblatt L 1997 Alternative medicine: a pediatric conundrum. Contemporary Pediatrics 14(8): 51–61

Stevensen C 2001 Nursing perspectives. In: Barraclough J (ed) Integrated cancer care holistic complementary and creative approaches. Oxford University Press, Oxford

Sumner J 2000 The natural history of medicinal plants. Timber Press, Oregon

Swayne J 1998a Homeopathic therapeutics: many dimensions or meaningless diversity? In: Vickers A (ed) Examining complementary medicine. Stanley Thornes, Cheltenham

Swayne J 1998b Homeopathic method. Churchill Livingstone, Edinburgh

Tiran D 2000 Complementary therapies for pregnancy and childbirth, 2nd edn. Baillière Tindall, Edinburgh

Tisserand R, Balacs T 1995 Essential oil safety: a guide for health care professionals. Churchill Livingstone, Edinburgh

Todd B 1990 Holistic nursing: a new paradigm for practice. NSNA/Imprint (September/October) 75–80

Treleaven J, Meller S, Farmer P 1993 Arsenic and Ayurveda. Leukemia and Lymphoma 10(4): 343–345

Tsen L, Segal S, Pothier M et al 2000 Alternative medicine use in presurgical patients. Anaesthesiology 93(1): 148–151

Ullrich S, Hodge P 1999 The Ullrich–Hodge alternative therapy assessment model: teaching students to evaluate patients for use, motivation and risks. Nurse Educator 24(6): 19–23

Vessey J, Rechkemmer A 2001 Pediatric Nursing 27(1): 61–67

Vickers A 1996 Massage and aromatherapy: a guide for health professionals. Chapman & Hall, London

Vincent C, Furnham A 1997 Complementary medicine: a research perspective. John Wiley, London

Warrior G 2002 Ayurveda. The right way to live. Carlton Books, London

Watson J 1985 Nursing: the philosophy and science of caring. Colorado Associated University Press, Colorado

Zagorsky E 1993 Caring for families who follow alternative health care practices. Pediatric Nursing (Jan/Feb) 19(1): 71–75

2 Clinical effectiveness, clinical supervision and legal and professional issues

CHAPTER CONTENTS

- **Clinical effectiveness** 33
  Evidence-based practice 33
  CAM and clinical effectiveness 34
  Integrating CAM 39
- **Clinical supervision** 40

- **Legal and professional issues** 41
- **References** 43

CLINICAL EFFECTIVENESS

Article 13 of the Human Rights Act refers to the right to an effective remedy. This has implications for nurses, who need to understand what constitutes an effective remedy. CAM remedies may be used if they are known to be effective, though this does not necessarily mean that the remedy used must demonstrate a higher level of effectiveness than a conventional medicine. One way of achieving effectiveness of interventions, treatment or remedies is to base practice on the evidence available.

Evidence-based practice

The move towards evidence-based practice began with the publication of Cochrane's *Effectiveness and efficiency* (1971), which stimulated discussion and examination of the clinical effectiveness of medical interventions. A key finding was that the supposed value of some of the most commonly used procedures and therapies was not borne out by research findings (Grayson 1997). Meanwhile Eddy and Billings (1993) had determined that only about 15% of medical practice was based on scientific research. The movement towards evidence-based practice was established on these foundations. Trinder (2000) summarised its emergence, giving four main reasons:

- The research–practice gap
- Information overload
- Reluctance to change practice even when existing practice is shown to be ineffective
- The poor quality of much of the research.

Evidence-based practice is central to audit and effectiveness, to professional accountability and to risk assessment, although critics of the movement have raised concerns about its application and its effect on resources, the suggestion being that it is over-simplistic and constrains professional autonomy (Trinder 2000).

What is evidence-based practice?

Sackett et al (1996) define evidence-based practice as: 'The conscientious, explicit and judicious use of current best evidence in making decisions about individual patients ... by integrating individual clinical experience with the best available clinical evidence.' By 'clinical experience' the authors mean the proficiency and judgement acquired through clinical experience and practice. Sackett et al (1996) go on to state that neither clinical experience nor the best external evidence is good enough on its own; they point out that, however excellent the external evidence might be, without clinical expertise, it might be inapplicable or inappropriate for an individual patient. Reynolds (2000) challenges the relevance of applying evidence-based medicine to individual patients whose values and expectations may not embrace the intervention planned. She suggests that the individuality of the patient is the greatest challenge to evidence-based medicine; after all, nurses nurse an individual patient, not a 'control group' or an 'experimental group'. There will be instances in this book where it is apparent that, whilst the results of a CAM intervention may not have achieved a level of statistical significance, a sub-group of subjects has been identified who appear to benefit from the intervention. Reason and Rowan (1981) have summed up the issue in their description of results as being 'statistically significant, humanly insignificant' which can, of course, be turned the other way round. As Reynolds (2000) points out, many methods of treatment may have no effect or even a negative effect on some patients.

CAM and clinical effectiveness

Is there the evidence for CAM to be regarded as clinically effective? Contrary to popular opinion, there is a wealth of research using a variety of methodologies and covering a wide range of therapies. Muir Gray (1997) lists the following criteria for evaluating a therapeutic intervention:

1 Effectiveness
2 Safety
3 Patient acceptability and satisfaction
4 Cost effectiveness
5 Appropriateness.

He goes on to list five categories of evidential strength:

1 Strong evidence from at least one systematic review of multiple, well-designed, randomised controlled trials.
2 Strong evidence from at least one properly designed, randomised controlled trial of appropriate size.
3 Evidence from well-designed trials, without randomisation, with single group pre- and post-test, cohort, time series or matched case-control studies.

4 Evidence from well-designed, non-experimental studies from more than one centre or research group.

5 Opinions of respected authorities based on clinical evidence, descriptive studies or reports of expert committees.

Sackett et al (1996) have suggested that evidence of efficacy may be gleaned from a number of sources, such as tradition, empirical evidence, research, reported observation and survey, which give validity to clinical experience and support the concept of evidential strength. Again, Muir Gray (1997) echoes this by stating that 'many health care decisions must be made for which there is no high quality evidence ... which does not make evidence-based decision making impossible, it simply requires the best evidence available'.

CAM and randomised controlled trials (RCTs)

The randomised controlled trial (RCT) is commonly held to be the 'gold standard' for research. However, this approach has frequently been challenged and the limitations of the RCT are described by Dove and Anthony (1987). They suggest that, whilst the method is particularly suited to laboratory animals, which are bred to be genetically similar and are fed, housed and treated in a similar manner, there are grounds for doubting that the results are applicable to humans, who have highly individual constitutions, predispositions towards illness and reactions to illness. As Cole and Shanley (1998) point out, clinical trials may be a very useful way of evaluating treatments and determining useful interventions when therapeutic outcomes are easily discernable, however they fail to accommodate the complexity of human nature and experience and, consequently, are a poor measure of human behaviour, which is impossible to reduce to quantifiable measures. Cole and Shanley (1998) further state that the RCT does nothing to address the complexity of the human condition and experiences which are the subject of the investigation. This is highlighted again in Section 3 in relation to CAM in health promotion. Other critics of RCTs include Liverani et al (2000) and Heron (1986), who have criticised the value of RCTs for conventional therapies by noting the limitation of the method, whilst Altman (1994) suggests that the use of quantitative research without a proper basis is deeply unethical since it involves volunteers and patients in clinical trials. Arguments that are frequently put forward against the use of RCTs with CAM include not only the individuality of the patients but also the uniqueness of the interventions, and the difficulty in designing a convincing placebo for therapies such as acupuncture, hypnosis or reflexology (Anthony 1987). In contrast, Resch and Ernst (1997) argue that, given the right outcome measures, even the most holistic approach can be evaluated through the use of RCTs.

An indication of the problems of undertaking research in CAM using RCTs can be obtained by examining the difficulties in investigating the efficacy of acupuncture as a treatment modality. A number of issues have been identified. The main problem is in trying to assess the therapeutic effect of acupuncture on a range of conditions when 'acupuncture' describes not just one, discrete therapy but a range of inter-linked techniques which have been described as a 'multi modal system of healing with complex explanatory models' (Birch 1998). It is a therapy that is constantly evolving in response to social and political pressures, and, in doing so, has developed a wide range of diagnostic and explanatory models and interventions (Birch 1998). This makes generalisation from specific investigations difficult if the type of theoretical model used is not clarified; consequently, the fact that 'acupuncture' in one instance does not 'work' does not mean that other models of the intervention will not. Birch (1998) points out that 'there is no scientific evidence to support the notion that one method of acupuncture is superior to any other', and suggests that to reflect and validate the wide range of acupuncture models, an equally wide range of research methodologies should be considered. Contrary to popular belief, not all acupuncture models use a holistic approach and, again, research methods should reflect this principle.

Another key problem in acupuncture research is the use of sham or placebo acupuncture as a research intervention and its use has been critically evaluated by Jobst (1995), Birch (1997), Hammerschlag (1998) and Ryan (1999). Birch (1997) points out that what is used as a sham or placebo intervention may, in fact, constitute an active treatment, which may be quite adequate to produce a therapeutic effect. In a group of studies reviewed by Schwartz (1988) it was shown that sham and 'real' acupuncture were almost equally effective.

CAM and systematic reviews

These two issues are also apparent when another technique used to assess evidence-based practice is applied to acupuncture. This technique involves the use of a systematic review and meta-analysis of the research data between a number of studies in order to determine whether, overall, the statistical power of the intervention is effective. The key principle in meta-analysis is the definition of inclusion and exclusion criteria for the studies under scrutiny, through the allocation of points to specific aspects of the research design. For example, points may be allocated according to the number of subjects studied, whether the subjects were randomised, and whether the study was blinded. Generally speaking, studies having a poor research design will be excluded from the analysis, even though their results may be positive, thus leading to a bias in the conclusions drawn from the meta-analysis.

An example of this, again relating to research into acupuncture, in this instance, for the treatment of chronic pain, is found in Ter Riet et al (1990a), who commented on the poor methodology used in the trials they reviewed. In analysing the papers, the authors weighted the methodology of each trial with points: for example, randomisation was awarded 12 points, and studies with groups of subjects over 50 in number were awarded 10 points. The larger the final total of points, the better the study. In spite of the poor methodology, acupuncture was credited with having a role to play in the treatment of chronic pain. However, other reviews of the efficacy of acupuncture have suffered from a negative conclusion because of the subjectivity of the inclusion and exclusion criteria. A fuller critique of the use of meta-analysis is offered by Bailar (1997), who cites problems with this technique as including the failure of the investigator to understand the basic issues of the intervention being reviewed. Again, using reviews of acupuncture effectiveness as an example, this criticism has been highlighted by Rampes and Mortimer (1997), who challenged the rigour of Ter Riet et al's (1990b) assessment of the role of acupuncture in treating addictions. In a letter to the editor of *Complementary Therapies in Medicine* Rampes and Mortimer (1997) challenged the validity of the scoring system employed on their study of electro-acupuncture for the relief of alcohol craving. They also pointed out that other researchers, in this case Lewith and Vincent (1995), had commented on the discussion section of Ter Riet et al's review, stating that it was muddled, and had challenged the credibility of Ter Riet et al to assess acupuncture as a clinical modality. This example illustrates the importance of reviewers having a sound understanding of the philosophy and methodology of the technique under scrutiny. In Ter Riet's review, the concept of sham (or placebo) acupuncture was totally misplaced and a false conclusion was drawn.

This casts doubt on earlier clinical trials using the Western research paradigm of acupuncture versus placebo and reduces the internal validity of trials included in many of the meta-analysis reviews. The use of the Western research paradigm in investigating acupuncture has also been challenged by Given (1998). He cogently urges a return to what he calls 'the sensitivity and subtlety of Traditional Chinese Medicine', deploring and rejecting the set protocol approach to addiction treatment, which he refers to as a 'one size fits all' approach. In a well argued paper, Lewith (1998) suggests that a better approach would be to compare the results of an intervention using a complementary therapy with conventional treatment rather than with a placebo. This approach has been commented on by Hammerschlag and Morris (1997) who, in their review of research on the use of acupuncture versus standard biomedical care, noted that there was an improvement, over time, in the quality of the research. They point out, however, that in spite of the low standard of research design, 20 of the 23 studies showed results in which acupuncture was at least as effective as standard medical care.

Of course, reviews of research can only be undertaken if the studies are published in the first place. The concept of publication bias has frequently been raised in discussion of both CAM and orthodox research. In a seminal piece of research by Resch et al (2000), the extent of the publication bias against CAM was glaringly revealed. Two identical research papers (in terms of design structure and results) were submitted on the treatment of obesity, one paper alleging that an orthodox drug treatment was used and the other a homeopathic remedy. When the papers were distributed to a range of suitable reviewers, results indicated overwhelmingly that the paper referring to the orthodox drug usage was accepted for publication and review on more occasions than the paper referring to the homeopathic remedy.

Other approaches

The traditional form of defining homeopathic efficacy has been the 'provings' mechanism by which Hahnemann identified the remedies. Hahnemann recruited health volunteers who took the remedy and reported on their reaction to it. The match between the reported reactions and the patients' symptoms indicated which remedy would be suitable in any particular instance. Proving, from the German *prufung* meaning test, is now known as homeopathic pathogenic trial (HPT), and involves administering the remedy under trial to a number of healthy individuals and noting their subsequent reactions. The remedy is then added to the homeopathic repertory.

The purpose of proving a homeopathic remedy is to seek the character of the remedy and test its qualities (Wieland 1998). Following the taking of a case history, each proving goes through a number of stages:

■ Probability – confirmation that the same symptoms are experienced by more than one subject

- Corroboration, where physiological effects are noted when the remedy is taken in its raw state
- Verification, when the remedy is tried out on different subjects, and
- Characteristic, when after lengthy verification the remedy is accepted as characteristic for the condition.

The validity of these provings has been assessed by Fisher (1998), who highlights issues around observer bias, lack of placebo control and no 'blinding' of the remedy. Elements of a minimum standard for provings have now been devised. However, because homeopathy is such an individualised treatment and success depends on the accurate matching of remedy and patient, other more general methods of research are particularly problematic.

Dantas and Fisher (1998), who reviewed homeopathic provings published between 1945 and 1995, looked at the reported effects, methodological rigour, reliability of design outcomes, and the assessment and interpretation of data. Data collected was submitted to a panel of practitioners for comment. They found that methodological quality was poor overall, clinical application was not outstanding and information on volunteer selection was poor. Furthermore, they suggested that it may not be appropriate to try out homeopathic remedies on healthy volunteers. Work by Walach (1993) indicates that the more rigorous the methodology, the fewer symptoms are reported. The concept of provings has been fundamental to homeopathy since its beginnings but is less applicable for other practitioners. However, all practitioners use their own clinical judgement as a basis for their prescribing methods, so because of this, and the individuality of homeopathic prescribing, an audit tool known as a systematic outcome correlation has been developed and used at the Royal Homeopathic Hospital, London. The tool, described by Fisher (1995), is based on conventional outcome audit but also includes measurements of objective and subjective parameters relating to diseases and quality of life. Computer analysis enables the practitioners to examine which patients using which treatments do well.

Research undertaken by Evans (1991) involved a survey amongst Anthroposophical doctors to ascertain their use and clinical evaluation of 18 Anthroposophical medications. The replies were analysed and the comparative efficacy of the medicines, based on clinical observations, was determined, whilst the value of the more negatively reported medications was reassessed. The researcher notes that: 'the nature of the evidence may be regarded as having an intermediate level of objectivity between the experience of the clinician and the objectivity of the randomised controlled trial'. He then goes on to suggest that the data has a high degree of detail and practice relevance and, since it is grounded in practice, has greater relevance than trials, which are undertaken in a more artificial situation. This is what Swayne (1998) refers to as 'informed empiricism', founded on experience and clinical judgement.

Similarly, a well-designed single case study can provide clear evidence of the efficacy of an intervention (Aldridge 1988, Ernst 1998), and as Leibrich (1990) points out in her critical evaluation of research methodologies for complementary therapies, there is nothing inherently unscientific about anecdotal evidence when published by a world authority, and it can yield valuable scientific information without the use of a randomised controlled trial. Leibrich (1990) also offers a well argued rationale for a range of scientific research methods which are suitable for complementary therapies, pointing out that no one method of evaluation should be expected to assess the effectiveness of all treatments. She goes on to suggest that the assumption that only one method of research is acceptable can lead to scientific stagnation. She proposes that there is a need for more research using trends within individual patients rather than differences between groups of patients. It is not always appreciated that the use of multiple methodologies was also supported by Cochrane (1972) when he stated that he did not want to give the impression that the RCT was the only technique of any value in medical research. The Research Council for Complementary Medicine emphasises that 'studies should not conflict with the best practices in the complementary discipline involved and that they should be planned so that the main sources of error and bias are avoided and provided that this rigour is sought, they need not conform to the traditional patterns of clinical trials methodology' (Aldridge 2000).

Notwithstanding the above, since the information contained in many complementary therapy text books is based on the opinion of an 'expert' in the field, questions are raised as to whether nurses should be prepared to accept such information at face value and, if difficulties arise, how far these 'experts' should be held accountable in a court of law. It is essential that practitioners should evaluate critically the research described in these texts and decide for themselves the evidential strength with which they feel comfortable.

As far as complementary therapies are concerned, it would seem unfair to reject any of the therapies as a treatment modality on the basis of reviews suggesting poor research and inappropriate design, especially since some of the research featured in some of the reviews of clinical trials was carried out over 30 years ago when, for example, the mechanics of sham acupuncture were not fully understood. Unfortunately, poor research design prevents justice being done to the many therapies that have stood the test of time, and the acceptance of CAM is thereby often unfairly hampered. Nurses should continue to keep an open mind in the light of this poor quality of research, and should assess the evidential strength of the research for themselves, as suggested by Muir Gray (1997). Blomfield and Hardy (2000) suggest that nurses risk becoming expert mimics if they uncritically adopt evidence-based practice, and they should not base their practice solely on one source of evidence, e.g. the RCT. Lewith (1998) puts it very well when he states that it is no longer valid or reasonable for a physician (this could equally apply to a nurse) to suggest that there is no evidence of efficacy within CAM. He goes on to agree that the evidence is sometimes conflicting and unclear, but suggests that this is entirely comparable with conventional medicine.

Integrating CAM

In spite of the problems with the evidence base of some of the therapies, there have been strong moves towards the integration of CAM into orthodox care. Fulder (1998) has suggested that orthodox medicine could learn a great deal from CAM about defining and measuring health. He suggests that orthodox medicine, with its emphasis on defining health as a freedom from obvious symptoms, has developed a population of patients who are, indeed, free from obvious symptoms but who are not fully well either. Adjusting the diagnostic focus from concrete symptoms to issues of vitality and constitution would result in a more meaningful understanding of the patient's health status. Peters (2000) suggests that the increased interest in CAM by members of the public is a useful indication of how health needs and health beliefs are changing. He points out that healthcare systems are not, and should not be, static but should continue to evolve as new and different needs come to light, and we develop the capabilities to deal with them. Jobst (1998) offers a persuasive argument for the economic advantages of integrating CAM with orthodox care and suggests that the emphasis on wellbeing and self-help that is a central feature of CAM will result in a healthier population and reduce the need for medicine and state welfare. He suggests that integrating appropriate therapies into health care would reduce the levels of morbidity and the need for expensive orthodox treatment. This would reduce the pressures on hospitals, allowing them, in turn, to offer patients more individualistic care. However, much of CAM is at present provided by the private sector and the implication of Jobst's paper is that people will have the financial resources to access these treatments, which is not necessarily the case. This is echoed by Fox (2001) who, arguing for the integration of CAM into the NHS, suggests that the more disadvantaged members of the community, who could most benefit from CAM, will not be able to access its benefits if there is no local NHS provision. There is a danger that, unless true integration of CAM into the NHS is achieved, we will further extend the health divide between the upper and lower economic classes.

Nurses who wish to integrate CAM into their practice need to be completely clear as to why they are planning to implement these interventions and should take into account the following factors: the amount of time involved in administering the therapy; the cost implications; and the attitudes of other members of staff who may not be sympathetic to the new initiative. They should also consider which therapies may be deemed to be appropriate to the clinical area, and the qualifications of the therapists considered to be acceptable for practice (Mantle 1997, Rankin-Box & McVey 2001). Nurses might then seek to identify common problems within their sphere of practice, such as insomnia, constipation or mobility problems, for which procedures from a range of therapies would add to their range of nursing interventions.

In conclusion, The Prince of Wales Foundation for Integrated Health (formally the Foundation for Integrated Medicine) was set up in 1995 to steer the use of CAM into mainstream health care, and since its inception in 1997, has worked towards an integrated healthcare system. Its agenda covers issues relating to training, research and regulation of the various therapies.

CLINICAL SUPERVISION

Clinical supervision is an area that may be of some concern to managers who support or may wish to support the integration of CAM into their clinical areas. Mackereth (2001) has eloquently addressed this issue in relation to CAM, noting that whilst clinical supervision is a place to provide a supportive environment in which nurses can reflect on their practice and professional development, it can be open to organisational differences. There are a number of models of clinical supervision, but it is probably best described as an 'exchange between practising professionals to enable the development of professional skills' (Faugier & Butterworth 1994). This may be appropriate in the normal nursing context but it raises the question of what constitutes supervision if one person has qualifications and practices not shared by the other. How can supportive reflection take place if the nursing practice to be discussed includes interventions which are not mutually understood?

Mackereth (2001) suggests that nurses using CAM may find that opportunities for support and guidance may be hard to obtain, but goes on to offer some valuable guidelines in setting up clinical supervision in CAM, suggesting networking with other CAM practitioners, not only for one-to-one peer supervision to share experiences and skills but also to create the opportunity for analysis of their own work.

His list of potential benefits of particular value in clinical supervision in CAM includes:

- Clarifying professional and personal issues and boundaries
- Clinical risk management tool
- Guidance and support in fulfilling professional potential.

These three points address issues such as assessing how far a therapy should be taken in addressing a patient's needs, and identifying where additional training in the same or an additional CAM would enhance patient care in the specific clinical area. Such supervision would also supply valuable data on any risks involved in the therapy and so add constructively to the debate on CAM use.

LEGAL AND PROFESSIONAL ISSUES

Much of what follows will be familiar to nurses from their own nurse education, but there are a number of points which are particularly relevant to complementary therapies. Explaining the role of the UKCC (as it was then), Darley (1995) notes that the council does not have the expertise to decide on the efficacy of individual therapies and does not plan to register complementary therapy qualifications in the near future. At the time of writing no further statements have been made by the new Nursing and Midwifery Council. However, the council feels that its own *Code of Professional Conduct* (2002) and *Scope of Professional Practice* (1992) provide a professional framework within which nurses can offer complementary therapies safely and responsibly for the benefit of their patients. Key points from these documents are acting in the best interests of the client (NMC 2002) and knowledge and competence (including limitations of practice) (NMC 2002). Readers are also referred to paragraphs 8–11 in the Scope of Professional Practice document (UKCC 1992). In addition, nurses will acknowledge their accountability within a range of legal parameters, including accountability to the patient underpinned by common law and legal responsibility in civil law, accountability to the employer enshrined within the practitioner's contract of employment and job description, and accountability to the public in general through criminal law. It is particularly important in relation to CAM therapies that the child and parent are fully appraised of any possible side effects or reactions, such as the healing crisis which occurs with many CAM interventions, and that no unsubstantiated claims are made about the healing properties of any therapy, particularly in relation to TB and cancer. In the case of cancer, the Cancer Act (1939) makes it a criminal offence for anyone who is not suitably qualified to advertise (including by word of mouth) and offer to treat a person for cancer, to prescribe a remedy for cancer, or to give any advice in connection with their cancer treatment. Nurses also need to ensure that patients' questions are answered fully and truthfully. Under vicarious liability, an employer is liable for any harm that may occur to a client and, therefore, is liable for any compensation claimed by the client. However, the employer may redefine the parameters of nurses' practice for which they are willing to accept liability. Employees must then ensure that their practice is authorised under these policies, otherwise they will be liable themselves. This demonstrates the importance of clear policy development.

Use of CAM falls into the same legal framework as other therapeutic interventions. Of particular relevance to the paediatric nurse is the provisions of the Children Act (1989) with regard to consent to treatment and the duty of parents or guardians to ensure that children in their care receive appropriate treatment for any illness or condition they may have. This would be of particular relevance to practitioners if it came to their notice that parents or guardians had rejected a known and effective orthodox treatment and were relying on the use of CAM solely and inappropriately for their child. Failure to obtain medical treatment would be grounds for neglect and, if necessary, removal of the child from their care. Rodgers (2000) cites the example of the parents of a diabetic child, who in 1993 were convicted of manslaughter when the child died after being given homeopathic treatment rather than conventional medication.

The Children Act (1989) would also apply if practices were undertaken, such as fasting or inappropriate dietary restrictions, within the CAM treatment, which would adversely affect the child's welfare. There is a precedent for this concern. Some years ago, a consultant paediatrician initiated the removal of two children from their parents. One was being subjected to a macrobiotic diet and the other to a fruitarian diet, to the detriment of their health (Dr Richard West, personal communication 2002). Parents and guardians have a duty to ensure that children receive adequate nutrition according to their developmental needs.

Dimond (1996) states that consent to CAM treatment by children follows exactly the same principles as consent for any other intervention, for example Gillick competent children can give consent in their own right. Patients and clients allow nurses and other health professionals to invade their personal space in order to carry out nursing procedures. Within the hospital setting this consent is usually 'implied'. A patient holding out his arm for the nurse to take his pulse tacitly gives the nurse permission to touch him. Since most patients are familiar with the procedure there is little chance of misunderstanding. With less familiar procedures informed consent is required, although this normally falls within the bounds of common courtesy. However, with procedures which are unusual, such as CAM interventions, a fuller explanation is needed. This involves giving the patient enough information to make an informed decision about receiving the therapy and should include information about benefits, side effects and contraindications.

Much debate has been generated as to whether written consent is needed before complementary therapies can be integrated into patient care. Initially, when therapies were first introduced into the health service, it seems to have been a wise precaution. However, it could be argued that if therapies and, specifically, techniques from the therapies are to be a part of normal nursing care, then we need to move beyond this rather inhibiting, paternalistic approach. A more autonomous approach would be to allow nurses to use their clinical judgement and interpersonal skills to negotiate their CAM nursing care with their patients as they do with other nursing interventions. This will involve courageous innovation for practitioners, but is a vital move if the integration of complementary therapies into nursing is to make progress.

A number of other Acts of Parliament relate to the practice of complementary therapies. The Control of Substances Hazardous to Health Regulations Act (1988) basically deals with noxious substances and danger of infection, and in CAM would relate mostly to acupuncturists. The Supply of Goods and Services Act (1982) maintains standards of care in the delivery of services. The Consumer Protection Act (1987) is relevant to herbalists, homeopaths and aromatherapists in that the Act requires them to use products which are safe and calls them to account if this requirement is not met. The Data Protection Act (1984) covers access to patients' medical records.

So what of the future? With nursing in a state of constant evolution, and nurses undertaking new tasks, new roles and new methods of working, the way is wide open for the development of CAM in nursing, both as a practical intervention and as a theoretical discipline. The debate as to whether nurses should be using CAM is over. Nurses and patients are already using CAM, patients need information about its use and efficacy, and nurses are in the best position to give this. Research is now accepted as an integral part of nursing development and not something which is confined to academia. Hopefully this fact will encourage practitioners to verify their practice; in so doing they will be seizing the opportunity to retain the nurturing role of CAM and prevent it becoming medicalised and lost.

REFERENCES

Aldridge D 1988 Single case study research designs. Complementary Medical Research 3(1): 37–45

Aldridge D 2000 Guidelines for clinical research in complementary medicine. Journal of Alternative and Complementary Medicine 8(3): 254–251

Altman D 1994 The scandal of poor medical research. British Medical Journal 308: 283–284

Anthony H 1987 Some methodological problems in the assessment of complementary therapies. Statistics in Medicine 6: 676–771

Bailar J 1997 The promise and problems of meta analysis. New England Journal of Medicine 337(8): 559–560

Birch S 1997 Issues to consider in determining an adequate treatment in a clinical trial of acupuncture. Complementary Therapies in Medicine 5: 8–12

Birch S 1998 Diversity and acupuncture: acupuncture is not a coherent or historically stable tradition. In: Vickers A (ed) Examining complementary medicine. Stanley Thornes, Cheltenham

Blomfield R, Hardy S 2000 Evidence based nursing practice. In: Trinder L, Reynolds S (eds) Evidence based practice: a critical appraisal. Blackwell Science, Oxford

Children Act 1989 HMSO, London

Cochrane A 1972 Effectiveness and efficiency: random reflections on health services. Nuffield Provincial Hospital Trust, Oxford

Cole A, Shanley E 1998 Complementary therapies as a means of developing the scope of professional nursing practice. Journal of Advanced Nursing 27: 1171–1176

Consumers Protection Act 1988 HMSO, London

Control of Substances Hazardous to Health (COSHH) Regulations 1988 HMSO, London

Culpeper N 1653 Complete herbal: a book of natural remedies for ancient ills. Wordsworth Editions, Hertfordshire

Dantas F, Fisher P 1998 A systematic review of homeopathic pathogenic trials ('provings') published in the United Kingdom from 1945–1955. In: Ernst E, Hahn E (eds) Homeopathy: a critical appraisal. Butterworth-Heinemann, Oxford

Darley M 1995 Complementary therapies: the position of the UKCC. Complementary Therapies in Nursing and Midwifery 1(4): 106–109

Data Protection Act 1984 HMSO, London

Dimond B 1996 The legal aspects of child health care. Mosby, London

Dove C, Anthony H 1987 The patient as individual and statistic: introduction. Proceedings of the 2nd Conference of Research Methodology of the RCCM. Complementary Medical Research 2(1): 48–52

Eddy D, Billings J 1993 The quality of medical evidence and medical practice. Paper prepared for the National Leadership Commission on Health Care.

Ernst E 1998 Single case studies in complementary/alternative medicine research. Complementary Therapies in Medicine 6(2): 75–78

Evans M 1991 On the efficacy of anthroposophical medicine. Complementary Medical Research 5(2): 71–78

Faugier J, Butterworth T 1994 Clinical supervision: a position paper, published by the School of Nursing Studies, University of Manchester, Manchester

Fisher P 1995 The development of a research methodology in homeopathy. Complementary Therapies in Nursing and Midwifery 1(6): 168–174

Fisher P 1998 Is homeopathic prescribing reliable? In: Vickers A (ed) Examining complementary medicine. Stanley Thornes, Cheltenham

Fox M 2001 Access to complementary health care: why the NHS is the key. Complementary Therapies in Nursing and Midwifery 7(3): 123–125

Fulder S 1998 The basic concepts of alternative medicine and their impact on our views of health. Journal of Alternative and Complementary Medicine 4(2): 147–158

Given S 1998 Understanding addiction the Chinese way. International Journal of Alternative and Complementary Medicine 16(2): 26–30

Grayson L 1997 Evidence based medicine. The British Library, London

Hammerschlag R 1998 Methodological and ethical issues in clinical trials of acupuncture. Journal of Alternative and Complementary Medicine 4(2): 159–171

Hammerschlag R, Morris M 1997 Clinical trials comparing acupuncture with biomedical standard care: a criteria based evaluation of research design and reporting. Complementary Therapies in Medicine 5(3): 133–140

Heron J 1986 Critique of conventional research methodology. Complementary Medical Research 1(1): 12–22

Jobst K 1995 A critical analysis of acupuncture in pulmonary disease: efficacy and safety of the acupuncture needle. Journal of Alternative and Complementary Medicine 1: 57–85

Jobst K 1998 Complementary and alternative medicine: essential for the future of effective, affordable healthcare? (editorial) The Journal of Alternative and Complementary Medicine 4(3): 261–265

Johnson G 1995 Complementary therapies in nursing: implications for practice using aromatherapy as an example. Complementary Therapies in Nursing and Midwifery 1(5): 128–132

Leibrich J 1990 Measurement of efficacy: a case for holistic research. Complementary Medical Research 4(1): 21–25

Lewith G 1998 Misconceptions about research in complementary medicine. In: Vickers A (ed) Examining complementary medicine. Stanley Thornes, Cheltenham

Lewith G, Vincent C 1995 Evaluation of the clinical effects of acupuncture. A problem re-assessed and a framework for future research. Pain Forum 4: 29–39

Liability of Suppliers of Services Directive 1991 EC

Liverani A, Minelli E, Ricciuti A 2000 Subjective scales for the evaluation of therapeutic effects and their use in complementary medicine. Journal of Alternative and Complementary Medicine 6(3): 257–264

Mackereth P 2001 Clinical supervision. In: Rankin-Box D (ed) The nurse's handbook of complementary therapies: a guide for nurses and the caring professions, 2nd edn. Baillière Tindall, Edinburgh

Mantle F 1997 Implementing evidence in practice. British Journal of Community Health Nursing 2(1): 36–39

Muir Gray J 1997 Evidence based health care: how to make policy and management decisions. Churchill Livingstone, Edinburgh

NMC 2002 Code of professional conduct. Nursing and Midwifery Council, London

Peters D 2000 From holism to integration: is there a future for complementary therapies in the NHS? Complementary Therapies in Nursing and Midwifery 6(2): 59–60

Rampes H, Mortimer A 1997 Letter to the editor. Complementary Therapies in Medicine 5(3): 178–179

Rankin-Box D, McVey M 2001 Policy development. In: Rankin-Box D (ed) The nurse's handbook of complementary therapies: a guide for nurses and the caring professions. Baillière Tindall, London

Reason, Rowan A 1981 Human inquiry: a sourcebook of new paradigm research. Wiley, Chichester

Resch K, Ernst E 1997 Research methodologies in complementary medicine: making sure it works. In: Ernst E (ed) Complementary medicine: an objective appraisal. Butterworth-Heinemann, Oxford

Resch K, Ernst E, Garrow J 2000 A randomised controlled study of reviewer bias against an unconventional therapy. Journal of the Royal Society of Medicine 93: 164–167

Reynolds S 2000 The anatomy of evidence based practice: principles and methods. In: Trinder L, Reynolds S (eds) Evidence-based practice: a critical appraisal. Blackwell Scientific, Oxford

Rodgers M 2000 The child patient and consent to treatment: legal overview. British Journal of Community Nursing 5(10): 494–498

Ryan D 1999 Toward improving the reliability of clinical acupuncture trials: arguments against the validity of 'sham acupuncture' as controls. American Journal of Acupuncture 27(1/2): 105–109

Sackett D, Rosenberg W, Muir Gray J et al 1996 Evidence based medicine: what it is and what it isn't. British Medical Journal (13th Jan) 312: 71–72

Schwartz J 1988 Evaluation of acupuncture as a treatment for smoking. American Journal of Acupuncture 16: 135–142

Supply of Goods and Services Act 1982 HMSO, London

Swayne J 1998 Homeopathic therapeutics: many dimensions or meaningless diversity? In: Vickers A (ed) Examining complementary medicine. Stanley Thornes, Cheltenham

Ter Riet G, Kleijnen J, Knipschild P 1990a Acupuncture and chronic pain: a criteria based meta analysis. Journal of Clinical Epidemiology 43(11): 1191–1199

Ter Riet G, Kleijnen J, Knipschild P 1990b Meta analysis of studies into the effect of acupuncture on addiction. British Journal of General Practice 40: 379–382

Trinder L 2000 Introduction: the context of evidence based practice. In: Trinder L, Reynolds S (eds) Evidence-based practice: a critical appraisal. Blackwell Scientific, Oxford

UKCC 1992 Scope of professional practice. UKCC, London

Walach H 1993 Does a homeopathic drug act as a placebo? Journal of Psychosomatic Research 37: 851–860

Wieland F 1998 The role of drug provings in the homeopathic concept. In: Ernst E, Hahn E (eds) Homeopathy: a critical appraisal. Butterworth-Heinemann, Oxford

Section

2 0–11 years

SECTION CONTENTS

Chapter 3 Problems related to breathing 49

Chapter 4 Problems related to rest and sleep 70

Chapter 5 Problems related to pain 79

Chapter 6 Problems related to eating and drinking 94

Chapter 7 Problems related to elimination 109

Chapter 8 Problems related to mobility 118

Chapter 9 Problems related to washing and dressing 134

INTRODUCTION

This section looks at the contribution CAM can offer in a range of paediatric problems, both nursing and medical, which for convenience sake, have been grouped under the categories of Roper et al as described in the preface. These include problems related to breathing, sleeping, pain, eating and drinking, elimination, mobility and washing and dressing. As Roper has said in the preface to the 4th edition of Roper et al (1988), all the activities of living are interconnected and a certain amount of overlap is acknowledged, so Roper's category of working and playing could be regarded as the synthesis of all these nursing activities.

THEORIES OF CHILDHOOD DEVELOPMENT

The span between birth and 11 years covers Piaget's developmental periods from sensorimotor to concrete operations, and Erikson's from trust versus mistrust to industry versus inferiority. These developmental periods are also reflected in other cultures. In traditional Chinese culture, the Five Element theory divides childhood into four developmental phases, three of which are contained within this time period, although the transition from one stage to another is neither sudden nor complete. At each stage the child exhibits behaviour from at least two Elements at the same time, although the behaviour relating to one Element is more pronounced at any one time. The first stage is Metal transition to Water (the Element Metal is the mother of Water), and this stage lasts up to the age of 2–3 years. This corresponds to Piaget's sensorimotor stage and Erikson's trust versus mistrust and autonomy versus shame and doubt stages. At this point, the dominant emotion is fear of all kinds, from fear of hunger to fear of abandonment. Vulnerable organs at this stage are Lungs and Kidney. The next stage is Water transition to Wood, which lasts up to the age of about 7 years. This roughly corresponds with Piaget's preoperational stage and Erikson's initiative versus guilt stage. In Chinese terms, Piaget's egocentricity is shown in the Water characteristics of the child. It is suggested that in water, children are all powerful, but they still have a need to feel solid earth underneath their feet. Mother (Earth) is still the most important person in the child's life. If the mother is too overpowering, the child will become like land-locked water, unable to move and flow under its own direction. However, if the mother is not nurturing enough, the Water child is without boundaries and 'flows' everywhere, looking for guidance. The last stage before adolescence is Wood transition to Fire and corresponds with Erikson's industry versus inferiority. In this stage the child absorbs its cultural norms and learns basic skills, both manual and social, thereby acquiring a sense of personal competence and ability to participate in society. This stage also corresponds with Piaget's stage of operational thinking, in which the child's thinking is logical and linear. The Wood phase child is described as a young tree with its roots firmly planted under the earth, thereby identified with Mother Earth. Heaven is identified with the father, who provides guidance and direction for the child, so that the child can learn right from wrong. If family relationships are poor at this stage, the child will not be able to root properly and will lack a solid inner stability and sense of self, which may lead to behavioural problems.

Anthroposophical medicine divides childhood into two periods of 7 year cycles, based on the theory that the body totally renews itself every 7 years. In the small child the disproportionately large head represents the cephalic pole. Steiner states that in spite of this large head, the child is unable to intellectualise. It is suggested that this is because it is from the head that the growth forces arise that will shape the rest of the body, and until the body has reached a certain level of development, these forces are not available for thinking. These etheric forces are repetitive and rhythmic, and as the child's development proceeds they take on other tasks, and connections with the other elements change. During these years, children love to imitate, and of particular importance at this stage are the examples set by the child's family and associates. During this time the child's etheric body remains united with the maternal etheric body until at 7 years, these separate and the child has a body which is totally its own. This liberation of part of the etheric body allows for the development of memory, and intellectual learning can start. This also allows for the development of the emotional life, which continues through the next 7 years, during which time the child becomes capable of friendships. In the second 7 years of life, the astral body takes the lead and the child begins to develop a social sense. At about 9 years, the ego connects with the metabolic pole and if this is unsuccessful, metabolic type disorders can develop.

REFERENCE

Roper N, Logan W, Tierney A 1988 The elements of nursing, 4th edn. Churchill Livingstone, Edinburgh

3

Problems related to breathing

CHAPTER CONTENTS

- **Introduction** 49
- **Therapeutic approaches** 50
  Herbalism 50
  Aromatherapy 51
  TCM 52
  Ayurvedic medicine 53
- **Upper respiratory tract conditions** 53
  Colds 53
  Allergic rhinitis 55
  Sinusitis 57
  TCM and upper respiratory tract conditions 57

- **Asthma** 58
  Hypnosis 59
  Massage 60
  Ayurvedic medicine 61
  Homeopathy 62
  Herbalism 63
  Anthroposophical medicine 64
  TCM 64
  Reflexology 65
- **Acute respiratory distress** 66
  The ventilated patient 66
- **References** 67

INTRODUCTION

Respiratory disease is the fifth most common cause of death in children after accidents, cancer, central nervous system problems and congenital abnormalities, whilst respiratory infections and asthma constitute the most common reasons for GP consultations. Children are particularly vulnerable to respiratory problems because of their relatively high need for oxygen, their higher metabolic rate for growth, the immaturity of their lungs and their fewer alveoli. Problems are often age-related and the presentation of the infection will change in different age groups.

Most upper respiratory tract infections are self-limiting and so the use of antibiotics is of limited value. Most respiratory infections in children are viral and antibiotics are not indicated, although a variety of organisms, such as *Streptococcus pneumoniae, Haemophilus influenzae, Staphylococcus aureus* and *Mycobacterium tuberculosis,* can be responsible for superimposed infections in children, particularly those with chronic conditions such as cystic fibrosis. Taylor (1999) points out that, whilst the advent of antibiotics in the early part of the 20th century contributed enormously to the health and welfare of the population, the extensive and often inappropriate use of antibiotics has led to a number of organisms becoming resistant to their effect. He suggests that one approach to addressing this problem is for nurses to educate the public about the appropriate use of antibiotics, specifically to clarify the differences between bacteria and viruses, thus weaning patients away from expecting a prescription at every consultation. A number of CAM therapies have a valuable role to play in supporting treatment or relieving symptoms, therefore, this chapter will describe preventative and supportive therapies aimed at increasing resistance to infection before going on to address specific respiratory conditions.

THERAPEUTIC APPROACHES

Herbalism

In common with other complementary therapy practitioners, a medical herbalist's approach to respiratory conditions would aim at increasing the body's resistance to infection by boosting the immune system. This would be achieved by the use of a herb such as echinacea (*Echinacea augustifolia*) (Mills 1993). This herb, native to North America and known as the purple cone flower, has been used by Native Americans for centuries for a range of infectious conditions, and can be taken internally or applied externally. Recent research has supported its claim as an immunostimulant, although there are only a few controlled trials looking into its use. The root of the echinacea herb is traditionally used as an anti-infective agent and research into its efficacy has indicated that it has antiviral properties (Wacker & Hilbig 1978), demonstrating a 24-hour resistance to herpes, influenza and vesicular viruses. Its immunostimulant properties are being investigated and, to date, phagocytosis enhancement has been noted in vitro (Bauer 1985) and tissue cultures have yielded immunologically active polysaccharides (Wagner 1988). Antibacterial activity has been noted against *E. coli*, *Staphylococcus aureus* and *Proteus mirabilis* when echinacea is mixed with other herbal preparations, the response against *Staphylococcus aureus* and *Proteus mirabilis* being attributed to the echinacea (Westendorf 1982).

More recent research by Sun et al (1999) has indicated the prophylactic role of echinacea in ameliorating viral infections. The research was done on mice, who were fed extract of echinacea root daily for 1–2 weeks with the aim of establishing a possible mechanism for the action of the herb. After only 1 week of the trial there was a significant increase in natural killer (NK) cells and monocytes in both the bone marrow and spleen. Both monocytes and NK cells are mediators of nonspecific immunity and well-demonstrated killers of virus containing cells. This trial demonstrates the specific action of the echinacea, since there was no demonstrable change in size of the haemopoietic and immune cells in either spleen or bone marrow. Sun et al (1999) suggest that this significant elevation of two fundamental immune cell populations indicates a prophylactic role for the herb.

It is suggested that echinacea should not be taken by patients who are deliberately immunosuppressed (Barnes et al 2002) and the German commission E monographs, a guide for German doctors who routinely prescribe orthodox medication and herbal remedies together (Blumenthal 1998), caution against its use in progressive systemic diseases such as MS or TB, though this is challenged by Bone (1997), who suggested, following a detailed analysis of the data, that these restrictions are not supported. The German commission E monographs support the use of echinacea for the treatment of colds and chronic respiratory conditions, although Fetrow and Alvila (2001) suggest that the evidence for the use of echinacea is still conflicting and that further clinical trials should be conducted. It is possible that parents of children with illnesses such as leukaemia, which suppress the immune system and increase susceptibility to infections, may seek to use echinacea in an attempt to reduce the risk of superimposed infections.

Although not a herb, propolis is sometimes prescribed by herbalists for respiratory problems. The role of propolis as an anti-infective agent has been supported in a number of studies, both in animals and humans. In his review, Bone (1994) states that propolis appears to be particularly effective in upper respiratory tract infections such as tonsillitis and sinusitis, especially in children, and a prophylactic effect has been demonstrated in a clinical trial. A Bulgarian study described by Bone (1994), which involved administering propolis to mice prior to infection with *Haemophilus influenzae*, noted that untreated mice died within 5 days of infection compared with a 40% survival rate in mice given oral propolis and a 60% survival rate in mice injected with propolis. The research suggests that the effect was due to the activation of macrophagic phagocytic activity. Research done at the National Heart and Lung Institute by Grange and Davey (1990) demonstrated the efficacy of propolis against *Staphylococcus aureus* (completely inhibited growth), *Pseudomonas aeruginosa* and *E. coli* (partly inhibited growth) and *Klebsiella pneumoniae* (no effect). However, in general, it has been shown that propolis is more active against Gram-positive than Gram-negative bacteria.

This effect was confirmed by Dobrowolski et al (1991), who investigated the use of propolis against *Staphylococcus aureus, Streptococcus pyogenes, Streptococcus viridians, Diplococcus pneumoniae* and *E. coli*. Three preparations of propolis were used and compared with standard antibiotic treatment. The findings of the study showed that propolis preparations exhibited antibacterial activity (especially against Gram-positive bacteria).

Aromatherapy

The consensus of professional opinion indicates that most essential oils are to some extent antiviral and antibacterial and can be used either during an acute infective phase or prophylactically, this being an area in which patients can help to treat themselves. An aromatherapy approach to respiratory disorders would involve the use of oils that are particularly noted for having these antibacterial and antiviral properties, such as cinnamon, clove, thyme and marjoram (Deans & Ritchie 1987). In their research, Deans and Ritchie (1987) tested 50 plant essential oils against 25 organisms, including *Klebsiella pneumoniae, Pseudomonas aeruginosa, Staphylococcus aureus, Streptococcus faecalis* and *E. coli*. Thirty-three oils were inhibiting to 10 or more of the 25 test organisms. The 10 essential oils which displayed greatest inhibitory properties were angelica, bay, cinnamon, clove, thyme, almond, marjoram, geranium, lovage and pimento. Both Gram-positive and Gram-negative bacteria were susceptible to the essential oils. The botanical origins of the oils were not stated. Lis-Balchin et al (1996) examined the effects of a number of essential oils on 25 bacterial species. Of the oils studied, camphor inhibited 25 species and cinnamon, frankincense and tea tree each inhibited 24. Research on patented inhalations using, variously, camphor, eucalyptus or menthol for the treatment of respiratory infections indicated that they are of value (Cohen & Dressler 1982).

Singh et al (1995) noted the role of cinnamon bark oil (*Cinnamomum zeylanicum*) against fungi causing respiratory tract mycoses, specifically three species of candida. Baratta et al (1998) tested essential oils of coriander (*Coriandrum sativum*), laurel (*Laurus nobilis*), oregano (*Origanum vulgare*), rosemary (*Rosmarinus officinalis*) and sage (*Salvia officinalis*) against 25 bacterial and 1 fungal species. Oregano demonstrated the broadest and highest activity, having strong action against 19 bacteria and the fungus. Coriander, laurel and rosemary demonstrated significant activity against 7 species, including *Staphylococcus aureus*, whilst sage affected most bacteria, but to a lesser degree in comparison with other oils.

The most popular over-the-counter antiseptic oil in current use is tea tree oil (*Melaleuca alternifolia*) and its antimicrobial action has been demonstrated in a number of papers. Tea tree oil is an aboriginal traditional medicine and is used for bruises, insect bites and skin infections. Research started into its therapeutic properties during the 1930s, but with the advent of antibiotics, its use fell into decline. With people's increased resistance to antibiotics, its use as an antimicrobial agent has resurfaced. Carson and Riley (1993, 1994) have conducted two reviews into the use of tea tree oil. In their 1994 paper they reviewed its action against *Pseudomonas aeruginosa*, *Candida albicans*, *Escherichia coli*, *Staphylococcus aureus* and *Clostridium perfringens*. Of these, only *Pseudomonas aeruginosa* was resistant to the oil. Cox et al (2000) suggested that the mode of action of tea tree essential oil was due to the disruption of the cell membrane permeability and the resultant loss of chemiosmotic control. They also considered the possibility that the oil in some way altered the metabolism within the microorganism.

From their own experiments, Budhiraja et al (1999) concluded that the antiseptic activity of tea tree oil appeared to be due, in part, to white blood cell activation. The most recent review of the antimicrobial and fungal actions of essential oils is that of Chao et al (2000), who reviewed the action of 45 essential oils on eight bacteria (four Gram-negative and four Gram-positive), two fungi and one yeast. They found that, in general, the oils were more effective against Gram-positive bacteria; however, cinnamon bark (*Cinnamomum zeylanicum*), savory (*Satureia montana*) and rosewood (*Aniba rosaeodora*) oils were equally effective against Gram-positive and Gram-negative bacteria. Oils which showed the greatest overall antifungal activity were coriander (*Coriandrum sativum*), cinnamon bark, lemongrass (*Cymbopogon flexuosus*), savory and rosewood. They concluded that overall, cinnamon bark and tea tree oils showed the strongest effect against all test organisms.

Nicholls (1998) expresses surprise that the anti-infective properties of essential oils are largely unknown in medical circles and has reviewed these properties and their mode of action. The possible role of certain essential oils, specifically tea tree, as a prophylactic treatment for children with chronic respiratory conditions such as cystic fibrosis would seem to be well worth investigating and submitting to clinical trial.

TCM

Traditional Chinese Medicine views prophylaxis as playing a vital role in the treatment of disease, and focuses on adherence to dietary recommendations, suitable lifestyle, the regular use of acupuncture to tonify the immune system and maintain the balance of the internal organs, along with Qigong breathing exercises. Children of all ages are given tonifying acupuncture at regular intervals in much the same way as Western medicine suggests regular check ups. Parents are also taught how to do meridian, abdominal and Shu point massage. Parents are seen as active partners in their children's medical care.

Ayurvedic medicine

Similarly, the whole focus of Ayurvedic medicine is prevention of illness and the maintenance of wellbeing, which is achieved through the practice of a healthy regime and the maintenance of balance within the body. As with TCM, this involves diet, exercise, good sleeping patterns and rest and relaxation. In addition, Ayurvedic medicine uses herbal formulations called rasayanas, which promote overall health. Although they can be used for specific conditions, they are generally used to stimulate the immune system. Rasayanas are ancient formulae originating many thousands of years ago and few modern doctors are aware of their composition. One such formula is amrit kalash, which is available in two formulations, one a herbal concentrate, the other a herbal tablet. Between them the rasayanas consist of 24 different herbs and fruits. There is a specific procedure for the creation of these rasayanas and two formulae have been dispensed, MAK 4 and MAK 5. These substances have been subjected to research which shows that both MAK 4 and MAK 5 increase the responsiveness of lymphocytes, while MAK 5 increases the responsiveness of macrophages (Sharma and Clark 1998).

UPPER RESPIRATORY TRACT CONDITIONS

Colds

The common cold is usually caused by the rhinovirus, though other viruses may be implicated, and children typically suffer between two and eight colds per year. Treatment includes supportive measures and, where necessary, the use of decongestants in the short term.

Herbalism

Specific herbs used in the treatment of chronic catarrhal conditions such as colds might include the root or leaf of the marshmallow plant (*Althaea officinalis*), a demulcent which has a long tradition of use in herbal medicine for its soothing and healing properties and for the fact that it loosens the respiratory secretions. Antimicrobial activity by marshmallow against *Pseudomonas aeruginosa, Proteus vulgaris,* and *Staphylococcus aureus* has been documented (Recio 1989). Marshmallow has no recorded side effects or toxicity; however, Barnes et al (2002), caution that it may interfere with hypoglycaemic therapy. The German commission E monographs (Blumenthal 1998) approve of its use for irritated oral and pharyngeal mucosa and cough. Elderflower (*Sambucas nigra*), also known as black elder, European elder or sambucas, is another herb which has a long history of medicinal use in respiratory disorders, and has been called the 'medicine chest of the country people' (Hollis 1994). It is said to reduce fever and is an expectorant, being used for chronic catarrh, influenza and sinusitis. Research by Serkedjieva (1990) noted that, in conjunction with infusions of St John's wort (*Hypericum perforatum*) and soapwort (*Saponaria officinalis*), it demonstrated antiviral activity against influenza types A and B and herpes simplex type I. It has no documented contraindications although it may interfere with immunosuppressive therapy (Barnes et al 2002).

Homeopathy

Another supportive treatment which parents or child may be using is homeopathy. For a cold, for example, the prescription might include: Nat. mur (*Natrum muriaticum*) or Aconite (*Aconitum napellus*) with Gelsemium (*Gelsemium sempervirens*), Bryonia (*Bryonia alba*) or Ferrum phos (*Ferrum phosphoricum*), depending on how the symptoms develop. Nat. mur for example, which is based on sodium chloride obtained from rock salt, is the homeopathic remedy for the early stages of a cold, when the cold starts suddenly with sneezing and a blocked nose, with the possible onset of cold sores. The remedy Gelsemium, on the other hand, is prescribed when the cold presents as more flu-like, with aching limbs, shivering and a general feeling of heaviness. Gelsemium or yellow jasmine has been used medicinally since the 1840s as a fever cure in herbal medicine; the homeopathic remedy is prepared from the root. The remedy Bryonia is useful for the headaches which so often accompany colds or flu and, in particular, those that are made worse by coughing, thirst and dry mouth, whilst Ferrum phos is used if the cold is of slow onset.

It can be seen from these descriptions of homeopathic remedies that a cold is not simply a cold to the homeopath, but rather a syndrome of interdependent features from the illness and from the patient, all of which need to be taken into consideration. De Lange de Klerk et al (1994) investigated the effect of individually prescribed homeopathic treatments, compared with placebo, on upper respiratory tract infection in 170 children. The results showed small but consistent differences between the two groups: the treatment group had fewer courses of antibiotics than the placebo group.

Anthroposophical medicine

Anthroposophical medicine describes the symptoms of the common cold as symptoms of the metabolic type and ascribes the cause of colds to the person being 'run down' or 'chilled'. This chilling is seen as the foreign element or outer coldness. The Anthroposophical approach to colds would be to let the infection take its course, with perhaps the use of a chamomile or eucalyptus inhalation. Common childhood diseases are part of the body's learning process, when it learns how to react appropriately to further infections. Anthroposophical medicine also considers that the illness contributes to the child's developing maturity, and that following feverish childhood illnesses the child will undergo an acceleration in development, since the speeding up of the metabolic processes results in the active reshaping of the physical body. An interesting survey by Alm et al (1999) looked into the incidence of atopy in children of families following an Anthroposophical lifestyle. These families used fewer antibiotics, had fewer immunisations and ingested higher levels of live lactobacilli than the control group. The researchers noted that the prevalence of atopy was lower in children from Anthroposophical families and suggested that lifestyle factors may reduce the risk of atopy in childhood. Support for the use of probiotics in the prevention of atopy in childhood has been offered by Kalliomäki et al (2001), who noted that the incidence of atopy in an at-risk group of babies was lower when they were administered lactobacilli via their mother 2–3 weeks before birth and for 6 months after birth. The incidence of eczema in the probiotics group was half that in the placebo group.

The immune system develops over time and develops differently for atopic and non-atopic people. In the non-atopic person, Th1 type immunity, which is directed against infections, predominates whilst in the atopic individual, Th2 type immunity is predominant. Th2 type immunity is associated with the production of IgE antibodies and its predominance leads to continuous IgE production. When such an individual encounters an allergen, atopic disease occurs.

Allergic rhinitis

Allergic rhinitis or hay fever is the bane of many people's lives and, typically, is at its peak during exam time. It is characterised by sneezing, nasal itching and discharge, watering eyes and nasal congestion. It can be seasonal or perennial, the seasonal variety being caused by allergens produced at certain times of the year, grass pollen being the main cause followed by tree pollen. Rhinitis is defined as a non-infective nasal disorder of more than 8 weeks duration which is characterised by inflammation of the nasal mucosa (Scadding et al 1995).

Seasonal allergic rhinitis is one of the most chronic conditions, affecting 16–23% of the population (ISAAC 1998). It has a particular impact on school work, with absences from school and lack of sleep due to nasal congestion and mouth breathing (leading to snoring) adding to already existing exam stress.

Homeopathic treatment

The homeopath sees allergic rhinitis as a range of conditions, and treatments include constitutional as well as specific remedies. Lockie (1990) lists 16 symptom categories, a sample of which are given here.

- Constant sneezing, heavy swollen eyes, dizziness and shaking
- Itching nose and sneezing but with no discharge, roof of mouth and ears very itchy
- Eyes smarting, sensitivity to light, stuffy nose, obstructed breathing, irritated eustachian tubes
- Constant sneezing, stuffy or streaming nose, watery, swollen eyes.

In treating a rhinitis, the homeopath would first address the client's constitutional background and then give nosods or relevant pollens as a long-term treatment. Clients should expect the treatment to take a couple of seasons before the condition can be cured. Although there are very few published randomised controlled trials, as opposed to 'provings', of homeopathy, two trials make interesting reading. The first is a well designed, double-blind placebo controlled study using a homeopathically prepared dilution of house dust mite allergens, which was given to 144 patients with active allergic rhinitis. The result was a significant reduction of symptoms and a halving of the need for antihistamines (Reilly et al 1986). This study compares with another trial the previous year when Wiesenauer and Gaus (1985) compared Galphimia potentiation D6 with a placebo. Again, this was a well designed, double-blind trial with a large sample which resulted in the Galphimia offering no significant benefit over placebo, though the results indicated a trend in favour of homeopathy.

Anthroposophical medicine

The anthroposophical goal in the treatment of hay fever is to strengthen the astral forces in relation to the upper respiratory tract, since the allergic reaction is seen as a violent attack similar to an abnormal emotional response to an external stimulus, and the emotions are seen as astral functions. The usual remedy is a mixture of quince pulp and lemon juice called Gencydo which acts on the mucous membranes and which is given as an inhalant or a subcutaneous injection. Other remedies might include the homeopathic remedies of Gelsemium, mixed pollen, Nat. mur or Pulsatilla (*Pulsatilla nigricans*). One additional treatment involves giving the child a spoonful of honey (including the wax), locally produced since this contains local pollen, for a year as a desensitisation remedy. The role of honey in relation to wound care will be discussed further in the chapter on washing and dressing.

Herbalism

Herbal preparations which might be used in the treatment of rhinitis traditionally include golden rod, golden seal (*Hydrastis canadensis*), which contains the antibiotic berbine as well as other related alkaloids, and ground ivy (*Nepeta hederacea*). Research supports some of ground ivy's traditional herbal uses: specifically, its anti-inflammatory activity has been reported by Mascolo (1987), and it is reported as having antiseptic and astringent properties. However, it is contraindicated in epilepsy and existing renal disease and it may be irritant to the gastro-intestinal mucosa (Barnes et al 2002). Golden rod has anti-inflammatory properties and is anticatarrhal, whilst golden seal has documented antihistamine activity (Preininger 1975) and its constituents are active against a range of bacteria, such as *Staphylococcus*, *Streptococcus*, *Pseudomonas aeruginosa* and *Diplococcus pneumoniae* (Barnes et al 2002).

Aromatherapy

Two pieces of research using essential oils indicate their place in reducing the mould of allergens in the home. Chaumont and Leger (1992) describe the use of essential oils of Bourbon geranium, citronellol, geraniol and citral as a vapour aimed at reducing or eliminating spores of aspergillus, geotrichum, mucor, penicillium, rhizopus, trichothecium, scropulariopsis, wallemia and cladosporum. Fungicidal activity was not demonstrated but all exhibited significant fungistatic activity. The researchers concluded that using the vapours of these essential oils in human environments could help to slow down the proliferation of moulds that are of potential risk to immunosuppressed children at home. Similarly, Tovey and

McDonald (1997) described a washing procedure using eucalyptus oil for controlling house dust mites and their allergens in clothing and bedding (the botanical source was not indicated). First, live house dust mites (*Dermatophagoides pteronyssinus*) were immersed in 0.05–0.4% eucalyptus oil in liquid detergent for periods up to one hour, washed and then left to dry. Secondly, the effect of 100 mL of eucalyptus oil dispersed in 15 mL of detergent against mites in woollen blankets was determined. The solution was added to 50 L of warm water in a washing machine and the blankets left to soak for 30–60 minutes before the washing cycle. Results for the first experiment indicated that 80% of mites were killed, whilst in the second experiment, survival on the eucalyptus soaked blankets was 0.6%, compared with 97.6% on untreated blankets. The authors concluded that the low concentration of eucalyptus oil (0.2%) needed to achieve the acaricidal effect was achievable in most households and removed the need for hot washes.

Sinusitis

The pain and discomfort of chronic sinusitis, caused by the inflammation of the mucous membranes of the sinuses as a result of viral or bacterial infection, is familiar to many people and is usually treated with antibiotics, decongestants and analgesics. However, this condition is typical of the type of long-term problem which responds well to homeopathy.

Homeopathy

Treatment will depend upon the presenting symptoms and since sinusitis is a chronic problem, the homeopath might use a constitutional remedy or address the presenting symptoms. For a throbbing, tearing pain felt deep in the facial bones Silicea is used. The source of this remedy is flint and the mineral silica is essential for growth and bone development. For yellow catarrh, when the face feels very tender and sensitive and the person feels chilly, *Hepar. sulphuris calcareum* is used. *Hepar. sulphuris calcareum* is made from calcium sulphide, which is obtained from the lining of oyster shells and flowers of sulphur. For sticky mucus, pain over the root or bridge of the nose, red eyes and frontal pain that is worse for pressure, Cinnabaris is used. For yellow catarrh with pain above the eyes, a stuffed up nose that is worse out of doors, affecting the front and right maxillary sinuses, and neuralgic type of pain, *Pulsatilla nigricans* is used.

TCM and upper respiratory tract conditions

Upper respiratory tract conditions such as colds, allergic rhinitis and sinusitis have been addressed together because in TCM they are deemed to have a common origin which, according to the traditional diagnosis, is due to the invasion of Wind that can be either Cold or Heat with Qi deficiency. This concept relates to Western medicine in that the external Cold pathogen is transmitted by Wind, i.e. droplet infection. Wind in TCM is seen as a Yang pathogenic influence and Wind disharmonies often have a sudden onset, such as in a cold or sinusitis. Heat is also a Yang pathogenic influence, leading to fevers and inflammation. In TCM the Lungs are responsible for distributing Defensive Qi (Wei Qi) throughout the body and preventing invasion by external pathogenic factors such as Cold, Wind and Damp, so when this Qi is depleted, the body is open to infection. Treatment is supportive and there is evidence that acupuncture is effective in treating the common cold (Hu 2000), whilst massaging acupoints was found to be effective in relieving symptoms and improving immune function (Zhu et al 1998). Anti-allergy herbs used in TCM include Minor Blue Dragon, which is a combination preparation consisting of licorice (*Glycyrrhiza glabra*), cinnamon (*Cinnamomum cassia*), ginger (*Zingiber officinale*), ma huang (*Ephedra sinica*) and peony.

Acupuncture is well documented to be an efficacious remedy in the treatment of respiratory conditions. In addition, there is good evidence for the use of acupuncture in the treatment of allergic rhinitis. Lau et al (1975) conducted a trial of 22 subjects which showed that 11 were symptom free after six treatments, 8 experienced moderate reduction in symptoms and 3 had no significant relief. Laboratory results noted a concurrent drop in absolute numbers of eosinophils and a percentage of nasal eosinophils. IgE level decreased in 64% of the subjects in the trial at the completion of the acupuncture treatment and in 76% at the 2-month follow-up. This coincided with a reported significant decrease in subjective clinical rating of symptoms but unfortunately there was no control group in this study with which to compare the results. Further work was done by Williamson et al (1996) in a randomised, controlled, single blind study using 102 patients over 16 years of age suffering with moderate to severe symptoms. Participants were divided into two groups, one of which received standard Western acupuncture and the other sham acupuncture. Not surprisingly, the results were inconclusive since 39% of the treatment group and 45.2% of the sham group reported remission of symptoms, with 16 patients in the treatment group and 14 of the patients in the sham group feeling that their treatment had an excellent or very good effect on their hay fever. Although this study involved a large sample, it is a good example of the type of research problem discussed in Chapter 2 in relation to the use of sham acupuncture. Although an attempt was made to conduct a controlled trial, the application of acupuncture was open to criticism because key elements relating to the philosophy of acupuncture were not addressed and the trial could have reached a false conclusion.

ASTHMA

Of all the allergic conditions the one which concerns school nurses and health visitors the most is asthma, the incidence of which is increasing at an alarming rate. In the 1960s there were around 100 000 cases per year. Now there are an estimated 3 million people with asthma, of whom 1 million are children (Hunt 1997). Hunt goes on to suggest that part of the problem is the drugs that are prescribed for asthma, which in 1994 cost the NHS £380 m. Asthma is the reversible obstruction of the bronchi and bronchioles of the lungs due to inflammation of the airways and the constriction of the muscles in the walls. There are many causes of asthma, including allergy (particularly in childhood), exercise, emotion, bronchitis or bronchiolitis, and it is treated conventionally with bronchodilators and steroids. Psychological factors have long been known to play a role in asthma and many children with asthma are described as anxious, shy, dependent and feeling that they lack control over their condition. Some children, however, can and do use their asthma as a convenient weapon, and family circumstances need to be taken into account when planning treatment. Other important psychological factors in the aetiology of asthma are expectation and suggestibility. From this description it can be seen that hypnosis is a potential intervention in treating asthma.

Hypnosis

The use of hypnosis in the treatment of chronic asthma is illustrated by Morrison (1988) and by Ewer and Stewart (1986). These two studies show how everyday suggestions, given under hypnosis, can have a powerful therapeutic effect. In the latter study there was a 26.2% reduction in the use of bronchodilators following a 6-week course of hypnotherapy. Morrison (1988) treated 16 chronic asthmatics and, after 1 year of therapy, admissions to hospital had fallen from 44 to 13. Prednisolone was withdrawn in six cases and reduced in a further eight and there were no increases in prednisolone dosages. Treatment approaches include therapeutic suggestion, ego strengthening and relaxation, all of which have a beneficial effect for many asthma sufferers. Ben-Zvi et al (1982) gave asthma sufferers positive therapeutic suggestions under hypnosis prior to exercise on a treadmill, and under these conditions there was a 15.9% decrease in forced expiratory volume compared with 31.8% in the no-treatment group. The authors concluded that hypnosis can therapeutically alter bronchospasm after exercise in asthmatic patients.

Other studies have noted that self-hypnosis can lead to significant improvement in younger patients who are not heavily dependent upon steroids and where emotional factors play a part. In their review of the use of hypnosis in treating children with asthma, Olness and Kohen (1996) note that, because of the complexity of asthma aetiology, the exact role of hypnosis is difficult to determine. However, self-hypnosis is very valuable in addressing underlying emotional aspects of asthma and re-establishing a patient's control over the condition.

In their review of the role of hypnosis in the treatment of asthma, Hackman et al (2000) discuss a number of studies which have been conducted on children and conclude that non-randomised controlled studies have shown significant effects of hypnosis regarding asthma, although the duration of hypnosis treatment may be a factor in differing results and it has been suggested that more than 1 month is necessary to achieve efficacy with hypnosis. Kohen et al (1984) evaluated the efficacy of using relaxation mental imagery (RMI) for asthma. This form of hypnosis is self-administered and requires practice at home. Using this intervention in the treatment of a number of clinical conditions, Kohen et al noted that among the asthma sufferers (n = 40) 70% attained either complete resolution or more than 50% reduction in symptoms. Those who attained a >50% improvement in symptoms also had reduced school absences and fewer visits to physicians or the emergency room.

Two further studies were conducted, concentrating on asthma alone. The first, again using RMI, studied a group of children aged 7–12 years (n = 28). Outcome measurements included pulmonary function tests, forced expiratory volume, forced expiratory flow, emergency room visits and missed school days. The RMI group had significantly fewer missed school days than the control group and rated their asthma as significantly better (Kohen, 1996). In the second study, of children aged 2–5 years, all the children received seven sessions of RMI. Asthma-related visits to physicians were significantly reduced and symptom severity scores were improved. However, there were no changes in the frequency of asthmatic attacks nor in pulmonary function tests (Kohen & Wynne 1997).

Of particular interest is the use of hypnosis during an acute attack of asthma. A number of hypnosis scripts are available for use during an acute attack (Hammond 1990). This use of hypnosis is controversial and it has been suggested that it should not be used on its own for an attack unless conducted within a clinical setting with resuscitation equipment available. However, when Ferreiro (1993) evaluated the use of hypnosis in 50 children aged between 5 and 14 years, who arrived in hospital during an acute asthma attack, 80% of the subjects needed no medication after hypnosis, suggesting that hypnosis is safe to use during an asthmatic attack.

Massage

Field et al (1998) undertook a study into the role of massage in the treatment of childhood asthma, following previous studies which indicated that massage reduced levels of anxiety and levels of cortisol in children. They had a sample of 32 asthmatic children aged 4–16 years, with 16 in the massage group and 16 in the control group. The subjects' asthma had been classified as mild (22%), moderate (58%) or severe (20%). The children were divided into two age groups, 4–9 years and 9–14 years. All were on medication. The massage therapy group were given a 20-minute massage by their parents every night before bedtime, whilst the control group did progressive relaxation. Pre- and post-anxiety levels were measured, using cortisol levels, the State Anxiety Scale and the State Anxiety Scale for Children, and physical measurements of peak expiratory flow rates were recorded daily by the parents, along with forced vital capacity and forced expiratory volume. Results indicated that in the younger age group massage was more effective than relaxation. Their anxiety levels decreased after the first day and their cortisol levels were reduced after the first and last days of the study. Their attitude towards their asthma improved and parents of both the massage and relaxation groups reported reduced anxiety levels. In addition, the massage group reported increased peak flow rating over the 30 days of the experiment and improved pulmonary function: forced vital capacity, a 24% increase; average flow rate, a 57% increase; peak expiratory flow rate, a 30% increase. However, in the older group there were only two measures of improvement: there was a greater improvement in attitude towards asthma and average flow rate increased by 52%. Field suggests that these differences might be attributed to less compliance on the part of the parents and children, either because they were busier, with increased social activities, or because the older children were less comfortable than the younger children with being massaged.

The therapeutic value of massage in reducing anxiety in both parents and children appears to be worth further investigation. Field particularly highlights the importance of the parents having a positive interaction with and effect on their child's asthma. The appropriateness of massage as an intervention in older children is discussed in the chapter on adolescence.

Ayurvedic medicine

The Ayurvedic approach to medical conditions in general involves addressing emotional states, but this is particularly the case in relation to respiratory conditions, where emotions are a factor. For example, the negative emotion associated with the lungs is sadness and grief. Diseases are also defined in terms of their dosha type and the person's constitutional dosha will determine their propensity to certain illnesses. For example, a number of respiratory conditions discussed in this chapter, such as sinusitis, asthma and bronchitis, are kapha conditions. Kapha will obstruct the movement of vata in the chest, resulting in the vata leaking out of its normal channels, carrying with it the kapha dosha. This results in the three major channels in the chest becoming blocked and dysfunctional. At this stage an asthma attack can occur. Treatment is aimed at clearing lung congestion through therapeutic vomiting and pacifying the vata and kapha doshas. Prior to treatment, excess kapha is stimulated by using calamus root, which is an antispasmodic, and chest decongestant, or licorice (*Glycyrrhiza glabra*).

The effect of calamus root is supported by evidence, although it is classified as an unsafe herb by the Federal Drug Administration (FDA) (Gerson 1995, Barnes et al 2002). Bielory and Lupoli (1999), in their review of herbs used for allergy and asthma in both Ayurvedic and Traditional Chinese Medicine, describe the use of a number of medicines used for asthma in Ayurveda. *Tylophora asthmatica* or *Tylophora indica* are Ayurvedic medicines used to treat respiratory conditions in which mucus accumulation is a symptom. Shivupuri et al (1968, 1969, 1972) conducted several studies on the treatment of asthma using this preparation and noted that, compared with a placebo group, the medication offered a moderate to complete relief of symptoms, in some instances lasting 8–12 weeks. Gore et al (1980) compared tylophora with isoprenaline and demonstrated a significant improvement in lung function test results in asthmatics. Another herb used in respiratory conditions is cinnamon (*Cinnamomum cassia*), which is used in herbal medicine as an antispasmodic and antimicrobial, and which completely suppresses the growth of E. *coli, Staphylococcus aureus* and *Candida albicans* (Barnes et al 2002), although Fetrow and Avila (2001) do not recommend its ingestion other than as a spice. The antimicrobial activities of garlic, which is anti-kapha and also good for sinus headaches, are well documented. Bacterial species known to be sensitive to garlic include *Staphylococcus, Candida albicans, E. coli*, influenza type B and herpes simplex type 1 (Adetumbi & Lau 1983, Tsai 1985, Hughes 1989). Garlic (*Allium sativum*) was known and used in ancient times, and was fed to the slaves who build the pyramids. Licorice (*Glycyrrhiza glabra*), which is also used in Western herbalism and TCM, has antimicrobial properties against *Staphylococcus aureus* and *Candida albicans*, and turmeric and purified ashes of tin are good for asthma. Tin is also used in the form of *Stannum metallicum* in homeopathy for asthma and bronchitis.

In Ayurvedic medicine the patient's diet would also be adjusted to balance the dosha. To reduce kapha, the patient would be advised to eat fruits and vegetables such as apples, apricots, cherries, cranberries and mango, sprouts, cabbage, carrots, mushrooms and peas, as well as chicken, turkey or eggs. For a full account of dietary indications see Lad (1983). Complementary to the practice of Ayurvedic medicine, which is the science of the body, is the practice of yoga, which is regarded as the science of union with the Ultimate Being. The type of yoga used is determined by the individual's constitution as well as their specific disorders; for example, the fish posture is suitable for bronchitis, asthma and sinusitis. Other asanas include headstand, plough and half wheel for bronchitis, boat, plough and breath of fire for sinus congestion and half wheel, bow, cobra and palm tree for asthma. In addition, breathing exercises or pranayama are undertaken.

As with yoga, there are many forms of pranayama and the type is dictated by the person's constitutional type. Pitta individuals should do left nostril breathing (inhaling through the left nostril and exhaling through the right), kapha individuals should do right nostril breathing and vatas alternate nostril breathing. Pranayama brings cleansing and healing if done correctly, but can in itself cause disease if practised incorrectly. These aspects of Ayurvedic medicine are important to bear in mind when looking at the research that has been undertaken in the use of yoga and transcendental meditation (TM) in the amelioration of asthma. For example, Singh et al (1990) investigated the effects of pranayama on asthma in a controlled study in which subjects were taught pranayama breathing on a 1:2 inspiration/expiration rate and compared with a control group who used a placebo exerciser, which imposes a slowing of breathing, again at a 1:2 ratio. It is not clear what form of pranayama was used. Results, however, indicated that pranayama exercises may lead to an overall improvement in people with mild asthma.

A controlled study using yoga for bronchial asthma (Nagarathna & Nagendra 1985) included breathing exercises, meditation and physical postures. The results showed a highly significant reduction in the number of weekly attacks and a reduction in drug treatment. The authors concluded that yoga seemed to stabilise and reduce excitability of the nervous system and noted that the deep physical and mental relaxation seemed to have a stabilising effect on bronchial activity, making vagal efferents less excitable. In none of these studies is it indicated that the yoga asanas were related to traditional Ayurvedic medicine as applied to asthma, nor which forms of pranayama were used, which raises the question of whether the subjects were getting the full effect of the yoga or only the relaxation effect.

Homeopathy

Homeopathy has a great deal to offer in the treatment of asthma, and many children and their parents may turn to it as a treatment, but it must be used on a long term basis to be effective.

Since asthma is a chronic problem, the treatment is developed constitutionally where possible, i.e. by assessing the patient's constitutional type and treating that, with the addition of other remedies. For example, if the asthma is caused by an allergen, the homeopath will prescribe a diluted allergen as a treatment. Common medicines used by homeopaths in the treatment of asthma include Kali. carb for when the asthma is at its worst between 2 and 4 a.m., with a pale, tired patient who complains of feeling chilly, Nux vomica for when the attack follows a digestive upset and is at its worst around 4 a.m., and Aconite, which was mentioned earlier. These examples of remedies (there are others) show, yet again, the importance of the individuality of the prescriptions and the types of factors homeopaths take into consideration when prescribing a remedy. An illustration of the kind of commitment to treatment a patient might need to make in seeking a homeopathic cure was demonstrated by Castellsagu (1992), who treated 26 cases of bronchial asthma with homeopathy. Many patients in the study needed more than 3 years of homeopathic treatment to stabilise their condition; previous treatment with steroids complicated and prolonged the treatment. What was interesting in this study was that a high percentage of patients were cured (1 year without an asthmatic attack) by using only one homeopathic medicine.

In a review of over 100 published trials of homeopathy, Kleijnen et al (1991a) noted that 77% showed a positive effect for the use of homeopathy and suggested that 'this would be sufficient for establishing homeopathy as a regular treatment for certain conditions'.

One trial by Reilly et al (1994) consisted of 28 patients with allergic asthma, most of them being sensitive to house dust mite. The design was a randomised, double-blind assessment of two parallel groups, one receiving homeopathic treatment based on allergen material, the other a placebo. Treatment was assessed by using a visual analogue scale of overall symptom intensity. Pulmonary function tests were performed at the beginning of the trial and results from the visual analogue scale indicated that 9 of the 11 patients in the treatment group improved, the patients with the most severe initial symptoms showing the greatest improvement. The results of the pulmonary function tests elicited that 7 of the 9 patients on homeopathic treatment showed improvement, compared with 4 of the 11 in the placebo group, demonstrating that results of homeopathy differ from those of placebo. This trial, and the previously quoted study by Reilly into homeopathy and allergic rhinitis (Reilly 1986), both used the isopathic rather than the classical approach and this may be significant to their results.

Herbalism

Herbs used in the treatment of asthma would include the antispasmodic remedies such as lobelia, also known as Indian tobacco or asthma weed, which has been traditionally used in the treatment of bronchitic asthma and chronic bronchitis. Lobelia (*Lobelia inflata*) contains the alkaloid constituent lobeline, which has effects on the central nervous system similar to those of nicotine and is also used in anti-smoking preparations. Lobelia has the same toxicity effects as nicotine and, generally, it is only dispensed by a professional herbalist (Barnes et al 2002). Specific to the treatment of asthma is the herb ephedra (*Ephedra sinica*), also known as ma-huang, which is native to Northern China and used in TCM for the treatment of asthma. The alkaloid of ephedra contains ephedrine, which acts as a bronchial dilator, an expectorant and a diuretic. Since its toxicity has not been established, its use is confined to professional practitioners.

Of equal value is the herb euphorbia (*Euphorbia capitata*), which, again, is antispasmodic, anti-asthmatic, expectorant and anticatarrhal. It has antibacterial properties against Gram-positive and Gram-negative bacteria. There are no reported contraindications and it does not appear to be toxic (Barnes et al 2002). As with other therapies, the herbalist will seek to ascertain the fundamental causes of the asthma and treat them accordingly. For example, if the presenting asthma is associated with stress, preparations of lemon balm (*Melissa officinalis*), chamomile (*Matricaria recutita*) or lime flowers (*Tilia cordata*) might be prescribed. It was originally believed that lemon balm could completely revive a person since its ability to dispel melancholy has long been recorded by herbal writers (Bremness 1995). Chamomile, both Roman (*Chamaemelum nobile*) and German (*Matricaria recutita*), has a long history of therapeutic use and was known to the Egyptians, who dedicated it to the sun because of its healing properties. It was also known to the Greeks, who christened it the 'earth apple' because of its scent. Chamomile is renowned for its soothing and healing properties, is traditionally used as an anti-emetic and antispasmodic, and is known to be mentally relaxing. However, it should not be taken by anyone who has a known allergy to ragweed, chrysanthemums and other members of the compositae family, since anaphylactic reaction has been reported in these instances (Benner & Lee 1973, Casterline 1980). Lime flowers (*Tilia cordata*), act as a peripheral vasodilator and are recommended in cardiovascular conditions where tension or anxiety are a factor, such as hypertension or atherosclerosis (Mills 1989). They are an effective relaxant, especially for children. Barnes et al (2002) suggest that lime flower should be avoided by people suffering from existing cardiac disorders.

Anthroposophical medicine

In Anthroposophical medicine the aetiology of asthma is similar to that of rhinitis. It is regarded as an astral disorder, the too intense union of the astral body and the lungs resulting in the secretion of plugs of mucus which impede respiration. Steiner proposed three basic remedies for the treatment of asthma, Gencydo, Nicotiana and Blackthorne, to be administered by subcutaneous injection.

TCM

In TCM, asthma is diagnosed as being caused internally by disharmonies of the Lungs, Spleen and Kidneys and externally by Wind/Cold or Wind/Heat invasion. The Wind/Cold invasion correlates to viral infections and airborne allergens. The Spleen in TCM is concerned with the transportation of fluids and a deficient Spleen results in the accumulation of fluids, resulting in Damp and Phlegm leading to airway obstruction. Children are constitutionally Spleen deficient and if the child is eating a diet which increases Phlegm, i.e. high in dairy produce, which is common in the modern diet, this will increase the Spleen deficiency. One of the roles of Spleen is to extract Qi from food and convert it into Nutritive Qi and Defensive Qi (Wei-Qi). If the Spleen is weak there will be a deficiency of Defensive Qi. Asthma resulting from Wind/Heat invasion may be the result of a bacterial infection. Chronic asthma is due to the child's Lung deficiency/Kidney deficiency. Lung deficiency impedes Lung-Qi descending, resulting in rebellious Qi causing wheezing and cough. Lungs send the Qi downwards to the Kidneys, which have the function of holding the Qi down, thus facilitating breathing. If Kidney function is impaired, the Qi will move back upwards and cause breathing difficulties. Babies and young children are in the Water stage of development, when their Kidneys are most vulnerable. Older children, who are in the Wood stage of development and for whom emotional factors are more likely to provoke an asthma attack, are also more susceptible to Liver disharmonies. Treatment is dependent on cause and would involve diet reform if necessary, rebalancing the disharmonies and, more importantly, instigating a programme of prevention, involving the parents massaging the relevant acupoints and administering herbal mixtures.

Zang (1990) noted that in 192 cases of bronchial asthma, the use of two specific acupuncture points (Lu 6 and Lu 10) had an immediate total effect rate of

98.9%, and a clinical remission plus marked improvement rate of 76.5%, which was effective for all age groups. In particular, effects on Cold type (according to TCM) and allergic type (according to Western medicine) were the most pronounced. However, in a review of 13 clinical trials Kleijnen et al (1991b) concluded that claims that acupuncture is effective in the treatment of asthma are not based on the results of well-designed clinical trials. Specifically, this completely valid criticism centred around the fact that the studies had too few subjects, lacked randomisation and lacked follow-up and, further, the use of concurrent medication was not assessed. However, as was discussed in Chapter 2, poor clinical trials do not necessarily mean that the treatment is ineffective. Of the five highest scores in the Kleijnen review, three had a positive result and two were negative. Since this review, further, better designed research has yielded more encouraging results. In one of the few trials to use individualised, traditional acupuncture methods, Joshi (1992) points out that acupuncture has a limited role in the treatment of acute attacks but that, long term, it has an excellent prophylactic effect in exercise-induced asthma; this confirms similar results obtained by Fung et al (1986) on the prophylactic treatment of exercise-induced asthma.

In a review of the use of acupuncture in pulmonary disease, Jobst (1995) suggests that its use in bronchial asthma, chronic bronchitis and chronic disabling breathlessness can facilitate the reduction of medication and that it might be safer than prolonged pharmaceutical maintenance therapy. The use of exercise for long-term self-help for respiratory conditions might include the ancient Chinese arts of t'ai chi and Qigong, involving breathing exercises as well as a full range of slow, controlled movements that raise the Qi within the body, are calming, and give the patient a feeling of control and relaxation.

Reuther and Aldridge (1998) conducted a pilot study into the value of Qigong in the management of asthma. The study was conducted over 1 year with 30 participants being taught Qigong and asked to practise on a daily basis. In addition, they undertook measurements of peak flow, use of medication, incidence of cough, sleep disturbance, expectoration, dyspnoea and general wellbeing. Results indicated that there was a statistically significant difference between the exercisers (n = 17) and the non-exercisers (n = 13) in peak flow variability, hospitalisation rates, sick leave and reduced antibiotic use, all leading to reduced treatment costs. Results also noted the potential of Qigong for the relief of acute symptoms in experienced exercisers. Although this investigation was performed on adults, the value of the findings for paediatric asthmatics is encouraging.

Herbal intervention would involve the use of anti-allergy preparations such as those indicated for allergic rhinitis, as well as ma huang (*Ephedra sinica*) and licorice (*Glycyrrhiza glabra*), which moistens the lungs and prevents coughing and wheezing. Specific for childhood asthma is the preparation Shinpi-To, which consists of seven plants. Hamaski et al (1997) studied the effects of Shinpi-To on IgE loaded basophilic leukaemia-2H3 cells and results indicated that Shinpi-To inhibited the release of LTC4 and LTB4.

Reflexology

According to research done in Denmark where reflexology is used extensively, therapists indicated that respiratory problems were one area in which they obtained the best results (Launso 1995). Some physiotherapists have now incorporated reflexology into their normal practice and frequently use it prior to treating with chest physiotherapy. This therapy, and techniques relating to it, could certainly be used by nurses and taught to parents of children with cystic fibrosis, where daily physiotherapy is required.

ACUTE RESPIRATORY DISTRESS

One of the most distressing problems with difficulty in breathing is the accompanying stress and anxiety, both for patients and for their relatives. Of particular value is the gentle effectiveness of homeopathic remedies to ease the immediate distress and to alleviate anxiety in the longer term. This breaks up the vicious cycle of distress, leading to difficulty in breathing, which leads to an even greater distress. Immediate care can be offered by giving the patient the remedy Aconite (*Aconitum napellus*). *Acon* is the Latin name for arrow and the plant, which is also known as blue monkshood, blue aconite or wolfsbane, is highly poisonous, having been used in the past as an arrow poison. The homeopathic remedy is prepared from the whole fresh plant and was first 'proved' by Hahnemann in 1805. It is traditionally used for states of acute or chronic tension and is particularly indicated for instances of extreme fear, such as fear of dying (Lockie 1990, Lockie & Geddes 1996). The homeopathic remedies mentioned earlier in this chapter can be given quite safely to anyone in an emergency situation.

The ventilated patient

One of the most traumatic situations for both patients and relatives is being ventilated and although patients are unconscious, many are very aware of what is going on around them. For this reason the use of guided visualisation has a valuable place in the care of these patients. Helen Passant has described her use of guided visualisation in relation to her care of the elderly: '… we use visualisation techniques to take a walk through bluebell woods or in spring rain … the mind can move anywhere, even though the body may be immobile' (Passant 1990). Other scenarios which might be developed in conjunction with the patient's relatives include reliving a special day or revisiting places which involve happy and positive memories for the patient. Since nurses and relatives are encouraged to talk to unconscious patients, such a therapy could be conducted during routine nursing care and need not take any time away from other patients.

Ongoing stress and anxiety need to be addressed at a deeper level and should involve care of the family as well as of the patient. Stevensen (1994) noted that using neroli essential oil in a massage reduced anxiety in highly dependent cardiac patients, and in her review of the use of massage in intensive care units, Hill (1995) noted that, overall, the results were very positive.

Chlan et al (2001) undertook a descriptive pilot study into the effectiveness of music therapy for alert patients undergoing mechanical ventilation. Over a 3-day period, patients indicated their music preference. Frequency and length of listening and outcome measurements of anxiety, heart rate, respiratory rate and blood pressure were noted. Music preferences, which were administered through earphones, included, alternative rock, classical/Mozart, instrumental hymns, guitar and classical and religious instrumental. Physiological indicators of blood pressure, heart rate and respiratory rate, as well as anxiety, were seen to decrease.

REFERENCES

Adetumbi M, Lau M 1983 Allium sativum (garlic) a natural antibiotic. Medical Hypotheses 12: 227–237

Alm J, Swartz J, Lilja G et al 1999 Atopy in children of families with an anthroposophic lifestyle. Lancet 353(9163): 1485–1488

Baratta M, Dorman D, Deans S 1998 Chemical composition, antimicrobial and antioxidative activity of laurel, sage, rosemary, oregano and coriander essential oils. Journal of Essential Oil Research 10(6): 618, 627

Barnes J, Anderson L, Phillipson J 2002 Herbal medicines: a guide for health care professionals, 2nd edn. Pharmaceutical Press, London

Bauer R 1985 Structure and stereochemistry of new sequiterpene esters from Echinacea purpurea. Helvetica Chimica Acta 68: 2355–2358

Ben-Zvi S, Spohn W, Young S 1982 Hypnosis for exercise induced asthma. American Review of Respiratory Diseases 1: 392–395

Benner M, Lee H 1973 Anaphylactic reaction to chamomile tea. Journal of Allergy and Clinical Immunology 52: 307–308

Blumenthal M (ed) 1998 The complete German commission E monographs therapeutic guide to herbal medicines. American Botanical Council, Austin, Texas

Bone K 1994 Propolis: a natural antibiotic. Australian Journal of Medical Herbalism 6(3): 61–65

Bone K 1997 Echinacea: when should it be used? Alternative Medical Review (Dec) 2(6): 451–458

Bremness L 1995 Herbs. Dorling Kindersley, London

Budhiraja S, Cullum M, Sioutis S et al 1999 Biological activity of Melaleuca alternifolia (tea tree oil). Journal of Manipulative Physiological Therapy 22(7): 447–453

Carson C, Riley T 1993 A review: antimicrobial activity of the essential oil of Melaleuca alternifolia. Letters in Applied Microbiology 16: 49–55

Carson C, Riley T 1994 The antimicrobial effect of tea tree oil. Medical Journal of Australia 160: 236

Casterline C 1980 Allergy to chamomile tea. Journal of the American Medical Association 4: 330–331

Castellsagu A 1992 Evaluation of 26 cases of bronchial asthma with homeopathic treatment. British Homeopathic Journal 81: 168–172

Chao S, Young D, Oberg C 2000 Screening for inhibitory activity in essential oils on selected bacteria, fungi and viruses. Journal of Essential Oil Research 12: 639–649

Chaumont J, Leger D 1992 Elimination of allergenic moulds in dwellings. Antifungal properties of vapours of essential oil of 'bourbon' geranium, citronellol, geraniol and citral. Annales Pharmaceutiques Francaises 50(3): 156–166

Chlan L, Tracy M, Nelson B, Walker J 2001 Feasibility of a music intervention protocol for patients receiving mechanical ventilatory support. Alternative Therapies (Nov/Dec) 7(6): 80–83

Cohen B, Dressler W 1982 Acute aromatics inhalation modifies the airways. Effects of the common cold. Respiration 43: 285–293

Cox S, Mann C, Markham J et al 2000 The mode of action of antimicrobial action of the essential oil of Melaleuca alternifolia (tea tree oil). Journal of Applied Microbiology 88: 170–175

Deans S, Ritchie G 1987 Antibacterial properties of plant essential oils. International Journal of Food Microbiology 5: 165–180

De Lange de Klerk D, Blommers D, Kuik D et al 1994 Effect of homeopathic medicines on daily burden of symptoms in children with recurrent upper respiratory tract infections. British Medical Journal 309 (Nov): 1329–1332

Dobrowolski J, Vohora S, Sharma K et al 1991 Antibacterial, antifungal, antiamoebic, antiinflammatory and antipyretic studies on propolis bee products. Journal of Ethnopharmacology 35: 77–82

Ewer T, Stewart D 1986 Improvement in bronchial hyper responsiveness in patients with moderate asthma after treatment with a hypnotic technique. A randomised controlled trail. British Medical Journal 293: 1129–1132

Ferreiro O 1993 Hypnosis: its use in acute attacks of bronchial asthma. Hypnosis 20: 236

Fetrow C, Avila J 2001 Professional's handbook of complementary and alternative medicines. Springhouse, Pennsylvania

Field T, Henteleff T, Hernandez-Reif M 1998 Children with asthma have improved pulmonary function after massage therapy. Journal of Pediatrics 132: 854–858

Fung K, Chow O, So S 1986 Attenuation of exercise induced asthma by acupuncture. Lancet 2(8521/2): 1419–1421

Gerson S 1995 Ayurvedic specific condition review: asthma. The Protocol Journal of Botanical Medicine (Autumn) 1(2): 108–109

Gore K, Rao K, Guruswamy M 1980 Physiological studies with Tylophora asthmatica in bronchial asthma. Indian Journal of Medical Research 71: 144–148

Grange J, Davey R 1990 Antibacterial properties of popolis (bee glue). Journal of the Royal Society of Medicine 83: 159–160

Hackman R, Stern J, Gershwin M 2000 Hypnosis and asthma: a critical review. Journal of Asthma 37(1): 1–15

Hamaski Y, Kobayashi I, Hayasaki R 1997 The Chinese herbal medicine, shinpi-to, inhibits IgE-mediated leukotriene synthesis in rat basinophilic leukemia-2H3 cells. Journal of Ethnopharmacology 56(2): 123–131

Hammond D 1990 Handbook of hypnotic suggestions and metaphors. Norton, London

Hill CF 1995 Massage in intensive care nursing: a literature review. Complementary Therapies in Medicine 3(2): 100–104

Hollis S 1994 The country diary herbal. Bloomsbury Books, London

Hu J 2000 Acupuncture treatment of the common cold. Journal of Traditional Chinese Medicine 20(3): 227–230

Hughes B 1989 Antiviral constituents from Allium sativum. Planta Medica 55: 114

Hunt L 1997 The big wheeze. Nursing Times 93(7): 32–33

International Study of Asthma and Allergy in Childhood (ISAAC) Steering Committee 1998 Worldwide variation in the prevalence of symptoms of asthma, allergic rhinoconjunctivitis and atopic eczema. Lancet 351(9111): 1225–1232

Jobst K 1995 A critical analysis of acupuncture in pulmonary disease: efficacy and safety of the acupuncture needle. Journal of Alternative and Complementary Medicine 1: 57–85

Joshi YM 1992 Acupuncture in bronchial asthma. Journal of the Association of Physicians of India 40(5): 327–331

Kalliomäki M, Salminem S, Arvilommi H et al 2001 Probiotics in primary prevention of atopic disease: a randomised placebo-controlled trial. Lancet 357: 1076–1079

Kleijnen J, Knipschild P, Ter Riet G 1991a Clinical trials of homeopathy. British Medical Journal 302: 316–323

Kleijnen J, Ter Riet G, Knipschild P 1991b Acupuncture and asthma: a review of controlled trials. Thorax 46(11): 799–802

Kohen D, Colwell S, Heimel A 1984 The use of relaxation/mental imagery (self hypnosis) in the management of 505 pediatric behavioural encounters. Journal of Developmental and Behavioural Pediatrics 5(1): 21–25

Kohen D 1996 Relaxation/mental imagery (self hypnosis) for childhood asthma: behavioural outcomes in a prospective controlled study. Australian Journal of Clinical and Experimental Hypnosis 24: 12

Kohen D, Wynne E 1997 Applying hypnosis in a pre school family asthma education program: uses of story telling, imagery and relaxation. American Journal of Clinical Hypnosis 39: 169

Lad V 1983 Ayurveda: the science of self healing: a practical guide. Lotus Press, Wisconsin

Lau BH, Wong DS, Slater JM 1975 Effect of acupuncture on allergic rhinitis: clinical and laboratory evaluations 3(3): 263–270

Launso I 1995 A description of reflexology practice and clientele in Denmark. Complementary Therapies in Medicine 3(4): 206–211

Lis-Balchin M, Hart S, Deans S 1996 Comparison of the pharmacological and antimicrobial action of commercial plant essential oils. Journal of Herbs, Spices and Medicinal Plants 4(2): 69–86

Lockie A 1990 The family guide to homeopathy. Penguin Books, Middlesex

Lockie A, Geddes N 1996 The complete guide to homeopathy, the principles and practice of treatment. Dorling Kindersley, London

Mascolo N 1987 Biological screening of Italian medicinal plants for anti-inflammatory activity. Phytotherapy Research 1: 28–31

Mills S 1989 The complete guide to modern herbalism. Thorsons, London

Mills S 1993 The essential guide to herbal medicine. Penguin Books, Harmondsworth

Morrison J 1988 Chronic asthma and improvement with relaxation induced by hypnotherapy. Journal of the Royal Society of Medicine (Dec) 81: 701–704

Nagarathna R, Nagendra H 1985 Yoga for bronchial asthma: a controlled study. British Medical Journal 291: 1077–1079

Nicholls C 1998 Aromatic medicine in the treatment of infections. British Journal of Phytotherapy 5(1): 40–47

Olness K, Kohen D 1996 Hypnosis and hypnotherapy with children. Guildford Press, London

Passant H 1990 A holistic approach in the ward. Nursing Times 86(4): 26–28

Preininger V 1975 The pharmacology and toxicology of the papaveraceae alkoloids. In: Manske R, Holmes H (eds) The alkoloids, vol 15. Academic Press, New York

Recio M 1989 Antimicrobial activity of selected plants employed in the Spanish Mediterranean area, part II. Phytotherapy Research 33: 77–80

Reilly D, Taylor M, McSharry C et al 1986 Is homeopathy a placebo response? Controlled trial of homeopathic potency, with pollen in hay fever as a model. Lancet 2: 881–886

Reilly D, Taylor M, Campbell J et al 1994 Is evidence for homeopathy reproducible? Lancet 344: 1601–1606

Reuther I, Aldridge D 1998 Qigong yangsheng as a complementary therapy in the management of asthma: a single case appraisal. The Journal of Alternative and Complementary Medicine 4(2): 173–183

Scadding G, Drake-Lee A, Howard P et al 1995 Rhinitis management guidelines. British Society for Allergy and Clinical Immunology, London

Serkedjieva J 1990 Antiviral activity of the infusion (SHS-174) from flowers of Sambucus nigra, aerial parts of Hypericum perforam and roots of Saponaria officinalis against influenza and herpes simplex virus. Phytotherapy Research 4: 97

Sharma H, Clark C 1998 Contemporary Ayurveda. Churchill Livingstone, Edinburgh

Shivupuri D, Menon M, Parkash D 1968 Preliminary studies in Tylophora indica in the treatment of asthma and allergic rhinitis. Journal of Association of Physicians of India 16(1): 9–15

Shivupuri D, Menon M, Parkash D 1969 A crossover double blind study on Tylophora indica in the treatment of asthma and allergic rhinitis. Journal of Allergy 43(3): 145–150

Shivupuri D, Singhal S, Parkash D 1972 Treatment of asthma with alcoholic extract of Tylophora indica: a crossover double blind study. Annals of Allergy 30: 407–412

Singh H, Srivastava M, Singh A, Srivastava A 1995 Cinnamon bark oil, a potent fungitoxicant against fungi causing respiratory tract mycosis. Allergy 50(12): 995–999

Singh V, Wisniewski A, Britton J, Tattersfield A 1990 Effect of yoga breathing exercises (pranayama) on airway reactivity in subjects with asthma. Lancet 335: 1381–1383 (June 9)

Stevensen C 1994 The psychophysiological effects of aromatherapy massage following cardiac surgery. Complementary Therapies in Medicine 2(1): 27–35

Sun L, Currier N, Miller S 1999 The American coneflower: a prophylactic role involving non-specific immunity. Journal of Alternative Complementary Medicine (Oct) 5(5): 437–446

Tsai Y 1985 Antiviral properties of garlic: in vitro effects on influenza B, Herpes simplex and coxsackie viruses. Planta Medica 51: 460–461

Taylor D 1999 Antibiotic resistance: a concern for all. Nursing Times Clinical Monograph No 16. Emap Healthcare, London

Tovey E, McDonald L 1997 A simple washing procedure with eucalyptus oil for controlling house dust mites and their allergens in clothing and bedding. Journal of Allergy and Clinical Immunology 100(4): 464–466

Wacker A, Hilbig W 1978 Virus inhibition by Echinacea purpurea. Planta Medica 33: 89–102

Wagner H 1988 Immunologically active polysaccharides of Echinacea purpurea cell cultures. Phytochemistry 27: 119–126

Westendorf J 1982 Carito in vitro. Untersuchungen zum nachweiss spasmolytischer und kontraktiler einlusse. Therapiewoche 32: 6791–6797

Wiesenauer M, Gaus W 1985 Double blind trial comparing the effectiveness of the homeopathic preparation Galphimia potentiation D6 Galphimia dilution 10(-6) and placebo on pollinosis. Arzneimittelforschung 35: 1745–1747

Williamson L, Yudkin P, Livingstone R, Prasad K 1996 Hay fever treatment in general practice – randomised controlled trial comparing standard western acupuncture with sham acupuncture. Acupuncture in Medicine 14(1): 6–10

Zhu S, Wang N, Wang D et al 1998 A clinical investigation on massage for prevention and treatment of recurrent respiratory tract infection in children. Journal of Traditional Chinese Medicine 18(4): 285–291

Zang J 1990 Immediate anti asthmatic effect of acupuncture on 192 cases of bronchial asthma. Journal of Traditional Chinese Medicine 10(2): 89–93

4

Problems related to rest and sleep

CHAPTER CONTENTS

- **Introduction   70**
- **Sleep patterns   70**
- **Sleep disorders   71**
- **Therapeutic interventions   71**
  Homeopathy   71
  TCM   72

Ayurvedic medicine   74
Aromatherapy   74
Herbalism   75
Anthroposophical medicine   76
Hypnosis   76
- **References   77**

INTRODUCTION

The healing power of sleep has been acknowledged since ancient days although its exact function was not and is still not fully understood. Sleep was an integral part of the treatment at the temple-hospices of Aesculapius, as were diet, meditation and bathing.

This chapter reviews what sleep is and describes some of the types of insomnia; it then looks at some complementary therapies that can help to address the problem, and discusses in more detail some of the preparations that can help to induce and maintain sleep.

SLEEP PATTERNS

Sleep is divided into two types: light active rapid eye movement (REM) sleep, during which the majority of dreaming and healing occurs; and non-rapid eye movement (NREM) deep sleep, which some researchers further divide into four stages, the fourth stage being the deepest. This deep NREM sleep increases during the first year of life and reaches its highest levels in early childhood, decreasing by about 40% during adolescent development (Mindell et al 1999). It is difficult to wake a child during this period and the child is often confused and disorientated if so woken. In the newborn period, REM sleep is referred to as active sleep, and NREM sleep as quiet sleep. Babies divide their sleeping time equally between the two. In the neonate, REM occurs at sleep onset and waking, and sleeping is randomly distributed throughout the 24-hour cycle; however, by 3 months, babies enter NREM when they fall asleep. A normal night's sleep will consist of cycles of these different levels of sleep. The early part of the night will consist mainly of deep sleep with short bursts of REM sleep, whilst the second part of the night will consist mainly of REM sleep, the longest periods occurring just before waking. It is at this stage that nightmares are most likely to occur. People who are disturbed during REM sleep report that they feel more mentally exhausted, tense and irritable, and their lack of sleep can result in difficulties with concentration, learning and memory. The structure of sleep changes over the life span, children having longer periods of NREM sleep than adults.

SLEEP DISORDERS

Mindell et al (1999) identify two categories of sleep disorder, the dyssomnias, which involve difficulties in establishing and maintaining sleep, and the sleep parasomnias, which are disorders that interrupt sleep, including arousal, partial arousal, or sleep stage transitions. In her review of common sleep problems of babies and young children, Kerr (1997) describes difficulties in getting to sleep and frequent night wakening as the most common problems, and indicates that sleep problems in the preschool years are among the most common problems referred to health professionals.

Contrary to common belief, these problems are not transitory but can persist for 6 months to a year, causing significant stress within the family and leading to depression, anxiety, irritability and apathy as well as aggression (Errante 1985). It is not always completely clear why some children suffer from sleep disturbances, but predisposing causes have included separation anxiety and social problems (Kerr & Jowett 1994), whilst failure to establish a night time routine can have a significant effect.

THERAPEUTIC INTERVENTIONS

The complexities of both the symptoms and the treatment of insomnia are most eloquently addressed by both homeopathy and TCM and these traditions are presented first in this chapter.

Homeopathy

Homeopathic prescriptions for remedies used to address sleep problems should be tailored to match the precise symptoms presented by the patient. For example, if insomnia is caused by irritability and anxiety, particularly in babies who will not settle, Chamomilla, derived from the herb chamomile, is the treatment of choice.

For children who wake in the night and are unable to go back to sleep Arsen. alb (*Arsenicum album*) might be suggested, particularly if the patient is generally very anxious, is very fearful, becoming frightened when alone, or is afraid of the dark. This remedy is useful for children who have vivid imaginations and who may scare themselves with stories about ghosts etc. Arsen. alb is derived from the mineral arsenic oxide, which was originally used as a medication for syphilis and as a general tonic before its dangers were realised; however, it is safe in homeopathic doses.

Sulphur is indicated for children who wake early in the morning. Sulphur has been used medicinally for over 2000 years and is used for a range of conditions in homeopathy. In this instance it is prescribed for the mental stress that can lead to disturbed sleep and nightmares coupled with early wakening. A fine yellow powder called flowers of sulphur is extracted from the mineral sulphur.

Many children today lead extremely busy lives, attending many out-of-school activities alongside their school work; this may leave children over-stimulated and very tired, and switching off after a fairly long day might become a problem. For these children, Nux vomica (*Strychnos nux vomica*) is indicated.

When the inability to sleep is due to anxiety or over-excitement because of a forthcoming event, such as sitting an exam or performing in the school play, Gelsemium (*Gelsemium sempervirens*) is the remedy of choice. Nightmares are treated with Aconite (*Aconitum napellus*), which is the remedy for intense fear and shock, whilst night terrors might respond to Kali. brom (*Kali bromatum*). Clearly, other underlying causes of sleep problems must also be addressed, and readers are referred to Chapter 6 on eating and drinking for colic and teething remedies.

The remedies described here have been selected from a wide repertory, covering every facet of sleeplessness, and indicate the wide variety of issues that a homeopath would take into consideration when assessing the patient and prescribing a suitable remedy.

TCM

It is recognised in TCM, as in Western medicine, that there are multiple pathologies which can cause insomnia and multiple presentations of the condition, so that an individual approach to treatment is required. Sleep in TCM is related to the Heart, which is believed to house the person's spirit or Shen. Insomnia is caused by 'empty Heart fire', a concept in which the spirit is said to reside in the Mind during the day and in the Heart at night. Insomnia in children can be due to either an excess or a deficient state. Excess state insomnia may result in restless sleep with frequent wakening during the night, whilst deficient state insomnia leads to disturbed sleep rhythms and, if specifically Liver-Yin deficient, will result in night terrors, sleepwalking, talking in the sleep and excessive dreaming, these dreams being filled with anger, frustration and agitation. If there is Kidney-Yin deficiency, the dreams will be disturbing.

Sleep disorders in children are usually due to excessive Yang energy, which can prevent children going off to sleep. Since, as we have noted, Yin should balance Yang, the lack of Yin can cause interrupted sleep and early wakening since it is not able to stem the surge of Yang energy that is arousing the child.

Following diagnosis of the underlying problem by traditional diagnostic methods, treatment would be directed to rebalancing the disharmony. Patients who are suffering from insomnia are not sedated but are given a herbal remedy specifically formulated to address the presenting symptoms. Just as a hop pillow may be used in the West to induce sleep, so gypsum is used in China. A Chinese doctor might also demonstrate a do-it-yourself acupressure massage (MacNamara 1995). In this country, over-the-counter acupressure kits are available, consisting of a disposable stud called an isocone which is fixed to the acupuncture point Heart 7, situated on the wrist. Research using this acupuncture point was carried out with six healthy subjects (who were then monitored with EEG), using a randomised double blind trial with a placebo acupuncture point. Results showed a decrease in wakefulness and an increase in total sleep time due to an increase in NREM sleep (Buguet et al 1995). It was admitted by the researchers that, classically, there is no single treatment protocol for treating insomnia. However, this research was carried out addressing three possible acupuncture sites: Kidney 6, which soothes the mind and makes it easier to fall asleep, Heart 7, which, again, has a sedative effect and is very good for agitated sleep troubled with nightmares, and for psychological or emotional problems (this should be used in all cases of insomnia); and Master of the Heart 6, which has a sedative effect that soothes the Heart and mind (Shen). The results suggested that Kidney 6 was indicated if failure to fall asleep was the main problem, whilst Master of the Heart 6 was useful against early wakening and Heart 7 against chronic disorders, though the latter might take several months to have an effect. The isocones also worked well on children who presented with a number of sleep-related problems. Treatment would normally be individualised; however, since most children's sleep problems are psychological or emotional, Heart 7 was stimulated in this piece of research.

Two further pieces of research are of interest, although the practitioners used different acupuncture points. The first was a report of 13 cases of night crying in infants who were treated by stimulating the acupuncture points Sifeng (on the finger joints) and Pericardium 7. The effect of stimulating these points is to eliminate Heat and restlessness, regulating the channels and internal organs and their function (Zangfu). In each case, night crying ceased after the third treatment (Liu 1994). The second report involved the treatment of 50 cases of insomnia by stimulation of the points Baihui and Sishenchong, which are situated on top of the head and have the effect of pulling and holding the Qi upwards. Treatment was given daily for 10 days with a 3-day rest period between courses. Twenty of the subjects were cured, i.e. slept for over 6 hours per night; twenty-three had excellent results and slept for over 4 hours; five improved and two showed no improvement. According to Traditional Chinese Medicine, Baihui and Sishenchong calm the mind and clear the head and eyes and, since these points directly regulate cerebral cortex function, they correlate with the Western concept of insomnia (Wang 1992).

The sedative effect of acupuncture in the treatment of insomnia may be related to the fact that acupuncture raises the levels of serotonin. Low levels of serotonin are implicated in severe insomnia where both REM and NREM sleep are affected and which responds to 5-hydroxytryptophan. Mao et al (1980) investigated the effects of high versus low intensity acupuncture in the treatment of pain. Although it was a small study, a biochemical analysis showed clearly that low serotonin levels which were identified at baseline measurement in the experimental group (as opposed to normal serotonin levels in the control group) were raised to normal levels following high intensity acupuncture. Although this investigation was related to pain control, the fact that acupuncture can raise serotonin levels is of importance in the treatment of insomnia.

Remembering that one of the aims of Qigong (mentioned in Chapter 1 and discussed in greater detail in Chapter 8 on mobility) is to calm the mind, the practice of Qigong as an aid to sleep is of value. Mokone (2000) describes a Qigong visualisation technique that children would find very easy to follow, involving the person imagining the flow of water over their body. This can be used to induce relaxation and counter sleeplessness.

Ayurvedic medicine

Ayurvedic medicine lays great emphasis on a healthy daily routine which is linked with the three doshas. From sunrise to about 10 a.m. the environment is believed to contain qualities which are related to the dosha kapha. As the sun and temperature rise between 10 and 2 p.m., pitta predominates, whilst in the later part of the day, from 2 p.m. to 6 p.m., vata predominates. The cycle then starts again with kapha from 6 p.m. until 10 p.m., pitta from 10 p.m. to 2 a.m. and vata again from 2 a.m. until sunrise. It is suggested that if a person rises before sunrise, during the vata period, they will reflect aspects of vata, i.e. alertness and a feeling of lightness and energy; sleeping in until the kapha period results in a feeling of sluggishness and heaviness. This approach fits in beautifully with the sleep cycles described at the beginning of the chapter, with the kapha element (heavy and sluggish) being most conducive to the onset of sleep. The later a person goes to bed, the more difficult it will be for them to fall asleep.

Insomnia is seen as an imbalance of vata, the principle of movement, related to being overactive and displaying too much mental activity. Individuals require different approaches to sleep depending on their dominant dosha, which may vary slightly according to circumstance: kaphas should not sleep during the day since too much sleep increases kapha; vatas need plenty of rest to revitalise the nervous system and should avoid late nights and night shifts; whilst pittas generally sleep soundly and require less sleep than other people. Falling asleep easily but having difficulty in waking up indicates excess kapha, waking up around midnight is due to excess pitta, and difficulty in getting off to sleep, with frequent wakening, is due to excess vata. Rebalancing the doshas would include dietary adjustment. To reduce vata and increase kapha the patient would be encouraged to eat certain foods, such as bananas, avocado, chicken, turkey, beef or pork; these foods coincide with those known in Western medicine to contain the vitamins thiamine (B1) and pyridoxine (B6) and the essential amino acid tryptophan (Dunwell 1995).

According to Ayurvedic medicine, dreams will reflect the dominant dosha and changes in dream types may indicate a dosha imbalance. Vata dreams, as might be expected, are very active, involving chasing, falling etc. Pitta dreams are angry or violent, whilst kapha dreams are slow and gentle, featuring natural surroundings of lakes and mountains (Morrison 1994). It is suggested that children will benefit from a foot massage just before bedtime as this will stimulate the murma points for sound sleep. Other chapters of this book indicate the value of yoga and transcendental meditation as aids to calmness and relaxation, and yoga positions for inducing sound sleep include corpse, cobra and backward bend; in addition, milk or a chamomile drink is also recommended before bedtime.

Aromatherapy

Interest in the use of aromatherapy as a safe, cheap alternative to night sedation has been well documented and, traditionally, lavender oil is the oil of choice. Unfortunately, research on human subjects to date has suffered from a number of methodological flaws which render its results open to question. However, other very tightly designed research on mice does support the traditional use of lavender oil (*Lavandula augustifolia*) (Buchbauer et al 1991). Normal motor activity was identified for all the mice using an electronic sensor. During the time when the mice were at their most active, the experimental group was exposed to a stream of fragrance compounds. During this experimental phase, the mice ceased their normal exploratory and social behaviour and remained inactive and drowsy. These levels of inactivity were measured at 30, 60 and 90 minutes after inhaling the vapours. The activity of the control group remained the same.

Davis (1996) suggests that the therapeutic properties of lavender and chamomile overlap, the choice of oil depending on the situation, and that they can be blended together to treat insomnia. Chamomile essential oil is distilled from the chamomile plant, usually either Roman (*Chamaemelum nobile*) or German (*Matricaria recutita*) chamomile and, as Davis (1996) points out, although the chemical composition of the essential oil varies between different varieties, all the chamomiles are soothing, calming and anti-inflammatory. Chamomile is sometimes referred to as 'the children's oil' and Tisserand and Balacs (1995) confirm its safety.

Badia et al (1990) demonstrated that humans reacted behaviourally, anatomically and in their central nervous systems to olfactory stimuli presented during sleep. From this they concluded that it was possible that oils reported to be relaxing would enhance sleep quality. This was confirmed by Manley (1993) who, in an experiment conducted on a range of essential oils, noted that chamomile (type unspecified) was confirmed to have relaxing properties, and by Torii (1990), whose research identified the relaxing effect of lavender in humans.

Miyake et al (1991), investigating a number of essential oils and their effect on insomnia, noted (using electroencephalograph imaging) that the inhalation of bitter orange or neroli (*Citrus aurantium*) essential oil increased sleeping time significantly. It was thought that the oil affected the cortex, inhibiting excitation of the central nervous system and causing a sedative effect, and decreasing sleep latency. One very interesting study was conducted by Mehta et al (1998) into the effect of the use of the essential oil sweet orange (*Citrus sinensis*) on the induction and recovery characteristics of children undergoing anaesthesia for dental extraction. The control group received anaesthesia in the normal way, whilst the study group had a breathing filter impregnated with four drops of the essential oil placed between the breathing system and the mask. After taking two breaths the children were asked to rate the odour from horrid to pleasant. Afterwards, the children graded the acceptability of the induction. In comparison to the control group, the children in the experimental group were more relaxed and cooperative during induction; 72% of them graded the odour favourably and 82% said they would like to experience a similar induction again, compared with 23% and 55% of the control group.

Herbalism

The herb chamomile, which has a mild sedative effect, has traditionally been given to children to calm them and to help them to sleep. Surprisingly, the German commission E monographs (Blumenthal 1998) do not list this as an application for chamomile, and neither does Culpeper (1653), although he praised it for its healing properties. However, Mann and Staba (1986) noted that German chamomile (*Matricaria recutita*) could induce a deep sleep in subjects when administered prior to cardiac catheterisation. Viola et al (1995) noted that several fractions of aqueous extract of chamomile (*Matricaria recutita*) have demonstrated an affinity for the central benzodiazepine receptors. Of these extracts, apigenin has demonstrated clear anti-anxiety and slight sedation activity after intraperitoneal administration in mice.

Mills (1994) refers to lemon balm (*Melissa officinalis*) as being particularly good for children who suffer from anxiety states and excessive tension. Traditionally, it has been reported as having antispasmodic and sedative properties. Although there are no controlled trials to support this claim, the German commission E monographs (Blumenthal 1998) sanction its use for nervous sleep disorders. One double blind, crossover study of 27 subjects taking hops (*Humulus lupulus*), lemon balm and valerian (*Valeriana officinalis*), however, showed no effect with either the lemon balm or the hops but did report an improvement in sleep patterns with valerian (Lindahl & Lindwall 1989). Valerian is discussed in greater depth in Section 3.

Anthroposophical medicine

In Anthroposophical medicine, Steiner taught that sleep was a withdrawal of the ego and the astral body from the physical/etheric complex, i.e. from the nervous sense system. There are different levels of this withdrawal. Full withdrawal leads to deep, dreamless sleep; partial withdrawal leads to REM sleep; whilst a slight withdrawal results in daydreaming or a feeling of being 'half asleep', the latter being closely associated with insomnia. An Anthroposophical nurse would describe this as an ego/upper astral complex. It is suggested that this is due to the individual's natural rhythm being thrown out of order by the artificial nature of modern life and by being divorced from the natural rhythm of the day and of the seasons of the year, for example in having unlimited access to heat and light and a wide variety of foods. Steiner suggested that it arises from our alienation from the spiritual side of life and our unwillingness to enter the spirit world, part of which is manifested in our dreaming. In some cultures dreaming is considered to be an integral part of life and what a person has dreamed at night influences their activities during the following day.

Steiner advocated meditation exercises to facilitate connection with the spirit world, as well as the use of Anthroposophical medicine. Anthroposophical remedies might include Coffea tosta or Belladonna, or Avena Sativa, a remedy composed of herbal and homeopathic remedies designed especially for sleeplessness, which is a mixture of valerian (*Valeriana officinalis*), passion flower (*Passiflora incarnata*), hops, oats and coffea. Attention would also be addressed to lifestyle patterns for example not eating too late in the day.

Hypnosis

With its emphasis on relaxation and its ability to uncover underlying problems, hypnosis is probably the best therapy for the treatment of sleep problems. Olness and Kohen (1996) discuss how fear of sleep onset presenting at bed time represents childhood anxiety, while insomnia presents as a symptom of a more generalised anxiety. They list a number of case studies (Olness & Kohen 1996) which describe various techniques to deal with night time problems. A very simple hypnotic procedure is the use of prior rehearsal of a suitable bedtime routine under hypnosis. This would include suggestions of calm, relaxation, safety and warmth and would finish with the posthypnotic suggestion 'go to sleep'. Also of value is the 'safe place' technique, in which the subject is encouraged to experience positive feelings of safety, warmth and relaxation and then go to sleep. This can be taught as self-hypnosis, thus giving children a measure of control over their problem. Hypnosis is a valuable tool for the control of nightmares, night time terrors and sleep terror disorder. Children who suffer from these conditions are caught between deep (slow wave) sleep and full arousal. Core elements of these conditions include:

- A high arousal threshold
- Unresponsiveness to the environment
- Mental confusion.

The conditions may manifest themselves in a variety of ways but all will include quiet sleep walking, confusional arousal, and sleep terrors or night terrors. Hypnosis can be used with a dream-alerting method for nightmares, but because children do not remember night terrors, this method is not useful for that particular problem.

Hypnosis is of value in the identification of precipitating factors, which can then be addressed and, if possible, put aside using a range of closure techniques suitable for children, such as turning off an imaginary video. Other interventions might include suggestions to reduce the level of arousal and reduce awareness of outside sounds and sensations, together with suggestions of a restful night's sleep (Koe 1989). Howsam (1999) offers an excellent case study concerning an 11-year-old boy who suffered from insomnia, nightmares, night terrors and fear of the dark. This distressing collection of symptoms was the result of separation anxiety following hospitalisation after an accident, and the situation had not been helped by his seeing a film in which the villain attacked his victims via their dreams. Howsam's intervention included the use of imagery, using the cartoon character Bart Simpson (one of the boy's favourite characters) who would intervene and make his dreams safe. Together they searched for the one person who would scare the villain. This was followed by a rehearsal of scary dreams, with the villain being vanquished. Treatment concluded with ego strengthening, stressing confidence, and posthypnotic suggestions of safety and normal sleep. At a follow-up session 2 weeks later the boy had had only one nightmare, and at a subsequent session 4 weeks later he reported no further nightmares or night terror attacks, and was experiencing no sleeping problems.

Other techniques are described by Levine (1980), who shows how fairy stories may be individualised for each child, and Porter (1975), who describes the use of guided fantasy in treating the sleep problems of an 8-year-old girl. The value of hypnosis in treating childhood sleeping disorders lies in its concordance with relaxation and sleep, the flexibility of the interventions in enabling the therapist to address the specific problems the child presents with, the way in which it can accommodate parental input, and the child's ability to gain mastery of the problem with self-hypnosis.

REFERENCES

Badia P, Wesensten N, Lammers W et al 1990 Responsiveness to olfactory stimuli presented in sleep. Physiology and Behaviour 48(1): 87–90

Blumenthal M (ed) 1998 The complete German commission E monographs therapeutic guide to herbal medicines. American Botanical Council, Austin, Texas

Buchbauer G, Jirovetz L, Jager W 1991 Aromatherapy: evidence for sedative effects of the essential oil of lavender after inhalation. Zeitschrift der Naturforschung 4(c): 1067–1072

Buguet A, Sartre M, LeKerneau J 1995 Continuous nocturnal auto massage of an acupuncture point modifies sleep in healthy subjects. Neurophysiologie Critique 25(2): 78–83

Culpeper N 1653 Complete herbal: a book of natural remedies for ancient ills (Wordsworth edn 1995). Wordsworth Editions, Hertfordshire

Davis P 1996 Aromatherapy: an A–Z. CW Daniel, Saffron Walden

Dunwell F 1995 Insomnia and mental health. Nursing Times 91(37): 31–32

Errante J 1985 Sleep deprivation or post partum blues? Topics in Clinical Nursing 6: 9–18

Howsam D 1999 Hypnosis in the treatment of insomnia, nightmares and night terrors. Australian Journal of Clinical and Experimental Hypnosis 27(1): 32–39

Kerr S 1997 Sleep problems in babies and young children. Primary Health Care 7(4) (research supplement)

Kerr S, Jowett S 1994 Sleep problems in pre school children: a review of the literature. Child: Care, Health and Development 20: 379–391

Koe G 1989 Hypnotic treatment of sleep terror disorder: a case report. American Journal of Clinical Hypnosis 32(1): 36–40

Levine E 1980 Indirect suggestions through personalised fairy tales for treatment of childhood insomnia. The American Journal of Clinical Hypnosis 23(1): 57–63

Lindahl O, Lindwall L 1989 Double blind study of a valerian preparation. Pharmacology, Biochemistry and Behaviour 32: 1065–1066

Liu B 1994 Night crying in infants treated by acupuncture. Journal of Chinese Medicine 46: 38

MacNamara S 1995 Traditional Chinese Medicine. Hamish Hamilton, London

Manley C 1993 Psychophysiological effect of odor. Critical Reviews in Food Science and Nutrition 33(1): 57–62

Mann C, Staba E 1986 The chemistry, pharmacology and commercial formulations of chamomile. In: Mann C, Staba E (eds) Herbs, spices and medicinal plants: recent advances in botany, horticulture and pharmacology, vol 1. Oryx Press, Arizona

Mao W, Ghia J, Scott D et al 1980 High versus low intensity acupuncture analgesia for treatment of chronic pain: effects on platelet serotonin. Pain 8: 331–342

Mehta S, Stone D, Whitehead H 1998 Use of essential oil to promote induction of anaesthesia in children. Anaesthesia 53(7): 711

Mills S 1994 A complete guide to modern herbalism. Thorsons, London

Mindell JA, Owens J, Carskadon MA 1999 Developmental features of sleep. Child and Adolescent Psychiatric Clinics of North America 8(4): 695–725

Miyake Y, Nakagawa M, Asakura Y 1991 Effects of odors on humans (1). Effects on sleep latency. Chemical Senses 16(2): 183

Mokone S 2000 Qigong and t'ai chi in physical therapy. In: Charman R (ed) Complementary therapies for physical therapists. Butterworth-Heinemann, Oxford

Morrison J 1994 The book of ayurveda: a guide to personal well being. Gaia Books, London

Olness K, Kohen D 1996 Hypnosis and hypnotherapy with children. Guildford Press, London

Porter J 1975 Guided fantasy as a treatment for childhood insomnia. Australian and New Zealand Journal of Psychiatry 9: 169–172

Tisserand R, Balacs T 1995 Essential oil safety: a guide for health care professionals. Churchill Livingstone, Edinburgh

Torii S 1990 Effect of odor on contingent negative variation (CNV). In: Indo M (ed) The psychophysiological effects of odor, aromachology. Koryo, Japan

Viola H, Wasowski C, Levi de Stein M 1995 Apigenin, a component of Matricaria recutita flowers is a central benzodiazepine receptors ligand with anxiolytic effects. Planta Medica 62: 60–61

Wang Y 1992 An observation on the therapeutic effect of acupuncture in treating 50 cases of insomnia. International Journal of Clinical Acupuncture 3(1): 91–93

<table>
<tr><td>

5

</td><td>

Problems related to pain

</td></tr>
</table>

CHAPTER CONTENTS

- **Introduction** 79
- **Therapeutic interventions** 80
  Massage 80
  Hypnosis 81
  TCM 82
  Ayurvedic medicine 83
  Homeopathy 84
  Anthroposophical medicine 84
  Aromatherapy 85
  Music therapy 85
- **Headache and migraine** 85
  Symptoms and aetiology 86

  Herbalism 86
  Homeopathy 87
  TCM 88
  Anthroposophical medicine 89
  Ayurvedic medicine 89
  Massage 90
  Aromatherapy 90
  Hypnosis 90
  Reflexology 91
- **Conclusion** 91
- **References** 91

INTRODUCTION

One of the main causes of insomnia is pain, which is defined as an 'unpleasant sensory and emotional experience, associated with actual or potential tissue damage or expressed in terms of such damage' (International Association for the Study of Pain 1979). There are four types of pain:

- Nociceptive pain
- Neuropathic pain
- Sympathetically mediated pain
- Psychogenic pain.

In chronic pain disorders there may be some overlap between these four types.

Unrelieved pain is known to interrupt sleep in adults and it is suggested that this also occurs in children. Lack of sleep may lead to increased pain perception (Pfeil 1993). In her review of pain, Gillies (1995) acknowledges the complexity of pain and notes that, in children, the fear and anxiety that accompany medical procedures make the experience of pain worse. Perception of pain will also be affected by whether it is acute or chronic. Gauvain-Piquard et al (1987) identified that acute pain tended to be accompanied by anxiety and chronic pain by depression. Gillies (1995) also highlights the fact that a number of studies (e.g. Eland 1990) have noted that children do not receive a comparable level of analgesia to adults.

Until quite recently, it was assumed that babies' and young children's neurological systems were not sufficiently developed for them to feel pain. This and a number of other myths surrounding children and pain are challenged and disproved in

Whaley and Wong (Wong 1993). In their review of the literature, Duff et al (1999) noted that children described pain as the most distressing part of their illness, particularly when undergoing painful procedures. Furthermore, the authors noted that if children claimed to be pain free they were believed, but if they said they were in pain it was either ignored or disbelieved. In her paper describing the team approach to chronic pain control at the Royal Hospital for Sick Children in Glasgow, Aitkenhead (2001) lists a number of common problems associated with nursing and caring for a child in chronic pain including:

- Disruption of family life
- Disorder of family dynamics
- Depression and anxiety
- Mistrust of health professionals.

To address these problems, guidelines such as the clinical practice guideline for the *Recognition and Assessment of Acute Pain in Children* (RCN 1999) have been developed. The aim of the guideline is to improve the recognition and assessment of pain in children, and the objectives are to:

- Identify methods by which pain can be recognised in children
- Identify reliable and valid measures for assessing pain in children of different age groups and levels of development.

Children identified procedures such as lumbar punctures, dressing changes, bone marrow aspirations, venepuncture and injections as being painful and very stressful.

As Mairs (1995) points out, the quality and quantity of a person's experience of pain is the result of a variety of factors, which include the underlying cause of the pain, the patient's cultural background and the attitude of that culture to pain. In addition to the patient's previous experience of pain, other factors include their physical and emotional wellbeing, including physical tiredness, any actual illnesses from which they may be suffering, and the context in which the pain is experienced. Olness and Kohen (1996) note that children vary far more greatly in their ability to tolerate pain than do adults. A number of theories of pain have been put forward and for a review of these see Jackson (1995).

THERAPEUTIC INTERVENTIONS

A range of therapies have been identified as being beneficial, having either a direct or indirect effect on pain. These interventions are reviewed here and, where indicated, their use will be generalised to a range of painful conditions.

Massage

Massage is the most obvious and instinctive of these therapeutic interventions. In their review of the effects of massage Watson and Watson (1997) highlight a number of studies into the use of massage as pain relief, but confess that there is little agreement as to the mechanism involved. It is thought that endorphin levels (the body's natural analgesia) rise following massage (Nelson et al 1986).

According to Sunshine et al (1996), somatostatin is released, during deep sleep, inhibiting pain perception, whereas patients who are sleep deprived produce increased levels of substance P (a pain transmitter). This leads Field (1998, 2000) to suggest that since massage increases deep sleep, less of the neuropeptide substance P is produced. Another theory as to how massage relieves pain indicates raised serotonin levels after massage therapy and, since serotonergic drugs do relieve pain, it would seem possible that the body's own serotonin levels would have some beneficial effect. The relevance of massage to the gate theory of pain (Melzack & Wall 1965) is suggested by Malkin (1994), who proposes that massage stimulates the larger diameter beta nerve fibres and consequently can block pain, and by Miller (1990), who suggests that massage may close the gate peripherally by the stimulation of these fibres. In Section 3 the use of massage in alleviating anxiety and depression in adolescents will be examined, both of these emotions being concomitant with pain, particularly chronic pain. Field (2000) has reviewed the evidence for the effectiveness of massage in relieving pain in a number of clinical situations, all of which are also beneficial for children.

Hypnosis

Modern theories of pain and our increasing insight into the nature of pain indicate that psychological factors are extremely important in pain perception, suggesting that hypnotic interventions, when used properly, can modify the client's perception of pain in more than one of its components (Gibson & Heap 1991). In fact, Heap and Aravind (2002) suggest that the treatment of pain is one of the success stories of hypnosis, whether it is used as an intervention for immediate pain relief following injury, during painful medical procedures or for more long-term relief of chronic pain. The greatest contribution to the alleviation of pain made by hypnosis is in the treatment of anxiety. Heap and Dryden (1993) point out that it is not just the induction of very deep relaxation which influences pain perception and is instrumental in pain relief (although clearly this reduces tension), but the fact that hypnosis can help clients to manage their anxiety in a variety of very positive ways. Barber (1986) makes a bold statement about hypnosis, stating that '…no other psychological technique is as efficacious in creating comfort out of discomfort with none of the adverse side effects associated with medical treatment of equal efficacy'. Barber goes on to suggest that altering the perception of pain is the most important weapon in dealing with it and further suggests that it is a shift in consciousness which allows this to happen. Since the link between anxiety and pain is well established, any mechanism which reduces anxiety will help to reduce the pain.

How can hypnosis be applied?

Chaves (2002) lists a number of interventions which could be adapted to suit children of different ages for either acute or chronic pain, including:

- Numbness, i.e. suggesting that a painful part of the body is numb and insensitive (glove anaesthesia)
- Distraction, i.e. deflecting the patient's attention away from the pain, either to a special place or special activities, or simply by reading a story or engaging in a discussion with the patient

- Transfer, i.e. transferring the pain to another part of the body where it can be better tolerated
- Direct suggestion to reduce the pain
- Time distortion (useful if doing a dressing), emphasising pain-free periods, thereby making them appear longer than they are and making periods of pain seem much shorter in length
- Imagery, e.g. dimmer switch to turn the pain down, or thermal imagery, possibly using colours to reduce its intensity.

Heap and Aravind (2002) have suggested a range of imagery based on the gate control theory, including a telephone switchboard in which the switchboard operator (the child) switches off the pain messages to the brain.

Olness and Kohen (1996) note that the positive side effects of using hypnosis as pain relief for children include:

- Reduction in anxiety
- Enhancement of mastery and hope
- Increased cooperation
- Reduction of anxiety for the family and healthcare professionals.

Ewin (1999), a professor of surgery and psychiatry who has written about the use of hypnosis in the emergency department, has noted that patients coming into the department are in a trance-like state, ignoring their surroundings and focusing on their injury. Many patients recall feelings of dissociation following trauma, i.e. 'this cannot be happening to me', which should make them very receptive to hypnotic interventions to reduce pain and to enhance immediate healing. In his work with burns patients in particular, Ewin has reported pain reduction and better healing outcomes as a result of using hypnosis as early as possible after the traumatic event. In fact, he suggests that positive comments concerning pain and healing should be started by paramedics as they transport the patient to the emergency room (Ewin 1986).

TCM

In TCM pain may be classified as either stagnant Blood or stagnant Qi. Common causative factors of pain in TCM include:

- Stagnation of Liver-Qi leading to restriction and tension
- Stagnation of Blood leading to sharp stabbing pains
- Accumulation of Cold
- Accumulation of Heat
- Retention of Phlegm.

In TCM, pain is the result of either excess or deficiencies in the circulation of Blood and/or Qi. Excess is associated with stagnation of Blood or Qi. Pain may also result from deficiencies resulting in insufficient nourishment of Qi, Blood or of the organs and tissues in general.

The aim of treatment is to rebalance excess and deficiencies by the use of acupuncture or herbs and to address the underlying cause (Bensoussan 1991). The use of acupuncture for pain relief has been well supported by a number of studies, although the exact mechanism is still open to debate. The general consensus of opinion is that acupuncture results in the release of opioid-like endorphins and related neurohormones, which inhibit or modify the transmission of the pain signals at the cord, brainstem or cortical levels (Pearce 2000). Evidence to support this theory is the observation that opiate antagonists, such as naloxone, block acupuncture analgesia (Cheng & Pomeranz 1980). Over 20 neurotransmitters have been associated with this response to acupuncture, specifically serotonin (5HT), dopamine, noradrenaline and somatostatin. Serotonin levels are raised following acupuncture activity (Mao et al 1980). It was noted earlier that substance P is modified by somatostatin.

Sims (1997) has reviewed the mechanism of acupuncture analgesia noting the equivocal evidence, which is due in part to poor research methodology, and some of these issues have been highlighted in Chapter 2, specifically the adherence to the false premise of sham and placebo acupuncture. Sims (1997) concludes by suggesting that whilst acupuncture needling needs to be specific for therapeutic interventions, it would appear that this level of accuracy is less critical for acupuncture analgesia. This has been highlighted by Bensoussan (1991), who states that Western research into the use of acupuncture and pain does not do justice to TCM. Wilson (1997) points out that a number of studies indicate that acupuncture does not necessarily induce complete analgesia, some researchers suggesting it to be mild and comparable with the administration of 33% nitrous oxide, and that in addition, cultural background and patient preparation play a part in attaining clinically useful levels of analgesia.

However, as Ernst and White (1999) highlight, experimentally induced analgesia in the laboratory usually involves a one-off treatment and it has been demonstrated that the analgesic effects of acupuncture are accumulative. Dyrehag et al (1997) found that the first session of acupuncture increased sympathetic activity, whilst after a number of sessions this sympathetic activity was decreased. This effect has also been noted in animal studies (Han 1997). In addition, Ernst and White (1999), quoting Price et al (1984), noted that some patients experienced a delay in analgesia onset of between 1 and 12 hours, with the effect being prolonged for 10–14 days. They support the concept that the human response to acupuncture is variable, in accordance with Mairs (1995).

Ayurvedic medicine

In Ayurvedic medicine, vata is involved in all pain. If the flow of the vata dosha is unobstructed, there is no pain. Pain is classified according to the factors which obstruct the flow of vata, for example:

- Pain due to excess vata would be described as radiating, shooting, fluctuating or pulsating and would be made worse by cold and be associated with fear, anxiety and insecurity; the pain interferes with sleep.

- Pain due to excess pitta obstructing vata would be described as acute, burning, sharp, cutting, penetrating, intense or violent and may be accompanied by inflammation, raised temperature, nausea and vomiting; again, it interferes with sleep.

- Pain due to excess kapha obstructing vata would be described as heavy, dull, aching, throbbing or mild and is usually long standing chronic pain; it may not interfere with sleep.

Ayurvedic medicine acknowledges the role of the emotions in the disturbance of the doshas, which can be the root cause of the pain. In general, vata constituted people have more painful types of illnesses. Treatment would be aimed at rebalancing the doshas using yoga, diet and herbs.

Homeopathy

Just as pain presents itself in a variety of ways, so a variety of homeopathic remedies are selected to match the presenting painful symptoms. The examples described here have been chosen as being the most relevant to paediatric care and are those which nurses may find their patients using. For a burning, stinging pain with inflammation and swelling (the sort of pain which results from immunisations), Apis (*Apis mellifica*) is prescribed. Apis is made from the whole of the bee. For throbbing or shooting pains which start and end suddenly and are made worse by light, movement and pressure, Belladonna is indicated. Belladonna is made from the plant deadly nightshade (*Atropa belladonna*) and was traditionally used in witchcraft and magic during the Middle Ages, possibly because of its hallucinogenic properties. It was first proved by Hahnemann in 1799 to treat scarlet fever. Poisoning from deadly nightshade results in giddiness, sweating, confusion, dry mouth and throat with flushed face and throbbing headache and it is the pain presenting with these symptoms for which Belladonna is prescribed.

For shooting nerve pain following injury to a part of the body which is well supplied with nerves, i.e. finger tips, nail beds, spine, eyes etc., or for head injuries, puncture or crush wounds, Hypericum (*Hypericum perforatum*) is indicated. Hypericum, which is also known as St John's wort, is further discussed in Section 3 for its antidepressant role with adolescents, and in Chapter 9 for its healing powers. In making the homeopathic remedy, the whole fresh plant in flower is used. In addition, Aconite is always valuable in treating the shock and fright following injury or accident and will help to ease the pain. The Bach flower remedies might also be used to address underlying emotions related to the pain.

Anthroposophical medicine

In Anthroposophical medicine, pain is related to increased activity of the astral body, which corresponds with the old categorisation by Celsius of dolor (pain). Pain is an integral part of inflammation, which in turn is a vital part of the healing process. Whether it is due to illness or trauma, inflammation is described in anthroposophical medicine as activity of the:

- Ego (calor/heat)
- Ego–astral body (dolor/pain)
- Ego–astral–etheric body (tumor/swelling)
- Ego–astral–etheric body–physical body (rubor/redness)

Inflammation is, therefore, the manifestation of the four main elements and in inflammation the action of the ego is intensified, acting through the other three elements. The treatment of inflammation in Anthroposophical medicine is the homeopathic use of Apis and Belladonna, described above. The use of Apis to treat inflammation is indicated from the homeopathic point of view since a bee sting matches the presenting symptoms of inflammation, i.e. heat, pain, redness and swelling.

Aromatherapy

Anecdotal evidence suggests that certain essential oils, particularly lavender and chamomile, have topical analgesic effects. Dale and Cornwell's (1994) well-designed clinical trial supported the role of lavender in reducing postnatal perineal pain. Although the role of lavender as a healing agent was not supported, mothers in the experimental group did report less discomfort between the third and fifth postnatal days. Ghelardini et al (1999) demonstrated the local anaesthetic effect of lavender essential oil (*Lavandula augustifolia*) in an animal experiment, comparing it with two citrus oils using a reflex test. The lavender oil demonstrated a dose dependent anaesthetic activity. In addition, given the proven relaxant effects of both lavender and chamomile essential oils on anxiety and stress identified earlier, they would appear to have a contributory role in pain control.

Music therapy

Music has long been valued for its therapeutic effects and a survey of music therapists' use of music for pain control indicated that 95% used the music to induce relaxation, 91% used it for distraction and 75% used it as a mood altering modality (Michel and Chesky 1995). Krout (2001) describes the process and results of music therapy in a clinical effectiveness study on the use of music with hospice patients. The purpose of the study was to indicate the effectiveness of a single session intervention on patients' pain control, physical comfort and relaxation. Over a 3-month period, a total of 80 patients were included in the study and results indicated that even one session of therapy resulted in increased pain control, relaxation and physical comfort, as determined by both patient report and independent observation. Good et al (2000) noted that there were marked cultural differences in music chosen by patients for pain relief and suggested that culturally appropriate music should be selected if therapy is to be used.

HEADACHE AND MIGRAINE

One demonstration of the use of CAM interventions in pain control is in the area of headaches and migraine. These are a serious problem in childhood, owing to their debilitating nature and the frequency with which they are reported, and they can have a profound effect on the child's schoolwork and ability to take part in social activities (Collin et al 1985, Carlsson et al 1996). Migraine and tension headaches are the two most common types of headache reported in childhood (Williamson et al 1993). Data from research conducted in Sweden showed that by the age of 7 years, 40% of children had suffered from headaches, with true migraine occurring in 4% of the sample (n = 9000) and with 54% reporting tension headaches (Bille 1962).

Symptoms and aetiology

Childhood migraine symptoms mimic many of the symptoms found in adults, but childhood migraine appears to occur more frequently and is of shorter duration. Accompanying symptoms of gastrointestinal upset, diarrhoea, increased urination, sweating and thirst are present, although visual auras may not be as common in children as in adults. Although the exact cause of migraine is uncertain, a number of factors have been identified which may contribute to its development and these differ depending on the type of headache experienced (Williamson et al 1993). Contributing factors may include noise, lights, too little or too much sleep, over-use of computers, stress and anxiety or food triggers (Budd & Kedesdy 1989, King & Sharpley 1990). Of particular importance amongst the latter are foods containing monosodium glutamate or tyramine which are found in preserved foods such as beans, bacon, sausages, Spam, ham, hot dogs and pork pies.

A migraine classically develops in two stages, with intra- and extra-cranial vasoconstriction in the first stage and intra- and extra-cranial vasodilation during the acute headache stage. Tension headaches, however, follow the sustained contraction of the head, neck and facial muscles, although a number of hypotheses have been generated around the role of muscular activity in tension headaches (Martin 1993):

- The headache is the result of muscle tension.
- The headache is the result of excessive tension levels related to stress.
- The headache is the result of slow reduction of tension levels following stress.
- Headache sufferers have a low pain threshold from muscular tension pain.

Williamson et al (1993) have noted that a child's coping style has a significant effect on the reported pain and disability: the more passive the coping style the greater the reported pain. This is understandable, since unpredictability is in the nature of headaches, making them difficult to control, and this can seriously reduce the child's sense of self-control. As noted in Chapter 1, the philosophy behind CAM encourages the development of autonomy and self-help skills in the individual, and a number of CAM therapies can be used in a prophylactic way, helping to prevent or ameliorate headaches and migraine.

Herbalism

Addressing both the symptoms and the aetiology of the headache, the herbalist will take into account not only the presenting symptoms of the headache, but also the underlying and background issues relevant to the child's lifestyle, and will utilise the eliminative remedies as well as the muscle relaxants and sedatives.

Feverfew (*Tanacetum parthenium*) has been used as a migraine treatment since Roman times and Culpeper (1653) states that it is 'very effective for all parts of the head'. Feverfew has been noted to have an inhibiting effect on platelet aggregation, which has been associated with the aetiology of migraine. Its traditional use has been confirmed by a number of clinical trials. In a trial with 17 patients, 8 received two capsules per day of dried feverfew while 9 received a placebo. Prior to taking part in the trial, these patients had all been self-medicating with feverfew and had noted a significant reduction in the number of migraines. During the trial, the placebo group reported a significant increase in the frequency and severity of their headaches (Johnson et al 1985). However, the results of this trial have been challenged and it has been suggested that the placebo group were suffering from feverfew withdrawal symptoms, which has been identified as a specific syndrome.

A further randomised, double blind placebo controlled clinical trial showed a similarly impressive outcome when treatment with feverfew resulted in a 24% reduction in mean number of attacks and a significant reduction in the amount of vomiting during each assessment period (Murphy 1988). However, as Barnes et al (2002) point out, patients during the crossover period did not appear to suffer from feverfew syndrome. It would seem that for the best results, feverfew should be taken for at least 6 months; clinical trials lasting less than 6 months have failed to demonstrate a reduction in migraine (DeWeerdt et al 1996).

Surprisingly, a systematic review of clinical trials of feverfew before 1998 failed to find sufficient evidence to support its use as a migraine prophylactic (Volger et al 1998). In fact, feverfew is not cited in the German commission E monographs (Blumenthal 1998) for use as a migraine treatment or prophylactic. Mills (1993, 1994) offers an explanation for this discrepancy. He acknowledges that treatment is always complex and, following traditional herbalism, divides migraine into hot and cold presentations. Hot migraines, where there is no vasodilation, are more likely to respond to relaxants and sedative remedies, whilst cold presentations would benefit from circulatory stimulants and peripheral vasodilators such as feverfew. Fetrow and Avila (2001) conclude that for those for whom conventional treatment has failed, feverfew may offer a useful migraine prophylactic. In addition to feverfew, any herbs that reduce anxiety and tension, such as chamomile and lemon balm, would be a useful adjunct for headache and migraine prophylaxis.

Homeopathy

The idiosyncrasies of headache and migraine are well reflected in their homeopathic treatments:

- For headaches starting with emotional stress, which are worse for light or movement, with a hot, dry head, flushed red face, and pulsating pain which is better for firm pressure, the headache often starting in the afternoon and continuing throughout the night, Belladonna (*Atropa belladonna*) is indicated.
- For headaches which are precipitated by exposure to severe heat or cold or following an emotional crisis, with the patient becoming restless with the pain and with a feeling of congestion in the face and head, with severe throbbing, bursting or tearing pains, often made worse by noise, movement, light or heat, Aconite is the remedy of choice.
- For headaches which start during the night where the patient is only aware of them in the morning, which present as a dull deep aching in the forehead spreading through the head to the back, with pain behind the eyes and pain on using the eyes, the patient tending to feel chilly and irritable, and feeling better for lying still and cold applications, Bryonia (*Bryonia alba*) is suggested (Gemmell 1997). Bryonia was used by the Greeks and Romans for the treatment of epilepsy, vertigo, hysteria and paralysis. The homeopathic remedy was

proved in 1834 and its main therapeutic use is for ailments which build up gradually but are painful for the slightest movement (Lockie & Geddes 1996).

Specifically for migraine, Lockie (1990) suggests:

- For those migraines which start with blurred vision, right-sided pain and a tight feeling in the scalp, better for movement but accompanied by vomiting, Iris (*Iris versicolor*) is recommended.
- For migraines which are worse on the right side, when trying to concentrate makes the pain worse and with a feeling of dizziness, Lycopodium (*Lycopodium clavatum*) is indicated. Lycopodium is specific for right-sided complaints and for digestive disorders. It is made from the pollen dust of the herb *Lycopodium clavatum*, which the Arab physicians used for stomach disorders and kidney stones.
- For migraines which start at the back of the head and later shift to settle over one eye, made worse by cold and made better for local warmth, Silicea (*Silicea terra*) is indicated.

There are a number of other presentations for migraine within the homeopathic repertory.

TCM

TCM recognises a number of headaches although, traditionally, they are not subdivided into categories such as migraine versus any other type of headache, but are seen as secondary to an underlying medical condition. As in Western herbalism, the TCM practitioner recognises the role of other systems in the treatment of headache. Loo (2002) has proposed an integrated approach using conventional medicine and TCM and has classified children's headaches into two groups: acute, due to external causes; and chronic, due to internal factors.

Acute/external causes include:

- Wind/Cold viral syndrome
- Wind/Heat bacterial infection
- Wind/Damp
- Blood stasis head trauma.

Chronic/internal headaches are caused by internal organ imbalance, e.g. Liver-Yang rising, and may be due to poor lifestyle, poor or badly balanced diet, emotional stress or a constitutional vulnerability. Loo classifies these headaches depending on where they are located in the head:

- Tai Yang, occipital headache
- Shao Yang, lateral side of head, migraines
- Yang Ming, forehead
- Shao Yin, inside the brain
- Tai Yin, heavy and tight sensation
- Jue Yin, vertex.

Chronic recurrent headaches are usually caused by impaired Qi and Blood flow to the internal organs. This can be the result of excess stress or emotional upheaval. Herbal treatment would involve individual recipes for each syndrome, but central to the treatment of most headaches is the use of angelica (*Angelica dahurica*), peony (*Paeonia lactiflora*), chrysanthemum (*Chrysanthemum morifolium*), which is related to feverfew, and corydalis (*Corydalis yanhusuo*), as well as wild ginger (*Asarum sieboldii heteropoides*) and Chinese date. Ginger root (*Zingiber officinale*), used in Chinese and Indian medicine and recorded in Greek, Roman and Arabic medical literature, is used as an anti-emetic, stimulant, anti-inflammatory and anti-platelet. Mills and Bone (2000) extrapolate from this that it would be effective for migraine headaches.

Research into the use of acupuncture for migraine relief and prophylaxis has been reviewed by Baldry (1998). The mechanism resulting in this effect is unclear but Baldry observes that migraine patients have tender points on the muscles of the neck and scalp. Loh et al (1984), whilst comparing acupuncture with drug therapy, noted that in 34 out of 41 cases, patients exhibited these tender points. He also noted that it was only these patients who responded positively to the use of prophylactic acupuncture. Baldry (1998) goes on to suggest that one of the reasons patients may suffer from migraine is the build-up of nociceptor activity at tender points in the neck muscles. This hypothesis gains some credence with the observation that excessive needling at these points can result in an attack of migraine.

Anthroposophical medicine

In Anthroposophical medicine, migraine is seen as diminished activity of the astral body and ego at the upper pole. This can often be due to emotional conflicts, overwork and sensory overload. The specific remedy for migraine is Bidor which is an amalgamation of iron sulphate (ferrous sulphate) and quartz (silica). This is prescribed for the prevention and treatment of migraine and tension headache. The action of Bidor is to harmonise the imbalance of the nervous and metabolic systems that is the cause of the headache, rather than to have an analgesic effect (Evans & Rodger 2000).

Ayurvedic medicine

Headache in Ayurvedic medicine is seen as the result of the suppression of natural urges such as urination and defecation, inadequate sleep and exposure to cold or inhalation of smoke. An imbalance of any of the doshas can cause a headache although vata is the first to go out of balance. Vata type headache is caused by insomnia, cold, trauma, vomiting, sadness and fear. It presents as a frontal headache with burning between the eyebrows, dizziness and neck stiffness. Pitta headache is caused by expressing, withholding or feeling anger, or by excessive exposure to sun and heat. Kapha headache is comparable to a catarrhal headache and presents as a feeling of heaviness, malaise and tiredness, with loss of appetite. General treatment would include attention to diet, with a dosha balancing diet, breathing exercises (pranayama), meditation and yoga, specifically the cobra, fish, spinal twist and shoulder stand positions. Herbal remedies would include the triphala and the aforementioned ginger, for both the pain and the nausea. Other herbs would be dispensed as necessary to address specific headache syndromes.

Massage

Because massage has been shown to reduce stress and anxiety and to deepen and improve sleep, all of which contribute to pain relief, it is argued that it will have a significant effect on migraine headaches. Field (2000) reports one study involving a massage group and a control group. The first group had a 30-minute neck and base of skull massage twice a week for 5 weeks, while the control group continued with their normal medication regime. Measurements were taken pre-and post-session and in the first and last sessions. The massage group showed a decrease in pain intensity, lower stress hormone levels, fewer somatic symptoms and a lower anxiety score, as well as more headache-free days, with an overall reduction in analgesics. The massage group also had an increase in serotonin levels over the course of the study. Silberstein (1992) has proposed that migraine pain is influenced by serotonin neurotransmission and many medications for migraine increase serotonin levels, albeit with some side effects.

Aromatherapy

Davis (1996) suggests the use of peppermint (*Mentha piperata*) and lavender (*Lavandula augustifolia*) either separately or in combination for headaches, although she points out that once a migraine has started many people are unable to tolerate the smell of essential oils. She suggests that using these oils in cool compresses would be effective or, to encourage vasodilation, warm packs with marjoram essential oil (*Origanum majorana*), known for its warming action, could be used. A study by Gobel et al (1995) has demonstrated the spasmolytic effect of peppermint and eucalyptus oils (the botanical sources were not given) on 32 healthy volunteers. A significant analgesic effect was obtained with the use of peppermint alone following the induction of pain using pressure, thermal and ischaemic modalities. Although the use of eucalyptus and peppermint in combination had little effect on pain sensitivity, they did have a mental and muscle relaxing effect, which led to increased cognitive performance. Measurements were made using electromyographic activity. Exteroceptor suppression periods of temporal muscle were measured, and also mood states. The superior spasmolytic effect of peppermint versus rosemary and sage had already been demonstrated by Taddei et al (1988). The anti-spasmodic effect of lavender oil has been demonstrated by Lis-Balchin and Hart (1999).

Hypnosis

Of particular value in the prophylaxis of migraine headaches is the use of self-hypnosis. Olness and Kohen (1996) cite a number of studies indicating that children can benefit substantially from training in self-hypnosis. Although these studies were uncontrolled, Olness and Kohen's own study compared placebo, propanolol and hypnosis. The study was undertaken on children aged between 6 and 12 years, who had been diagnosed as suffering from classical migraine and who had had no previous treatment. Twenty-eight children were randomised into either the mediation or the placebo group and studied over a 3-month period. They then crossed over to the other study group for a further 3 months. Following this 6-month period, each child was taught self-hypnosis and this training was reinforced during five visits over a further 3-month period. Statistical analysis showed a significant association between decrease in headaches and the self-hypnosis training. Mean results were 13.3 headaches during the placebo period compared with 14.9 during the propanalol period and 5.8 during the self-hypnosis period, although the severity of the headaches was not affected. Olness and Kohen (1996) recommend that training in self-hypnosis is undertaken as soon as the child has been diagnosed with migraine and they have found that training requires three to four visits, with twice daily practice by the child, which later can be reduced to once a day. Although not addressed in this study, hypnosis can also be used to treat other underlying problems such as shyness or lack of confidence, which predispose to stressful situations that may precipitate a migraine attack.

Reflexology

In a recent study by Launso et al (1999) a total of 220 patients were seen by 78 reflexologists drawn from five alternative therapist organisations over a period of 6 months. The study was an exploratory prospective investigation using random sampling techniques. Although the approach of the therapists may have varied, at 3-month follow-up, 81% of the patients reported that they had been helped by the treatment or were cured of their headaches. Of those who had formerly taken drugs to control their headaches, 19% were able to stop medication.

CONCLUSION

The quest for pain relief is as old as time and through the ages many interventions have been used. It is one of the biggest challenges for nurses, who may often find that conventional medication is simply not enough to give children the relief they need. A combination of conventional treatment and some of these CAM techniques may provide a more effective intervention.

REFERENCES

Aitkenhead S 2001 Managing chronic pain in children. Nursing Times 97(29): 34–35

Baldry P 1998 Trigger point acupuncture. In: Filshie J, White A (eds) Medical acupuncture: a western scientific approach. Churchill Livingstone, Edinburgh

Barber J 1986 Hypnotic analgesia. In: Holzman A, Turk D (eds) A handbook of psychological treatment approaches. Academic Press, New York

Barnes J, Anderson L, Phillipson J 2002 Herbal medicines: a guide for health care professionals, 2nd edn. Pharmaceutical Press, London

Bensoussan A 1991 The vital meridian. Churchill Livingstone, Edinburgh

Bille B 1962 Migraine in school children. Acta Paediatrica Scandinavica 51 (suppl 136): 1–151

Blumenthal M (ed) 1998 The complete German commission E monographs therapeutic guide to herbal medicines. American Botanical Council, Austin, Texas

Budd K, Kedesdy J 1989 Investigation of environmental factors in pediatric headaches. Headache 29: 569–573

Carlsson J, Larsson B, Marks A 1996 Psychosocial functioning in school children with recurrent headaches. Headache 36: 77–82

Chaves J 2002 Hypnosis in pain management. In: Rhue J, Lynn S, Kirsch I (eds) Handbook of clinical hypnosis. American Psychological Association, Washington DC

Cheng R, Pomeranz B 1980 Electroacupuncture analgesia is mediated by stereo specific opiate receptors and is reversed by antagonists of type 1 receptors. Life Sciences 26: 631–638

Collin C, Hockaday J, Water A 1985 Headache and school absence. Archives of Disease in Childhood 60: 245–247

Culpeper N 1653 Complete herbal: a book of natural remedies for ancient ills (Wordsworth edn 1995). Wordsworth Editions, Hertfordshire

Dale A, Cornwell S 1994 The role of lavender oil in relieving perineal discomfort following childbirth: a blind randomised clinical trial. Journal of Advanced Nursing 19(1): 89–96

Davis P 1996 Aromatherapy: an A–Z. CW Daniel, Saffron Walden

DeWeerdt C, Bootsma H, Hendriks H 1996 Phytomed 3(3): 225–230

Dyrehag L, Widerstroem-Noga E, Carlsson S, Andersson S 1997 Effects of repeated sensory stimulation sessions (electro acupuncture) on skin temperature in chronic pain patients. Scandinavian Journal of Rehabilitation 29: 243–250

Duff L, Louw G, McClaryey M 1999 Clinical guideline for the recognition and assessment of acute pain in children. Paediatric Nursing 11(6): 18–21

Eland J 1990 Pain in children. Nursing Clinics of North America 25(4): 871–884

Ernst E, White A 1999 Acupuncture: a scientific appraisal. Butterworth-Heinemann, Oxford

Evans M, Rodger I 2000 Healing for body, soul and spirit: an introduction to anthroposophical medicine. Floris Books, Edinburgh

Ewin D 1986 Emergency room hypnosis for the burned patient. American Journal of Clinical Hypnosis 26: 9–15

Ewin D 1999 Hypnosis in the emergency room. In: Remes R (ed) Medical hypnosis: an introduction and clinical guide. Churchill Livingstone, Edinburgh

Fetrow C, Avila J 2001 Professional's handbook of complementary and alternative medicines. Springhouse, Pennsylvania

Field T 1998 Massage therapy effects. American Psychologist 53(12): 1270–1281

Field T 2000 Touch therapy. Churchill Livingstone, Edinburgh

Gauvain-Piquard A, Rodary A, Rezvani A, Lemerle J 1987 Pain in children aged 2–6 years: a new observational rating scale elaborated in a pediatric oncology unit–preliminary report. Pain 31: 177–188

Gemmell D 1997 Everyday homoeopathy. Beaconsfield Publishers, Beaconsfield, UK

Ghelardini C, Galeotti N, Salvatore G, Mazzanti G 1999 Local anaesthetic activity of the essential oil of Lavandula augustifolia. Planta Medica 65: 700–703

Gibson H, Heap M 1991 Hypnosis in therapy. Lawrence Erlbaum Associates, London

Gilles M 1995 Pain management. In: Carter B, Dearmun AK (eds) Child health care nursing: concepts, theory and practice. Blackwell Science, Oxford

Gobel H, Schmidt G, Dworschak M et al 1995 Essential plant oils and headache mechanisms. Phytomed 2(2): 93–102

Good M, Picot B, Salem S et al 2000 Cultural differences in music chosen for pain relief. Journal of Holistic Nursing 18(3): 245–260

Han J 1997 Physiology of acupuncture: review of thirty years of research. Journal of Alternative and Complementary Medicine 3 (suppl 1): s101–108

Heap M, Aravind K 2002 Hartland's medical and dental hypnosis, 4th edn. Churchill Livingstone, Edinburgh

Heap M, Dryden W (eds) 1993 Hypnotherapy: a handbook. Open University Press, Milton Keynes

International Association for the Study of Pain Subcommittee on Taxonomy 1979 Pain 8: 249

Jackson S 1995 Acute pain: its physiology and the pharmacology of analgesia. Nursing Times 91(16): 27–28

Johnson E, Kadam MP, Hylands DM et al 1985 Efficacy of feverfew as prophylactic treatment of migraine. British Medical Journal 291: 569–573

King N, Sharpley C 1990 Headache activity in children and adolescents. Journal of Paediatric Child Health 26: 50–54

Krout R 2001 The effects of single session music therapy interventions on the observed and self reported levels of pain control, physical comfort and relaxation of hospice patients. American Journal of Hospice and Palliative Care 18(6): 383–390

Launso L, Brendstrup E, Arnberg S 1999 An exploratory study of reflexology treatment for headache. Alternative Therapies 5(3): 57–65

Lis-Balchin M, Hart S 1999 Studies on the mode of action of the essential oil of lavender (Lavandula augustifolia). Phytotherapy Research 13: 540–542

Lockie A 1990 The family guide to homeopathy. Penguin Books, Middlesex

Lockie A, Geddes N 1996 The complete guide to homeopathy, the principles and practice of treatment. Dorling Kindersley, London

Loh L, Nathan P, Schott G et al 1984 Acupuncture versus medical treatment for migraine and muscle tension headaches. Journal of Neurology, Neurosurgery and Psychiatry 47: 333–337

Loo M 2002 Pediatric acupuncture. Churchill Livingstone, Edinburgh

Mairs D 1995 Hypnosis and pain in childbirth. Contemporary Hypnosis 12(2): 11

Malkin K 1994 Use of massage in clinical practice. British Journal of Nursing 3(6): 292–294

Mao W, Ghia J, Scott D et al 1980 High versus low intensity acupuncture analgesia for treatment of chronic pain: effects on platelet serotonin. Pain 8: 331–342

Martin P 1993 Psychological management of chronic headaches. Guildford Press, New York

Melzack R, Wall P 1965 Pain mechanisms: a new theory. Science 150: 971–978

Michel D, Chesky K 1995 A survey of music therapists using music for pain relief. The Arts in Psychotherapy 22(1): 49–51

Miller K 1990 Pain management techniques. Heart and Lung 19(2): 136–146

Mills S 1993 The essential guide to herbal medicine. Penguin Books, Harmondsworth

Mills S 1994 A complete guide to modern herbalism. Thorsons, London

Mills S, Bone K 2000 Principles and practice of phytotherapy: modern herbal medicine. Churchill Livingstone, Edinburgh

Murphy L 1988 Randomised double blind placebo controlled trial of feverfew in migraine prevention. Lancet 2(8604): 189–192

Nelson D, Heitman R, Jennings C 1986 Effects of tactile stimulation on premature infants' weight gain. Journal of Obstetric, Gynaecological and Neonatal Nursing. May–June: 263–267

Olness K, Kohen D 1996 Hypnosis and hypnotherapy with children. Guildford Press, London

Pearce L 2000 Acupuncture and related therapies. In: Charman R (ed) Complementary therapies for physical therapists. Butterworth-Heinemann, Oxford

Pfeil M 1993 Sleep disturbances at home and in hospital. Paediatric Nursing 5(7):14–16

Price D, Raffi A, Watkins L, Buckingham B 1984 A psychophysical analysis of acupuncture analgesia. Pain 19: 27–42

RCN 1999 Recognition and assessment of acute pain in children: recommendations. RCN, London

Silberstein S 1992 Advances in understanding the pathophysiology of headache. Neurology 42: 6–10

Sims J 1997 The mechanism of acupuncture analgesia: a review. Complementary Therapies in Medicine 5(2): 102–111

Sunshine W, Field T, Schanberg S, Quintino O et al 1996 Massage therapy and transcutaneous electrical stimulation effects on fibromyalgia. Journal of Clinical Rheumatology 2: 18–22

Taddei I, Giachetti D, Taddei E, Mantovani P 1988 Spasmolytic activity of peppermint, sage and rosemary essences and their major constituents. Fitoterapia 59(6): 463–468

Volger B 1998 Feverfew as a preventative treatment for migraine: a systematic review. Cephalgia 18(10): 704–708

Watson S, Watson S 1997 The effects of massage: an holistic approach to care. Nursing Standard 11(47): 45–47

Williamson D, Baker J, Cubic B 1993 Advances in pediatric headache research. In: Ollindick T, Prinz R (eds) Advances in clinical child psychology, vol 15. Plenum Press, New York

Wilson O 1997 Biophysical modelling of the physiology of acupuncture. Journal of Alternative and Complementary Medicine 3(suppl 1): s25–39

Wong D (ed) 1993 (ed) Whaley and Wong's essentials of pediatric nursing, 4th edn. Mosby, London, p 595

6 Problems related to eating and drinking

CHAPTER CONTENTS

- **Introduction   94**
- **Problems with CAM and diet   94**
  Diagnostic tests for allergies   95
  Dangerous diets   96
- **TCM and nutrition   97**
- **Use of CAM in postoperative nausea and vomiting   98**
  Herbalism   98
  Hypnosis   98
  TCM   99
- **Use of CAM in nausea and vomiting following chemotherapy   100**
  TCM   100
  Guided imagery and music therapy   100

Hypnosis   101
- **Use of CAM for motion sickness   101**
  TCM   101
  Herbalism   102
  Homeopathy   102
- **CAM and diabetes   102**
  Introduction   102
  Ayurvedic medicine   103
  TCM   103
  Herbal treatment   104
  Other considerations   105
- **CAM and weight gain in babies   105**
- **References   106**

INTRODUCTION

This chapter addresses some of the problem areas related to nutritional intake that may be encountered when using some CAM therapies, as well as highlighting the usefulness of other CAM interventions for nutrition related problems. First, problems with the diagnosis of food allergies and the deficiencies of consequently recommended dietary regimes are discussed, then some of the special diets recommended for cancer sufferers are reviewed. Second, an overall view of nutritional issues from the point of view of TCM is given. Third, the usefulness of CAM interventions in the areas of nausea and vomiting following anaesthetic, following chemotherapy and as a result of motion sickness are discussed. The next section of the chapter looks at the particular issues involved in the use of CAM interventions in people with diabetes, and, finally, the role of massage in helping to stimulate growth and development in pre-term and medically compromised babies is discussed.

PROBLEMS WITH CAM AND DIET

Practitioners need to be aware that in several CAM interventions, dietary manipulation is an integral part of the treatment, as has already been indicated when discussing Ayurveda and TCM. This will be expanded on later.

Diagnostic tests for allergies

A particular concern is the use of therapeutic diets which involve the exclusion of one or more entire food groups, on the basis of an identified 'allergy', usually to wheat or dairy produce. Many of the tests offered to identify these allergies are unproven, and nurses may come across children whose parents have put them on a severely restricted diet without appropriate medical supervision, in the mistaken belief that their child is allergic to a wide range of foods.

Hair analysis

A number of diagnostic tests have been devised and are used by CAM practitioners to ascertain the patient's allergy. Ernst and Hentschel (1995) have reviewed a number of these, including hair analysis. The rationale behind hair analysis is that the trace elements in the hair provide a valuable indication of a person's health, and that excesses or deficiencies of trace metals can be diagnosed by this method. Trace metal analysis is said to be a useful investigation for atopic disease (David 1987). When the hair of two individuals was submitted to 13 commercial hair testing laboratories, results indicated a marked variability in the results from the laboratories as well as variability between the same samples sent to different laboratories (Barre 1985). There did not appear to be any consensus as to what constituted normal or pathological levels. Of particular concern is the fact that medical interventions were advised by the laboratories as a result of these tests. In a further study, samples of blood and hair (including a duplicate sample) were submitted to five commercial laboratories that offered allergy diagnosis. The samples were donated by subjects who were allergic to fish (diagnosed by Guy's hospital, having shown a positive result for fish in a skin prick test) and by a control group (non-allergic subjects). Again, the results were grossly unreliable. None of the laboratories diagnosed the fish allergy, but some diagnosed a range of other allergies in the non-allergic control group. In addition, results for identical samples submitted independently were inconsistent (Sethi et al 1987).

Kinesiology

Another procedure which claims to be able to detect allergies is kinesiology. The theory behind this procedure is that a feedback loop exists between the body's inner organs and the muscles; if an organ fails to function properly, this will affect the related muscle, thereby causing muscle weakness. The claim is made that this method will also identify allergens.

The diagnosis is obtained by testing the patient's muscle resistance whilst they hold the offending allergen. In a double blind trial following kinesiology diagnosis of milk allergy in six subjects, when retesting the results in a double blind manner the results were distributed by chance. Following serial testing, reproducibility of the results in the six subjects was poor (Garrow 1988). A further study by Lüdtke et al (2001) confirmed Garrow's results.

Vega test

One further diagnostic test used by allergy practitioners is the Vega test, which purports to detect changes in the resistance to the flow of electricity over acupuncture points on the ends of fingers and toes. Potential allergens are identified if they cause a fall in conductivity. There is no evidence that the Vega test works as a diagnostic tool for allergens (Garrow 1988, Lewith et al 2001). As a result of these inappropriate diagnostic procedures, children may be diagnosed as having an allergy when they do not, and as a consequence they may be subjected to an unnecessarily restricted diet, in which they are often advised to exclude more than one entire food group.

Dangerous diets

Special diets that have been advocated in the treatment of specific illnesses, particularly cancer, are discussed next. A review of these diets is given by the American Cancer Society (1993).

Gerson diet

Perhaps the best known of these diets is the Gerson diet. Although it is mainly known as a cancer diet, it is also advocated for use in other degenerative diseases. The theory behind this diet is that these conditions are the result of body toxicity which, in turn, undermines the immune system, resulting in tumour formation. The aim of the Gerson diet is to detoxify the system, and it involves a regime of 8 weeks of eating only organic, raw, salad vegetables, soups and potatoes, with a later addition of yoghurt and cottage cheese. Additional supplements include the ingestion of mixed potassium salts, Lugol's solution (iodine/potassium iodide), thyroid extract, pancreatin, royal jelly and niacin. Thirteen glasses of vegetable juice are drunk each day. It is estimated by the Gerson Institute that it takes 40–50 hours per week for shopping and preparing the food, which cannot be made in advance and stored.

The aim of the treatment is to stimulate the liver and the production of bile. Of particular danger to children is the use of castor-oil and coffee enemas, administered as often as every 4 hours, and some deaths have occurred as a result of this (Eisele & Reay 1980). Green (1992) has reviewed the theoretical assumptions made for the efficacy of the Gerson diet in the treatment of cancer and found them to be completely unsubstantiated. This therapy is practised mostly in Mexico, but there are some practitioners in Britain.

One account of the use of Gerson therapy is given by Baldwin and Baldwin (2001), who undertook the diet following a diagnosis of breast cancer. The account is of interest for a number of reasons. The first is that the therapy was chosen in place of 'aggressive' chemotherapy because it was 'natural' and had 'no side effects'. Secondly, it confirmed the amount of time involved in preparing the diet. Thirdly, when the diet failed to prevent the tumour increasing when the Baldwins went to Mexico for further treatment, blame for the failure of the treatment was firmly placed on the Baldwins themselves. Apparently, it was suggested that the juices had not been fresh enough when consumed, and the wrong green vegetables had been used. In spite of a brief respite, the outlook remained poor and, subsequently, a raft of alternative therapies was tried, many of them of no proven value at all. It can be seen that if parents undertake this regime on behalf of their child and it fails to work, the level of parental guilt will be greatly increased.

Macrobiotic diets

Macrobiotic diets are part of a quasi-religious philosophical system and consist of a largely vegetarian diet relying heavily on whole grains, which make up 60% of each meal; vegetables make up 30% and soya beans 10%, with small amounts of white fish or meat once or twice a week. It is proposed as an aid to cancer treatment, but some adherents use it as a lifestyle choice. The diet has 10 stages, each becoming increasingly restrictive, the last stage consisting of brown rice and water. There have been a number of reported health problems, including nutritional deficiencies, and some deaths amongst those who have followed the diet (Metz 2000). Metz goes on to state that children should not be put on the diet since they will not obtain the required nutrients for growth and development, and that cancer patients may lose a significant amount of weight, making it harder to tolerate conventional treatment. Sometimes promoters of the macrobiotic diet advise patients to stop conventional treatment.

TCM AND NUTRITION

In Traditional Chinese Medicine the importance of food and diet cannot be overemphasised. Not only the content of the diet but also how and when it is eaten are important. Because Qi comes from living things, great emphasis is placed on the freshness of food. To preserve the Qi, food should, preferably, be grown locally and organically. In order to maintain the harmony of the internal organs, food from the five flavours (Sour, Bitter, Sweet, Spicy, Salty) should be balanced within the diet. In addition, there are four categories of tonic to address deficiencies:

- Yin tonic
- Yang tonic
- Qi tonic
- Blood tonic.

As children are considered to be constitutionally Yin deficient, they tend to suffer from recurrent infections which generate Yin depleting Heat. In addition, Qi can become deficient due to illness or inappropriate diet.

Foods are classified as Hot, Warm, Neutral, Cool or Cold. Hot and Warm foods are Yang, directing energy and fluids upwards, whilst Cool and Cold foods direct energy and fluids downwards. A good diet is a balance between the five categories. Organ dysfunction can result from bad eating habits as well as from emotional upsets.

In concert with Ayurveda, TCM places great store on the social function of food, advocating an unhurried approach to meal times and the importance of eating slowly to enhance the effect of Nutritive-Qi. Stomach-Qi digests the food whilst Spleen-Qi transforms food into Nutritive-Qi and distributes it around the body. Meals in China revolve around a 2-hour cycle, allowing each organ to operate at its maximum Qi. For example, Stomach-Qi is at its maximum between 7 and 9 a.m. and at its minimum between 7 and 9 p.m.; Spleen-Qi is at its maximum between 9 and 11 a.m. and at its minimum between 9 and 11 p.m. Poor eating habits can result in Stomach and Spleen deficiency, resulting in poor digestion.

USE OF CAM IN POSTOPERATIVE NAUSEA AND VOMITING

One of the biggest challenges in nursing care is the control of nausea and vomiting. Prolonged and excessive vomiting leads to dehydration, debility, metabolic disturbances and nutritional deficiencies (Troesch et al 1993), and the dangers of postoperative nausea and vomiting have been highlighted by Blinkhorne (1995).

Herbalism

Clinical trials using ginger root have shown its usefulness in this area. In a review of its use as a postoperative anti-emetic, a double blind, randomised, controlled trial was conducted in which patients were given capsules containing 1 g of ginger at the same time as their premedication, compared with a placebo group and a group given metoclopramide. Anaesthetic type and duration of surgery were comparable. Results showed that there were significantly more incidents of nausea in the control group than in the experimental group or the group given metoclopramide; the authors concluded that the ginger significantly reduced the incidence of postoperative nausea compared with the placebo, and it had the same effect as metoclopramide but without the dangers or side effects (Bone et al 1990). This effect was supported in a study by Phillips et al (1993). Ginger (*Zingiber officinale*) has been used as a spice and medicine for thousands of years and is recorded in Ayurveda and TCM. Traditionally, it is used for its effect on the gastrointestinal system for dyspepsia, colic and diarrhoea. It can be administered as a tea and is just as effective in the form of crystallised ginger confectionery and ginger biscuits.

Mills and Bone (2000) reviewed the role of peppermint (*Mentha piperita*) in the treatment of gastrointestinal disorders and noted that peppermint oil increased gastric emptying. It was associated with a significant reduction of postoperative nausea in gynaecological patients after they inhaled the oil in a placebo controlled trial (Dalvi et al 1991, Tate 1997). Chamomile, both Roman and German, has a relaxing effect on the viscera and is calming and relaxing, helping to soothe a tense child and relax the muscles.

Hypnosis

Another approach to the problem of postoperative vomiting involved the use of positive intra-operative suggestion during routine gynaecological surgery, using two well-matched surgical groups with similar type and length of anaesthetic. The suggestions were delivered using a personal stereo and audio tape. Suggestions of wellbeing and not feeling sick afterwards were given, including the injunction that the anti-emetic drug given during premedication (which was not, in fact, given) would be effective. The incidence of vomiting was significantly lower in the experimental group, 32% compared with 69% in the control group, whilst metoclopramide requirements were significantly less in the trial group (Williams et al 1994).

TCM

The use of acupuncture in the treatment and prevention of nausea and vomiting is well recorded in both traditional and Western acupuncture books and a number of points have been identified for their anti-emetic effects. The point most commonly referred to is Pericardium 6 (P-6) and this point has been used in clinical trials for postoperative nausea and vomiting, motion sickness and cancer chemotherapy. Good results have been reported in the use of this point preoperatively in adults, although a number of interesting variations in efficacy have been noted. For example, when acupuncture was performed on P-6 at the same time as premedication, there was a significantly reduced incidence of nausea in an acupuncture group compared with a control (Dundee et al 1986). A further study yielded positive results when Barsoum et al (1990) used P-6 stimulation with acupressure (Sea Bands) in 162 major operations. Patients received a variety of premedications and acupressure; dummy Sea Bands and prochlorperazine were administered randomly, with one group not receiving any treatment. Nausea scores were significantly lower in the two postoperative days in the acupressure group than in the two other groups. Vomiting was lower, but not significantly, in the acupressure group than in the other two groups. However, when Weightman et al (1987) stimulated P-6 after anaesthesia had been induced, this stimulation did not lead to a significant reduction in nausea and vomiting. The anaesthetic may have been having an inhibiting effect on the acupuncture, since local anaesthetic has been shown to block the anti-emetic effect of P-6 (Dundee & Ghaly 1991).

Three other studies of the use of P-6 stimulation for postoperative nausea in children provided negative results. The first by Lewis et al (1991), using a double blind design, compared the effects of acupressure on P-6 with placebo on children undergoing strabismus correction. The bands (either Sea Bands or bands without studs) were put in place 1 hour before the operation and remained in place until discharge from the hospital later in the day. No statistically significant difference was found between the two groups in terms of nausea and vomiting. Yentis and Bissonnette (1992) found no difference between the use of acupuncture at P-6 and the use of droperidol following strabismus repair. However, in this instance the acupuncture was administered after anaesthesia had been induced. This finding was confirmed by another study when P-6 was used to prevent nausea and vomiting postoperatively in children undergoing tonsillectomy. Using 45 children in two groups, one group were given 5 minutes of acupuncture needling after anaesthetic and before surgery. There was no significant difference in the two groups (Yentis & Bissonnette 1991).

A number of reviewers such as Ernst (1996) and Lee and Done (1999) have suggested that whilst the evidence for the use of P-6 stimulation in the treatment of postoperative vomiting is compelling, children do not benefit from the intervention. Filshie and White (1998) suggest that, given the high incidence of postoperative vomiting associated with these operations, the aetiology is multifactorial, i.e. not simply the result of the anaesthetic. In the case of the strabismus, the nausea may have been caused by the manipulation of the eye, with muscle stretching resulting in visual sensory disturbance; in the case of tonsillectomy, the nausea may have been caused by the blood swallowed at operation causing irritation of the stomach. They further suggest that, given the high incidence of vomiting associated with these operations, invasive acupuncture might have been more effective than the Sea Bands in the Lewis et al (1991) trial. However, TCM would consider the repression of the vomiting reflex as inappropriate, particularly in circumstances of what TCM refers to as 'stagnant blood', resulting in Stomach-Qi rebelling upwards. Therefore, P-6 may not be the most suitable acupuncture point in this instance and Ren 10 or 13 may be more appropriate. A more recent study by Wang and Kain (2002), a double blind, randomised, controlled trial on a group of 190 children undergoing anaesthesia and surgery, had a more positive result. The children were randomly assigned to one of four groups. Group A were given intravenous saline plus bilateral P-6 acupoint injections; group B were given intravenous droperidol plus bilateral P-6 sham acupuncture; group C had intravenous saline plus bilateral sham point injections; and group D received intravenous saline plus bilateral P-6 sham acupuncture. Anaesthesia was standard for all groups and the incidence of postoperative nausea and vomiting was evaluated during recovery and 24 hours post operation. Results indicated that the active intervention resulted in significantly lower incidences of nausea than the sham group, but not in comparison with the droperidol group. At 24 hours post operation there was no difference between the groups. The researchers concluded that bilateral P-6 acupoint injections are effective in prevention of postoperative nausea and vomiting in the early postoperative period.

USE OF CAM IN NAUSEA AND VOMITING FOLLOWING CHEMOTHERAPY

Nausea and vomiting following chemotherapy have been shown to respond to a variety of therapies.

TCM

Stannard (1989) used acupressure point P-6 and found that nausea was much reduced but not eliminated, however, further studies were undertaken by Dundee et al (1989) and Dundee and Yang (1990) on patients who had had serious nausea and vomiting during previous courses of chemotherapy. These patients, who were prescribed a range of anti-emetics, continued to take them during the acupuncture trials. A number of interventions were used, manual and electrical acupuncture (Dundee et al 1989) as well as non-invasive approaches to stimulation (Dundee et al 1991, McMillan & Dundee 1991), which were all employed before the start of the chemotherapy course. Among these techniques, the best results were obtained with invasive acupuncture, which benefited 90% of the patients. These beneficial effects were only slightly less for patients having highly emetic compounds.

Price et al (1991) compared Sea Bands with placebo acupressure to the ankle in a controlled crossover study. Those patients who had acupressure to P-6 had significantly less nausea and sickness compared with the placebo group.

Guided imagery and music therapy

Mastenbroek and McGovern (1991) reviewed the use of relaxation techniques in the control of chemotherapy-induced nausea and anticipatory nausea. Anticipatory nausea is when nausea arises simply by talking about chemotherapy or during follow-up visits to the clinic, whether or not chemotherapy is given (Neese et al 1980).

Troesch et al (1993) describe the use of guided imagery, which employs relaxation techniques and the visualisation of a positive experience, accompanied by soft tranquil music. This study was designed to see if the addition of guided imagery to standard anti-emetic treatment decreased the incidence of nausea and vomiting. There was no statistical difference between the control and experimental groups in relation to effect; however, the guided imagery group reported feelings of greater control, power and relaxation and described their chemotherapy experience more positively than the control group. A trial using music therapy and guided visualisation with 15 subjects undergoing treatment for a variety of malignancies, and being treated with a variety of chemotherapy agents, used a single group pre- and post-test design. Results showed a significant reduction in the perception of nausea and vomiting, i.e. the participants perceived the vomiting to be less severe after music therapy. The experience of nausea was unchanged (Frank 1985).

Hypnosis

In an interesting study of the use of hypnosis as an anti-emetic therapy in children receiving chemotherapy (Cotanch et al 1995), 22 children were randomly assigned to control or experimental groups. The experimental group was taught an individual self-hypnosis technique. Positive suggestions included feeling safe in hospital, experiencing comfortable and restful sleep, time passing quickly and wanting to eat and drink after chemotherapy. Results were encouraging. Children in the experimental group reported a significant decrease in frequency, severity, amount and duration of nausea, showing that hypnosis is an effective intervention in reducing post-chemotherapy nausea. The self-hypnosis gave the children a sense of control, which is important to children of all ages but is particularly important for adolescents, who have a high rate of non-compliance with regimes.

USE OF CAM FOR MOTION SICKNESS

TCM

Motion sickness can be a very real blight on the lives of many children, ruining school outings, holidays and excursions. Acupressure has been shown to be of value here, as it is in postoperative nausea and in chemotherapy, although most of the evidence is anecdotal. Three scientific investigations into the use of Sea Bands for motion sickness showed no evidence of efficacy. The motion sickness was induced in a laboratory and interventions included active and placebo drugs and acupressure combinations (Bruce et al 1990). Warwick-Evans et al (1991) compared Sea Bands with a no stud placebo. Neither of these trials indicated that using a Sea Band on P-6 prevented laboratory-induced motion sickness. However, it is not clear how violent the motion sickness was and the bands may well be worth trying on children who suffer from this condition.

Herbalism

Of more proven value is ginger, which has been shown to be useful as a prophylactic for seasickness. Powdered ginger root was compared with placebo in preventing seasickness in naval cadets. The incidence of nausea and vomiting was significantly reduced in the experimental group compared with the control group (Grontved 1988). Mowrey and Clayson (1982) compared ginger with dimenhydrinate 100 mg in the prevention of motion sickness induced by a rotating chair, with positive results for the ginger. Further studies have produced mixed results, indicating that motion sickness is particularly difficult to investigate in a controlled trial, owing to the variability of its intensity and aetiology, which can depend on the type of vehicle, length of journey and what food was previously eaten. Empirical observation may be more appropriate in deciding which intervention to suggest.

Homeopathy

Parents and children who opt for homeopathic treatment of motion sickness may be using one or more of the following prescriptions:

- For anxiety before the journey, Gelsimium, Ignatia, Argentum nit
- For children who are over-excited, Coffea cruda given before and during the journey
- For nausea and vomiting made worse by thinking about food or with the sight and smell of food (not easy to avoid on a coach full of children), Cocculus before and during the journey.

If the nausea and vomiting are accompanied by giddiness and made worse by cigarette smoke, Tabacum given before and during the journey is useful.

CAM AND DIABETES

Introduction

Diabetes is a condition that affects 30 million people worldwide and its prevalence is increasing. Its symptoms include excessive thirst, polyuria and hyperglycaemia. These symptoms have been noted in many ancient medical manuscripts and the physician Hippocrates advocated the treatment of diabetes with a sugar free diet. Diabetes presents as type 1, which is insulin dependent, and type 2, which is non-insulin dependent. The latter is more commonly a condition of older people and is a result of obesity. Diabetes in children used to be almost exclusively insulin dependent but, with the increased incidence of childhood obesity (discussed in Section 3), more cases of type 2 diabetes in children are coming to light.

Pieber et al (1995) emphasise the importance of educating children and their parents in diabetes management. The serious impact that diabetes can have on their lives may cause them to seek alternative help. However, in a survey investigating the levels of distress caused by diabetes, West and McDowell (2002) noted that type 2 diabetes was the more stressful and that the impact of the condition was not noted for some years after diagnosis. This is interesting since, in their cautionary paper on the use of CAM in diabetes, Gill et al (1994) noticed that subjects described in their case studies who had turned to CAM were in their twenties and had been diagnosed as diabetic for some years, indicating that education regarding the use of CAM should be included in initial education packages, but should also be part of ongoing care. It was indicated in Chapter 1 that the majority of patients who turn to CAM are those suffering from long-term chronic conditions, and diabetes certainly comes into this category. It is not surprising that patients turn to CAM for additional or alternative help. Yeh et al (2000) investigated the types of CAM used by diabetics in the United States, where about 6.7 million people use CAM to treat their condition. In a representative sample of 95 people, 16% used alternative lifestyle diets such as macrobiotics, 7% used herbal remedies and 27% of the respondents reported that they found CAM to be very helpful.

Ayurvedic medicine

In Ayurveda, diabetes is classified according to dosha type, i.e. vata, pitta or kapha, with long-term diabetes being of the vata type. The most difficult cases to control are the vata types, which include diabetes mellitus. Pitta types are moderately difficult to control and kapha are the more easily controlled. The subdivisions within these categories are difficult to relate to Western diagnosis, but each is treated with herbs and the diabetes mellitus with diet. Other treatments include the restriction of sugar and sweet consumption and the restriction of carbohydrates and fats (Qutab 1996). Regular exercise is recommended, together with the practice of yoga, which has been shown to induce glucose homeostasis (Monro et al 1992).

TCM

Although the incidence of diabetes is low in the Chinese population, the TCM approach to treatment has been included here because parents may look to TCM treatments for help with this chronic illness. Diabetes is rare in China because the Chinese are not genetically predisposed to develop it, and social factors that are prevalent in the West do not occur in China, e.g. obesity is not a problem and the normal Chinese diet helps to reduce blood sugar. However, the condition has been noted and it has been treated with herbs for at least 2000 years. Classified as 'emaciated thirst', it was said to have occurred amongst wealthy people, and the description appears to relate to type 2 diabetes. Two of the formulae most frequently used for diabetes today were first described around 200 years BC. One of these, called the Rehmannia Eight Formula, was prescribed for patients suffering from increased urine, weakness and fatigue (Dharmananda 1996).

Traditionally, diabetes mellitus is described as presenting in three stages. The first stage is caused by deficient Yin and excessive Heat. As the condition progresses, this Yin deficiency produces Dry Heat which then damages both Yin and Yang. In type 2 diabetes this progress takes a number of years, but in insulin dependent diabetes progression to stage three is rapid (Chen et al 1994). A number of trials have been conducted on the therapeutic effect of TCM herbs. For patients suffering from type 2 diabetes, Rehmannia Six Formula and Ginseng and Gypsum Combination are recommended and have been shown to have hypoglycaemic effects in laboratory animals. For insulin dependent diabetes a formula to tonify Qi and nourish Yin is given alongside insulin, and for type 2 diabetes the same mixture is given alongside tolbutamide, with which it works synergistically (Yao 1987). In one study (Gao 1989), when patients who had not responded to either Western medicine or TCM herbs were given the medications concurrently, significant improvements were noted in eight out of the ten patients. Specifically, ginseng is reported to reduce the dosage of insulin needed by patients and to prolong its action (Chang & But 1987). A similar effect has been noted by Hui (1995) in his review of the use of acupuncture in the treatment of diabetes. Hui noted that on its own, acupuncture for insulin dependent diabetes gave poorer results than when combined with insulin, but for type 2 diabetes acupuncture alone offered good therapeutic results.

Herbal treatment

A number of herbs have been identified as being hypoglycaemic. Marles and Farnsworth (1996) have conducted an extensive review of more than 1200 species of plants reported to have been used to treat diabetes or to have been investigated for anti-diabetic activity. They suggest that traditional herbal medicines for the treatment of diabetes were mainly directed towards addressing the symptoms of thirst and polyuria. More than 80% of these plants were shown to have hypoglycaemic activity and they demonstrate a very wide variety of mechanisms, not all of which are therapeutically useful. For example, it was noted by Dharmananda (1996) in relation to TCM decoctions that, in order to obtain a useful therapeutic level, the amount of herbs taken in some of the complex formulas often contain large amounts of sugar, resulting in raised sugar levels during the hour after they have been taken. This subsequently subsides, with a gradual and sustained decrease in blood sugar levels. The herb rehmannia (*Rehmannia glutinosa*), the key ingredient of Rehmannia Six Formula, has a high sugar content. A number of herbs, whilst not being of long-term proven value in the treatment of diabetes, do have mild to moderate hypoglycaemic effects which should be borne in mind if they are taken for other conditions. Day (1995) cites agrimony (*Agrimonia eupatoria*), burdock (*Actium lappa*), coriander (*Coriandrum sativum*), dandelion (*Taraxacum officinale*), ginger (*Zingiber officinale*), licorice (*Glycyrrhiza glabra*), nettle (*Urtica dioicia*), sage (*Salvia officinale*), tarragon (*Artemisia dranunculus*) and thyme (*Thymus vulgaris*) and reports that dietary adjuncts commonly used by immigrants to the UK include: cerasee (wild *Momordica charantia*), guava (*Psidium guajava*), karela (cultivated *Momordica charantia*), lychee (*Lycium chinense*), Indian cluster bean (*Cyamopsis tetragonolobus*), mistletoe (*Viscum album*) and paw paw (*Carica papaya*).

Berman et al (1999), in their discussion about herbal remedies and diabetes, point out that whilst some of these herbs appear to be of value in the short term, others have been identified as having serious side effects in the long term. They also point out that none of the herbal mixtures have so far negated the need for insulin therapy in type 1 diabetes. An additional concern is the possibility that certain CAM practitioners may suggest that patients discontinue their insulin therapy whilst undergoing CAM treatment, and this has indeed happened in some cases.

Other considerations

One other consideration that needs to be mentioned and identified by nurses working with diabetic patients and their families is that some therapies, such as massage, reflexology and acupuncture, have mild hypoglycaemic effects. Parents should be alerted to this if they are seeking CAM help for other conditions in their diabetic children, e.g. stress, which has been associated with poor metabolic control in diabetic children (Delamater & Cox 1994), or any of the other conditions discussed in this book. Massage and reflexology do reduce blood sugar levels (Field et al 1997) and this effect is also important in therapies such as reflexology and homeopathy, which can induce a healing crisis that may temporarily induce blood sugar instability. Blood sugar levels should therefore be tested following treatment.

CAM AND WEIGHT GAIN IN BABIES

There is more to healthy nutrition and development than just the ingestion of nutrients, and the provision of correct nutrients and calorific requirements does not always result in optimum results. For example, babies who are deprived of human contact gain weight at a slower rate than babies who are held and stimulated. This maternal deprivation and inadequate stimulation may result in an impaired metabolic rate. In her review of the use of massage on neonates needing special care, Porter (1996) reviews the use of formal and informal massage as a normal activity between mother and baby. She points out that without this stimulation and appropriate loving touch, even if other needs are met, babies will not thrive and develop normally (Russell 1993). McFadyen (1989) points out that parents often feel dissociated from their special care baby and massage is a way in which they are able to participate in the baby's care. In a series of studies (described below) Field and others have demonstrated the value of massage for weight gain in pre-term, full term and medically compromised babies. Research into the mechanism for this effect led the researchers to consider the role of vagal tone. Whilst the baby is being massaged, the vagal nerve slows the heart rate, enhances gastric motility and increases the release of food absorption hormones such as insulin.

Field et al (1986) showed that tactile-kinaesthetic stimulation (or massage) in pre-term babies could have a significant effect on their weight gain, the treatment group gaining 47% more weight than the control group; moreover, the treatment group were in hospital for 6 fewer days than the control group. Scafidi et al (1993) investigated which pre-term infants would benefit most from massage therapy and noted that babies who had experienced more complications before the study started gained more benefit from the massage. Studies conducted on full term babies of clinically depressed mothers (Field 1992), had shown that even a short 15 minute massage twice a week resulted in marked improvements in the babies' stress levels, as measured by salivary cortisol levels and serotonin levels, and by weight gain and alertness, compared with the control group. Although the difference in weight gain was not significant between the groups, it was important, because babies of depressed mothers have been shown to display growth delays by the age of 1 year (Field 1992). The babies in Field's study maintained their growth trajectory, indicating that massage was a good way for depressed mothers to enhance their children's development. Two further studies on medically compromised babies showed that massage could influence the outcome for babies exposed to HIV virus and cocaine (Scafidi & Field 1996, Scafidi et al 1996).

Although previous studies had shown no effect with massage, this was due to the type of massage used, which consisted of light strokes; Field used a deeper pressure technique, to which the babies appeared to respond in a very positive way. In the studies described, the intervention was conducted for 15 minutes in a variety of patterns; for example, for pre-term infants and cocaine-exposed infants, massage was done at the beginning of each of 3 consecutive hours per day over a period of 10 days, whilst the normal infants were massaged for 15 minutes a day, 2 days a week for 6 weeks.

REFERENCES

American Cancer Society 1993 Questionable methods of cancer management: 'nutritional' therapies. Cancer Journal for Clinicians 43: 309–319

Baldwin S, Baldwin E 2001 A new chance in life. In: Barraclough J (ed) Integrated cancer care: holistic, complementary and creative approaches. Oxford University Press, Oxford

Barre H 1985 Commercial hair analysis, science or sham? Journal of American Medical Association 254: 1041–1045

Barsoum G, Perry E, Fraser I 1990 Post operative nausea is relieved by acupressure. Journal of the Royal Society of Medicine 83: 86–89

Berman B, Swyers J, Kaczmarczyk J 1999 Complementary and alternative medicine: herbal therapies for diabetes. Journal of the Association for Academic Minority Physicians 10(1): 10–14

Blinkhorne K 1995 Prepared for a smooth recovery? Nursing Times 91(28): 42–44

Bone M, Wilkinson D, Young J et al 1990 Ginger root – a new anti-emetic: the effect of ginger root on post-operative nausea and vomiting after major gynaecological surgery. Anaesthesia 45: 669–671

Bruce D, Golding J, Hockenhull J, Pethybridge R 1990 Acupressure and motion sickness. Aviation Space Environmental Medicine 61: 361–365

Chang H, But P 1987 (eds) Pharmacology and applications of Chinese materia medica. World Scientific, Singapore

Chen D et al 1994 Clinical and experimental studies in treating diabetes mellitus by acupuncture. Journal of Traditional Chinese Medicine 14(3): 163–166

Cotanch P, Hockenberry M, Herman S 1995 Self-hypnosis as anti-emetic therapy in children receiving chemotherapy. Oncology Nursing Forum 12(4): 41–46

Dalvi S, Nadkarni P, Pardisi R et al 1991 Indian Journal of Pharmacology 35(3): 212–214

David T 1987 Unorthodox allergy procedures. Archives of Disease in Childhood 62: 1060–1062

Day C 1995 Hypoglycaemic plant compounds. Practical Diabetes International (Nov/Dec) 12(6): 269–271

Delamater A, Cox D 1994 Psychological stress, coping and diabetes. Diabetes Spectrum 7: 17–49

Dharmananda S 1996 Traditional Chinese specific condition review: diabetes. The Protocol Journal of Botanical Medicine 1(3): 141–148

Dundee J, Ghaly G 1991 Local anaesthesia blocks the anti-emetic action of P-6. Clinical Pharmacology and Therapeutics 50(1): 78–80

Dundee J, Yang J 1990 Prolongation of the anti-emetic action of P-6 acupuncture by acupressure in patients having cancer chemotherapy. Journal of the Royal Society of Medicine 83: 360–362

Dundee J, Chestnutt W, Ghaly R, Lynas A 1986 Traditional Chinese acupuncture: a potentially useful anti-emetic? British Medical Journal 293: 583–584

Dundee J, Ghaly R, Fitzpatrick K et al 1989 Acupuncture prophylaxis of cancer chemotherapy-induced sickness. Journal of the Royal Society of Medicine 82: 268–271

Dundee J, Yang J, McMillan C 1991 Non invasive stimulation of P-6 anti-emetic acupuncture point in cancer chemotherapy. Journal of the Royal Society of Medicine 84: 210–212

Eisele J, Reay D 1980 Deaths related to coffee enemas. Journal of American Medical Association 244(14): 1608–1609

Ernst E 1996 Acupressure for nausea: a best evidence analysis. European Journal of Physical and Medical Rehabilitation 6(1): 28–29

Ernst E, Hentschel C 1995 Diagnostic methods in complementary medicine. Which craft is witchcraft? International Journal of Risk and Safety in Medicine 7: 55–63

Field T 1992 Infants of depressed mothers. Development and Psychopathology 4: 49–66

Field T 1998 Massage therapy effects. American Psychologist 53(12): 1270–1281

Field T 2000 Touch therapy. Churchill Livingstone, Edinburgh

Field T, Schanberg S, Scafidi F et al 1986 Tactile/kinaesthetic stimulation effects on preterm neonates. Pediatrics 77: 654–658

Field T, Hernanadez-Reif M, LaGreca A et al 1997 Glucose levels decreased after giving massage therapy to children with diabetes mellitus. Diabetes Spectrum 10: 23–25

Filshie J, White A 1998 Medical acupuncture. A western scientific approach. Churchill Livingstone, Edinburgh

Frank J 1985 The effects of music therapy and guided visual imagery on chemotherapy induced nausea and vomiting. Oncology Nursing Forum 12(5): 47–52

Garrow J 1988 Kinesiology and food allergy. British Medical Journal 296: 1573–1574

Gao J 1989 Treatment of diabetes with Shen Qi Tao Hong Tang. Journal of Zhejiang Traditional Chinese Medical College 13(1): 15–16

Gill G, Redmond S, Gareett F, Paisey R 1994 Diabetes and alternative medicine: cause for concern. Diabetic Medicine 11: 210–213

Green S 1992 A critique of the rationale for cancer treatment with coffee enemas and diet. Journal of American Medical Association 268(22): 3224–3227

Grontved A 1988 Ginger root against sea sickness. A controlled trial on the open sea. Acta Otolaryngology 105: 45–49

Hui H 1995 A review of the treatment of diabetes by acupuncture during the last forty years. Journal of Traditional Chinese Medicine 15(2): 145

Lee A, Done M 1999 The use of nonpharmacologic techniques to prevent postoperative nausea and vomiting: a meta analysis. Anaesthesia and Analgesia 88: 1362–1369

Lewis I, Pryn S, Reynolds P 1991 Effect of P-6 acupressure on postoperative vomiting in children undergoing outpatient strabismus correction. British Journal of Anaesthesia 67: 73–78

Lewith G, Kenyon J, Broomfield J et al 2001 The vega test has no reliability or validity in diagnosing allergies. British Medical Journal 322: 131–134

Lüdtke R, Kunz B, Seeber N, Ring J 2001 Test–retest reliability of the Kinesiology muscle test. Complementary Therapies in Medicine 9: 141–145

McFadyen V 1989 Infant massage. Bantam, New York

McMillan C, Dundee J 1991 The role of transcutaneous electrical stimulation of Neiguan anti-emetic acupuncture point in controlling sickness after cancer chemotherapy. Physiotherapy 77: 499–502

Marles R, Farnsworth N 1996 Anti diabetic plants and their active constituents: an update. The Protocol Journal of Botanical Medicine 1(3): 85–111

Mastenbroek I, McGovern L 1991 The effectiveness of relaxation techniques in controlling chemotherapy induced nausea: a literature review. The Australian Occupational Therapy Journal 38(3): 137–142

Metz J 2000 'Alternative medicine' and the cancer patient: an overview. Medical and Pediatric Oncology 34: 20–26

Mills S, Bone K 2000 Principles and practice of phytotherapy: modern herbal medicine. Churchill Livingstone, Edinburgh

Monro R, Power J, Coumar A et al 1992 Yoga therapy for NIDDM: a controlled study. Complementary Medical Research 6(2): 66–68

Mowray D, Clayson D 1982 Motion sickness, ginger and psychophysics. Lancet i: 655–657

Neese R, Carli T, Curtis G 1980 Pre-treatment nausea in cancer chemotherapy: a conditioned response? Psychosomatic Medicine 42: 33–36

Phillips S, Hutchinson S, Ruggier R 1993 Anaesthesia 48(5): 393–395

Pieber T, Brunner A, Schnedl W et al 1995 Evaluation of a structured outpatient group education programme for intensive insulin therapy. Diabetes Care 18: 625–630

Porter S 1996 The use of massage for neonates requiring special care. Complementary Therapies in Nursing and Midwifery 2: 93–96

Price H, Lewith G, Williams S 1991 Acupressure as an anti-emetic in cancer chemotherapy. Complementary Medical Research 5: 93–94

Qutab A 1996 Ayurvedic specific condition review: diabetes mellitus. Protocol Journal of Botanical Medicine Winter p. 138–139

Russell J 1993 Touch and infant massage. Paediatric Nursing 5(3): 8–11

Scafidi F, Field T, 1996 Massage therapy improves behaviour in neonates born to HIV positive mothers. Journal of Pediatric Psychology 21: 889–898

Scafidi F, Field T, Schanberg S 1993 Factors which determine which pre-term infants benefit most from massage therapy. Journal of Developmental and Behavioural Pediatrics 14(3): 176–180

Scafidi F, Field T, Wheeden A et al 1996 Behavioural and hormonal differences in pre-term neonates exposed to cocaine in vitro. Pediatrics 97: 851–855

Sethi T, Lessof M, Kemeny D et al 1987 How reliable are commercial allergy tests. Lancet i: 92–94.

Stannard, D 1989 Pressure prevents nausea. Nursing Times 85(4): 33–34

Tate S 1997 Peppermint oil: treatment for post operative nausea. Journal of Advanced Nursing 26(3): 543–549

Troesch L, Rodehaver C, Delaney E, Yanes B 1993 The influence of guided imagery on chemotherapy-related nausea and vomiting. Oncology Nurses Forum 20(8): 1179–1185

Wang S, Kain N 2002 P-6 acupoint injection for prevention of postoperative nausea and vomiting in children. Department of Anesthesiology, Yale University School of Medicine, Connecticut, USA

Warwick-Evans L, Masters I, Redstone S 1991 A double blind placebo controlled evaluation of acupressure in the treatment of motion sickness. Aviation, Space and Environmental Medicine 62: 776–778

Weightman W, Zacharias M, Herbison P 1987 Traditional Chinese acupuncture as an anti-emetic. British Medical Journal 295: 1379–1380

West C, McDowell J 2002 The distress experienced by people with type 2 diabetes. British Journal of Community Nursing 7(12): 606–613

Williams A, Hind M, Sweeney B et al 1994 The incidence and severity of post-operative nausea and vomiting in patients exposed to positive intraoperative suggestions. Anaesthesia 49: 340–342

Yao Q 1987 Integrated Chinese and Western treatment of 53 cases of diabetes. Chinese Journal of Integrated Traditional and Western Medicine 7(6): 363–364

Yeh G, Davis R, Eisenberg D, Phillips R 2000 Complementary/alternative therapy use among persons with diabetes mellitus in a national survey. Beth Israel Deaconess Medical Center, Boston, USA

Yentis S, Bissonnette B 1991 P-6 acupuncture and postoperative vomiting after tonsillectomy in children. British Journal of Anaesthesia 67: 779–780

Yentis S, Bissonnette B 1992 Ineffectiveness of acupuncture and droperidol in preventing vomiting following strabismus repair in children. Canadian Journal of Anaesthesia 39: 151–154

7

Problems related to elimination

CHAPTER CONTENTS

- **Introduction   109**
- **Constipation   109**
  Ayurvedic medicine   110
  TCM   110
  Massage   111
  Aromatherapy, homeopathy and herbalism   112
  Hypnosis   112
- **Diarrhoea   112**
  TCM   113
  Homeopathy   113

Aromatherapy   114
- **Enuresis   114**
  Hypnosis   115
  Homeopathy and herbalism   115
  Reflexology   115
  TCM   116
  Anthroposophical medicine   116
- **Conclusion   116**
- **References   116**

INTRODUCTION

Robinson (1996) has stated that nurses have a unique role in helping patients to manage their bowel functions. In her excellent book, Bracey (2002) discusses the impact of soiling on child and family and notes that the sense of social isolation and personal humiliation can lead to a multitude of other social and psychological problems, particularly if parents and child feel too embarrassed to discuss the problem with healthcare professionals. Contrary to some medical and lay opinion, soiling is not just a temporary problem which will go away in its own time. Approximately 3% of 5-year olds have not achieved bowel control, although most children manage to establish it by their third or fourth year. Problems with bowel control account for 3% of general paediatric referrals and 25% of referrals to gastro-enterology clinics.

Maestri-Banks (1996) has suggested that nurses should incorporate complementary therapies into their treatment and care of patients with bowel problems, and this chapter reviews the contribution that some of these therapies could make in the treatment of constipation, diarrhoea and enuresis.

CONSTIPATION

The commonest cause of soiling is constipation with overflow, and Nurko (2000) suggests that 34% of children aged between 4 and 11 years suffer from constipation. There are a number of criteria for defining constipation but there is no doubt about the amount of distress that it can cause, particularly in children when it can result in overflow and soiling. Bracey (2002) points out that there are certain times during a child's development when constipation is more likely to occur and knowledge of the mechanism of bowel control development is therefore important for health professionals. Problem times include the changeover from breast to bottle milk, the introduction of solids, and the period when toilet training begins. Conventional treatment is aimed at addressing the underlying cause, be it diet, habit, physiological cause or psychological origin, and might involve the use of stool softening laxatives, bulk forming laxatives or osmotic laxatives. In addition, enemas may be used, and dietary changes, increased fluid consumption, increased exercise and general lifestyle issues will be addressed.

Ayurvedic medicine

In Ayurvedic medicine defecation is the result of the downward movement of vata and if this movement is blocked, constipation will occur. Since early morning is the vata time of day, this is the best time for elimination. Ayurveda regards the colon as the seat of vata and constipation may be connected to an increase of this dosha, however, the development of constipation may also be related to imbalances in other doshas, which may be the result of changes in routine, diet, exercise or emotional state, all of which are deemed to be contributing causes of poor elimination. Different doshas dominate at different times of the year. During the summer when the temperature is high, pitta (the dosha which is increased by heat) predominates. This excess of pitta can result in pitta-type constipation, which presents as hard, dry stools and is the sort of constipation seen in small babies during the summer if they have not been given enough fluid. In all aspects of Ayurveda much emphasis is placed on routine, so that constipation is seen as the repression of natural urges and the failure to respond promptly to the call to defecate.

Other Ayurvedic interventions include knee to chest exercises, abdominal massage, squatting twice a day and taking the triphala to balance the doshas. The triphala is taken at night and has a mild laxative effect without causing dependency. Yoga postures to aid elimination include backward bend, shoulder stand and corps.

Ayurvedic medicine also advocates the use of enemas for a number of conditions. Bracey (2002) highlights the need for practitioners to be aware of local policy on the use of enemas with children and to discuss the rationale of such policies with parents who use CAM-based enemas to treat constipation. Practitioners will, of course, need to be alert to any underlying intentions related to the use of an enema by parents.

Anthroposophical medicine also advocates the use of enemas (chamomile), under medical direction, as well as a change to a high fibre diet.

TCM

Traditional Chinese Medicine recognises more than one type of constipation, and treatment is adjusted to address the specific aetiology and the age of the child. TCM and Western medicine recognise a number of causes in common, for example lack of exercise or faulty diet, but where conventional medicine advocates a high fibre diet, TCM would advocate a diet to remove excess Phlegm, e.g. by reducing dairy produce.

There are three major diagnostic categories of constipation in TCM:

- Spleen-Qi deficiency
- Liver-Qi stagnation
- Yin deficiency.

Spleen-Qi deficiency is seen as the result of excess Phlegm, resulting from living in damp accommodation and eating a mucus-producing diet. It is also the result of excess mental and physical activity. In its depleted state the Spleen is unable to effect the normal flow of fluids around the body, resulting in a decrease in fluid in the large intestine, the formation of hard, dry stools, and the possibility of the development of encopresis. Treatment includes attention to lifestyle and tonifying Spleen, and for children in the Water stage of development, tonifying Kidney-Yin and addressing the child's diet. Lack of Kidney-Yin results in a reduction of fluids in the large intestine, giving rise to stools which are hard and difficult to pass. Liver-Qi stagnation can result from the blockage of Qi by Dampness from Spleen deficiency, resulting in the reduction of circulation of Qi. Liver-Qi is important in ensuring the smooth flow of Qi in every organ and the smooth movement of stools in the large intestine.

TCM recognises the role of the emotions in disease and Loo (2002) refers to the high levels of stress that children may be under. Emotions associated with Liver imbalance include anger, worry and frustration, leading to stagnant Liver-Qi, and children in the Wood stage of development are particularly prone to this type of constipation. This is the stage of development relating to Eriksons' industry versus inferiority stage, in which children are subject to the demanding pressures of adjusting to school, school work and developing relationships. Treatment is aimed at decreasing stress and expelling Damp as well as tonifying Spleen and promoting the flow of Liver-Qi (Loo 2002).

Kausland (1995) describes the treatment of constipation by the use of herbs chosen specifically to redress the underlying imbalance in the organs and to strengthen the Qi where appropriate.

Massage

Abdominal massage has been shown to be beneficial in the treatment of constipation. Using a case study approach, Emly (1993) described the use of abdominal massage in the treatment of constipation in a patient with cerebral palsy, whilst Richards (1998) developed a protocol and training programme for the use of abdominal massage by nurses in the community. She lists the benefits of massage as follows:

- It encourages peristalsis in the gut.
- It relieves flatulence.
- It can precipitate bowel opening.
- It can be used in a retraining programme.
- It is a safe, non-invasive and pleasant treatment for constipation.
- It can be learned by a carer or parent or be self-administered.

Richards' article is recommended for any practitioners who may want to learn abdominal massage and use it in their work.

Holey and Lawler (1995), using a single case study approach, compared the use of classic massage and connective tissue massage in the treatment of constipation. This latter form of massage is applied to the lumbosacral area, and the aim of the intervention is to stimulate visceral reflexes. By applying traction force at connective tissue interfaces, autonomic reflexes in the cutaneo–visceral direction are stimulated.

Aromatherapy, homeopathy and herbalism

The essential oils that have been shown to be antispasmodic, for example chamomile and lavender, may be helpful in the treatment of constipation.

Homeopathy recognises five kinds of constipation, depending on the type of stool and how difficult it is to pass. Remedies used by patients might include Bryonia (*Bryonia alba*) for hard, dry stools, Graphites for large stools that are difficult to pass, Nux vomica (*Strychnos Nux vomica*) for incomplete evacuation, Silica (*Silicea terra*) for large hard stools which slip back when only partly expelled, and Sulphur when the stool is hard, dry and painful to pass.

A number of herbs have the same physiological action as prescribed medicines, and it is important to ascertain if these have been used to treat the constipation and to ensure that they are discontinued if other medications are prescribed. Some examples of herbal remedies will be familiar to practitioners, for example senna (*Cassia senna*), cascara (*Rhamnus purshiana*), rhubarb root (*Rheum officinale*) and bulk laxatives such as agar, psyllium seed and linseed; many other herbs also have a mild laxative effect. A full assessment of the patient's use of CAM needs to be made before any treatment is started.

Hypnosis

Hypnosis has a particularly valuable role to play in the treatment of constipation resulting from an embarrassing incident or trauma, or resulting from a phobia, e.g. about toilets. Treatment would be aimed at putting aside the previously traumatic episode, using anxiety control interventions, such as anchoring, desensitisation and rehearsal for the future.

DIARRHOEA

Diarrhoea is characterised as an alteration in normal bowel movement, with increased water content and a frequency of more than three stools per day. Causes include, psychological distress, infections (the commonest being *E. coli*, salmonella and campylobacter), food reactions and allergies. One form of chronic diarrhoea (chronic non-specific diarrhoea or CNSD) is known as toddler diarrhoea, usually occurring between the ages of 6 months and about 3 years. The child passes up to six loose stools per day, containing undigested food and mucus. In spite of this the child remains well and develops normally. The cause is unknown but it is thought to be primarily a gut motility problem. It may be an early mani-festation of irritable bowel syndrome.

TCM

In TCM, acute infective diarrhoea is caused by External Cold Pathogenic Invasion. The Stomach and Intestines are prone to Cold invasion. The diarrhoea Cold pathogen enters via the faecal–oral route. This correlates with viral infections. Cold impairs the Yang function of the Stomach, which then affects the Spleen, which influences fluid absorption in the Large Intestine. Treatment is aimed at tonifying the Spleen, avoiding Cold foods and Phlegm-producing foods, and expelling Cold from the Large Intestine. Two home treatments can be taught to parents: acupressure and massage. In Tui Na massage, the lower vertebral column from L4 to the coccyx is massaged in a circular motion, with the aim of eliminating waste products and toxins from the system.

External Damp Heat Pathogenic Invasion correlates with bacterial infections and treatment is aimed at dispelling Damp and Heat. The diet is adjusted to exclude Hot and Phlegm-producing foods and massage is prescribed as described for Cold Invasion.

Chronic diarrhoea is due to Spleen deficiency which results in Spleen-Qi descending instead of rising, and food and fluids are not properly absorbed. This Spleen deficiency can be aggravated by Phlegm-producing foods and, for children in the Wood phase of development, by excess stress, worry and emotional upsets. Loo (2002) suggests that whilst the child may look normal and healthy to the Western paediatrician, TCM practitioners may notice Spleen deficiency signs of pallor and abdominal distension. In addition, Loo has noted that increased drink-ing of apple juice, which is high in sorbitol and has a high fructose to glucose ratio, has contributed to CNSD in children (Smith & Lifshitz 1994, Hoekstra et al 1995, Dennison 1996). Loo (2002) comments that modern children's diets consist of a large proportion of unhealthy foods, resulting in Spleen deficiency and occasion-ally Kidney deficiency and Liver-Qi stagnation, these imbalances resulting in a ten-dency towards episodes of diarrhoea. A number of studies have indicated the value of acupuncture in the treatment of diarrhoea (Lin 1987, Su 1992, Lin et al 1993).

Homeopathy

Homeopathy offers a range of therapies, depending on the aetiology of the prob-lem. For fretful babies with yellow stool or slimy, watery green stool which turns yellow on exposure to air, Chamomilla is recommended; for older children who are also vomiting, with no appetite and painful windy distension made worse after fruit and milk, China is recommended. Profuse, watery stools with undigested food are treated with Phos. ac (*Phosphoricum acidum*). The remedy China is made from Peruvian bark, which was the first substance that Hahnemann tested on himself. It is primarily used to treat exhaustion resulting from debilitating con-ditions, usually as a result of loss of body fluids. Similarly, Phos. ac is used for conditions which result in a general lethargy and listlessness, as a consequence of severe loss of fluids.

Aromatherapy

Essential oils known for their antispasmodic effect would be of value in helping a child with diarrhoea. Of these, peppermint oil (*Mentha piperita*) has been the subject of the most extensive research. Its use is discussed in greater detail in Chapter 14 in relation to irritable bowel syndrome. However, oils are also of value where the diarrhoea is of psychological origin, e.g. before exams or due to stress and overwork. Neroli, chamomile and lavender have been shown to have relaxing effects and can be safely used, as can other CAM interventions which address problems of anxiety and stress.

ENURESIS

Enuresis in a child aged 5 years or older has been defined as an involuntary discharge of urine by day or night or both, in the absence of a congenital or acquired defect of the central nervous system or urinary tract (Forsythe & Butler 1989). It affects up to three-quarters of a million children aged 7 years or over (Collins 1980). Although 1 in 7 children grow out of the condition, a significant number continue to wet the bed into adulthood (Pierce 1980).

Children with enuresis experience a number of social and psychological repercussions including social isolation, poor interaction with peers and a restricted social life (Harari & Moulden 2000). Longstaffe et al (2000) specifically noted that, compared with non-enuretic children, these children lacked self-esteem, which can lead to immediate and long-term psychological dysfunction (Von Gontard 1999). The effects of enuresis on the child and family include frustration, anger and resentment with negative perceptions about the child and the condition (Butler & Brewin 1986). The risk of physical abuse of children with enuresis is high (Frude 1991). A particularly worrying aspect noted by Morison et al (2000) was that several of the parents in their sample (16%) admitted that they were too busy to help their child with any treatments suggested by health professionals in the clinic.

In spite of beliefs to the contrary, there is considerable concordance in nocturnal behaviour between bedwetting and non-bedwetting children (Troupe & Hodgson 1971). For example, it has been noted that non-enuretic children are as difficult to wake as enuretic children (Boyd 1960), and that enuretic children sleep as deeply on the nights they do not wet the bed as on the nights when they do (Gillin et al 1982). Both enuretic and dry children are known to wake in response to important internal and external signals such as illness, loud noises or nightmares, but enuretic children do not wake in response to bladder signals (Butler 1994). The reason for this is unclear. Enuresis can present in a number of ways: children who wet both day and night, for whom some of the interventions described below may be appropriate; primary nocturnal enuresis, in which children wet the bed at night never having been dry; and secondary nocturnal enuresis, when a child who has attained dryness and for some reason, often emotional, starts to wet the bed again. Key to treating this is the identification of the underlying cause. Various therapies are useful in treating primary nocturnal enuresis.

Hypnosis

A method of treatment which is able specifically to access and activate the 'wake up' signal is hypnosis. Olness (1975) noted that this therapy has been demonstrated to be effective in the treatment of childhood enuresis when other traditional methods, such as drugs and alarm bells, have proved to be unsuccessful. A number of clinical trials have indicated the value of hypnosis as a treatment for enuresis. In a group of 40 children aged between 4 and 16 years who were taught hypnosis, 31 became dry, usually within 1 month of starting treatment (Olness 1975). Similar results were obtained from a group of 28 children aged between 7 and 18 years, where 20 of the children had stopped wetting the bed after between one and three sessions, and 15 of these children were still dry on follow-up after 1 year. Kohen et al (1984) reviewed the results of a study of 257 children with enuresis and found that 44% achieved complete dryness, with 31% having a significant improvement. Again, these improvements occurred after more conventional treatments had failed. A comparative study by Banerjee et al (1993) compared the efficacy of hypnosis with imipramine in a group of children aged between 5 and 15 years. This study was useful as it demonstrated that, initially, there was little difference between the two groups. However, at 6 months follow-up, the hypnosis group had maintained their improvement rate at 68%, compared with the imipramine group in which improvement had dropped to 24%. For a full review of the role of hypnosis in the treatment of enuresis see Mantle (1999).

Homeopathy and herbalism

Parents who have been seeing a homeopath for their child's enuresis may be giving them homeopathic remedies, depending on how the enuresis is presenting itself. For a child who wets the bed whilst dreaming, Equistium (*Equistium arvense*) (or horsetail) is prescribed. Belladonna is prescribed for wetting the bed early in the night. For wetting during the early part of the night but worse for coughing and dry clear weather, Causticum (*Causticum Hahnemann*) is given. However, since wet beds are mostly discovered in the morning, it may be difficult to pinpoint exactly when the child voids and so identify the correct remedy, in which case Plantago is indicated. These remedies can be used safely alongside conventional treatments.

In herbalism, the herb horsetail (*Equistium arvense*) is prescribed for problems relating to bladder irritability and is also used by medical herbalists for enuresis.

Reflexology

Reflexology is particularly useful in the treatment of elimination problems, both acute and long standing. Tiran (1996) has described the use of reflexology in midwifery and has demonstrated its use in post-partum retention of urine. Children who are being treated with reflexology for their enuresis will have relevant points for the pituitary, bladder, ureters and urethra stimulated, along with relaxation sequences for underlying stress and anxiety.

Part of the healing crisis that commonly occurs in reflexology treatments is a temporary increase in urine output. Parents of enuretic children need to be aware of this, whether their child is being treated for enuresis or any other underlying problem.

TCM

Traditional Chinese Medicine does not have an exact correlation with the Western diagnosis of nocturnal enuresis, but can explain it as Kidney-Yang and Kidney-Essence deficiency. Secondary nocturnal enuresis is seen as Spleen and Lung-Qi deficiency. Kidney-Yang enables the Bladder to hold and store urine. Kidney-Yang deficiency results in a cold Lower Energiser, so that Bladder cannot regulate and store urine well. As children are in the Water stage of development, their Kidney and Bladder are most vulnerable to imbalances. Acupuncture is used to tonify Kidney-Yin and Kidney-Yang, disperse Kidney Cold and tonify Lower Energiser. Other interventions include increase in ingestion of Warming foods. Secondary nocturnal enuresis may arise post illness or as a result of stress, which may be caused by school work, bereavement or family tensions. Qi is diverted away from the Lower Energiser towards the Upper Energiser where it is needed (Loo 2002). Other treatments include changes in lifestyle and dietary adjustment, i.e. excluding Phlegm-producing and Cold foods. The calming effects of Qigong may be useful.

Anthroposophical medicine

The Anthroposophical approach to enuresis is supportive and encouraging and Glöckler and Goebel (1990) suggest the use of hypnosis, using a metaphor technique.

CONCLUSION

Children with elimination problems suffer intense feelings of humiliation and loss of confidence, and will be well aware of an all-pervading odour surrounding them. Some children may take comfort in the use of the Bach flower remedies and nurses caring for these children will note that the prescription may include Larch for lack of confidence, Pine for feelings of guilt, Willow for resentment and Crab apple for the sense of uncleanliness.

REFERENCES

Banerjee S et al 1993 Hypnosis and self-hypnosis in the management of nocturnal enuresis: a comparative study with imipramine therapy. American Journal of Clinical Hypnosis 36(2): 113–119

Boyd M 1960 The depth of sleep in enuretic school children and non-enuretic controls. Journal of Psychosomatic Research 44: 274–281

Bracey J 2002 Solving children's soiling problems. A hand book for health professionals. Churchill Livingstone, Edinburgh

Butler R 1994 Nocturnal enuresis: the child's experience. Butterworth-Heinemann, Oxford.

Butler R, Brewin C 1986 Maternal views on nocturnal enuresis. Health Visitor 59: 207–209

Collins R 1980 Enuresis and encopresis. In: Woody R (ed) Encyclopaedia of clinical assessment. Jossey-Bass, San Francisco

Dennison B 1996 Fruit juice consumption by infants and children: a review. Journal of the American College of Nutrition 15(5) (suppl): 4s–11s

Emly M 1993 Abdominal massage. Nursing Times 89(3): 34–36

Forsythe W, Butler R 1989 Fifty years of enuretic alarms: a review of the literature. Archives of Diseases of Children 64: 879–885

Frude N 1991 Understanding family problems: a psychological approach. Wiley, Chichester

Gillin J, Rapoport J, Mikkelsem E et al 1982 EEG sleep patterns in enuresis: a further analysis and comparison with normal controls. Biological Psychiatry 17: 947–953

Glöckler M, Gobel W 1990 A guide to child health. Anthroposophical Press, Floris Books, Edinburgh

Harari M, Moulden A 2000 Nocturnal enuresis: what is happening? Journal of Paediatric Child Health 36: 78–81

Hoekstra J, van den Aker J, Ghoos Y et al 1995 Fluid intake and industrial processing in apple juice induced chronic non specific diarrhoea. Archives of Diseases of Children 73(2): 126–130

Holey L, Lawler H 1995 The effects of classical massage and connective tissue manipulation on bowel function. British Journal of Therapy and Rehabilitation 2(11): 627–631

Kausland A 1995 The treatment of constipation by Chinese medicine. Journal of Chinese Medicine 47: 17–22

Kohen D, Colwell S, Heimel A 1984 The use of relaxation/mental imagery (self hypnosis) in the management of 505 pediatric behavioural encounters. Journal of Developmental and Behavioural Pediatrics 5(1): 21–25

Lin Y 1987 Observations of the therapeutic effects of acupuncture treatment in 170 cases of infantile diarrhea. Journal of Traditional Chinese Medicine 7(3): 203–204

Lin Y, Zhou Z et al 1993 Clinical and experimental studies on shallow needling technique for treating childhood diarrhea.

Journal of Traditional Chinese Medicine 13(2): 107–114

Longstaffe S, Moffatt M, Whalen J 2000 Pediatrics 105(4): 935–940

Loo M 2002 Pediatric acupuncture. Churchill Livingstone, Edinburgh

Maestri-Banks A 1996 Assessing constipation. Nursing Times 92(21): 28–30

Mantle F 1999 Hypnosis in the treatment of enuresis. Paediatric Nursing 11(6): 33–36

Morison M, Pappin D, Staines H 2000 'You feel helpless, that's exactly it': parents' and young people's control beliefs about bed-wetting and the implications for practice. Journal of Advanced Nursing 31(5): 1216–1227

Nurko S 2000 Current Gastroenterology Reports 2: 234–240

Olness K 1975 The use of self-hypnosis in the treatment of childhood nocturnal enuresis. Clinical Pediatrics 14(3): 273–279

Pierce C 1980 Enuresis. In: Rutter M, Hersov L (eds) Child psychiatry: modern approaches. Blackwell, Oxford

Richards A 1998 Hands on help. Nursing Times 12(32): 69–75

Robinson Z 1996 Bowel management and nurse's hidden work. Nursing Times 92(21): 26–28

Smith M, Lifshitz F 1994 Excess fruit juice consumption as a contributing factor in non organic failure to thrive. Pediatrics 93(3): 438–443

Su Z 1992 Acupuncture treatment of infant diarrhea: a report of 1050 cases. Journal of Traditional Chinese Medicine 12(2): 120–121

Tiran D 1996 The use of complementary therapies in midwifery practice: a focus on reflexology. Complementary Therapies in Nursing and Midwifery 2(2): 32–37

Troupe C, Hodgson N 1971 Nocturnal functional bladder capacity in enuretic children. Journal of Urology 105: 129–132

von Gontard A, Lettgen B, Olbing H et al 1999 Behavioural problems in children with urge incontinence and voiding postponement – a comparison of a paediatric and child psychiatric sample. British Journal of Urology 81(3) (suppl): 100–106

8

Problems related to mobility

CHAPTER CONTENTS

- **Introduction 118**
- **Limited movement 118**
  CAM *and cerebral palsy* 119
  TCM 119
  Alexander technique 120
  Ayurvedic medicine 120
  Anthroposophical medicine 120
- **Abnormal movement 121**
  Epilepsy 121

Attention deficit hyperactivity disorder 124

- **Chronic fatigue syndrome 129**
  Nutritional strategies 130
  Herbal remedies 130
  TCM 131
  Massage 131
- **References 131**

INTRODUCTION

This chapter will address circumstances in which CAM interventions may be applicable across a range of restricted mobility conditions, as well as considering their application in the amelioration of conditions resulting in abnormal movement. A number of problems which can accompany restricted movement, such as constipation and pain, are addressed in other sections.

LIMITED MOVEMENT

As Dearmun and Taylor (1995) have pointed out in their book, a child's altered mobility, however acquired, will impinge on all areas of its subsequent development and involve the family, often in the long term, with very demanding care. One of the commonest causes of restricted movement is as the result of an accident, whether this results in profound disability or a temporary problem, such as a broken leg. Any admission via an emergency department is traumatic but particularly so for children. The use of CAM in the emergency department is not a ready concept but integration has been achieved very successfully, using CAM either as a direct intervention, as an adjunct treatment post trauma, or for health promotion (Kelly 1998, Milton 1998, Taylor et al 1998). Many of the therapies described in this book can easily be incorporated into the emergency department, particularly acupuncture (see Chapter 5), reflexology, hypnosis (Ewin 1986, 1999) and music therapy (Edwards 1999). Immediate help can be given, using the homeopathic remedy Aconite for fear and distress or the Bach flower remedy Rescue Remedy, without compromising any orthodox interventions.

CAM and cerebral palsy

Cerebral palsy which, as May and Carter (1995) point out, is a description and not a diagnosis, is defined by Meadows and Newell (2000) as 'a disorder of posture and movement resulting from a non-progressive lesion of the developing brain' and may result from ante-natal (85% of causes), peri-natal (10% of causes) and post-natal incidents (5% of causes). Presenting problems may include spasticity, rigidity, involuntary movements, ataxia, diplegia, hemiplegia or quadriplegia, all of which can result in pain, distress and sleep disturbances. There may, in addition, be associated handicaps such as learning difficulties, epilepsy, and hearing and visual defects. As we have seen in the last two chapters, CAM is particularly beneficial in inducing a profound and lasting sense of relaxation, reducing stress, aiding sleep and decreasing pain. Almost any of the body therapies would be of value in helping children with special physical needs such as cerebral palsy. Massage and aromatherapy have been shown to help with muscle spasm, pain and sleep.

TCM

Other therapies that have proven to be valuable in helping patients with mobility problems include TCM, a medical system that regards problems resulting in limited movement as being caused by deficient Kidney-Yin, since they result from problems with the central nervous system. A small but interesting study by Miller (1996) demonstrated the use of acupuncture to relieve muscle spasm (in this particular instance spasm resulting from multiple sclerosis). One patient's spasticity had decreased to such an extent that she was able to reduce her medication. Of particular value for problems of limited movement is the practice of Qigong, one of its aims being to develop strength and prowess.

There are two branches of Qigong, the self-healing style which evolved into t'ai chi and the style of healing provided by Qigong practitioners. Qigong takes a number of forms:

- Movement orientated, which restores the energy system through specific movement exercises
- Meditation orientated, which relaxes the mind, rebalances Qi and enables the mind to perform self-healing
- Breathing orientated, which emphasises the role of breathing in replenishing, releasing and storing Qi for health, and to promote health and healing (Lee & Lei 1999).

Mokone (2000) points out that Qi is a concept or a function, rather than a substance that can be measured, and is thought to work through the autonomic nervous system and enhance the regulating systems of the body to achieve homeostasis.

The basic principles of Qigong include:

- Motor control
- Postural awareness
- Relaxation
- Breath control
- Visualisation
- Meditation.

These are achieved by the practice of slow, controlled movements, by maintaining static postures, and by maintaining the direction of Qi using breath control and movement, together with massage, to stimulate the movement of Qi through the meridians.

T'ai chi is a form of Qigong, sometimes referred to as moving meditation, and it involves the use of more formal sequences known as forms. Although most of the research into the efficacy of t'ai chi as a therapeutic intervention has been conducted on more elderly populations, many of the issues addressed, such as the efficacy of t'ai chi in maximising restricted movement, increasing general mobility, increasing the range of joint movements, and promoting balance and flexibility, can be just as relevant to children with restricted movement (Tse & Bailey 1992, Sancier 1996, Wolf et al 1997).

Vickers (1993) reports patients saying that they feel more confident and more aware of their bodies, the slow gentle movements increasing not only their mobility but also their sense of relaxation and wellbeing. Forms of both Qigong and t'ai chi have been adapted for wheelchair users.

Alexander technique

To redress compensatory movements, the Alexander technique is of particular value. The Alexander technique is the art of postural re-alignment leading to the best use of the body, making it more balanced and coordinated and correcting any compensatory patterns of posture or movement, which are common in people with disabilities and can lead to muscle tension, exacerbated pain and increased mobility difficulties. The Alexander technique reconnects mind and body and brings movement into conscious thought. This is helpful since how we use our body affects its function.

Ayurvedic medicine

In Ayurvedic medicine, the vata dosha is responsible for all movements, large or small, through the stimulation of nerves and the transmission of sensory stimuli to initiate motor functions. All problems with mobility would be seen as an imbalance of vata. This would be addressed by a vata-stimulating diet, herbs and massage. For vata conditions, massage with sesame oil, which is warming and heavy, would be used to calm and balance the body.

Anthroposophical medicine

The Anthroposophical approach to children with special physical needs would be embraced by the education arm of Anthroposophical thought, which works in concert with the medical approach. Central to the philosophy of Anthroposophical medicine is the concept of predestination. According to Glöckler and Goebel (1990) the child would have sought this 'hard destiny' for itself and should not be denied, by abortion, the opportunity to experience this. This destiny is thought to be determined by past lives and past deeds. Each disease or condition provides a unique but hidden task and a unique learning opportunity. The Anthroposophical approach to care would include trying to determine what a child's destiny is and how they can learn from it. The special education and medical branches of Anthroposophical thought have set up special communities called the Camphill communities for people of all ages with special needs.

Eurythmy, an Anthroposophical intervention used for a variety of conditions, not all necessarily involving mobility, is delivered by a specially trained therapist under medical supervision. This therapy, which would be part of an individually tailored package of care for a patient, appears in a number of forms, one of which is curative eurythmy. Movements are repeated to help strengthen the body and counteract pathological tendencies. Each movement is devised so that a particular exercise strengthens an area of weakness or reduces over development, aiming to calm, harmonise or stimulate. This system of exercise is also used to treat physical disability and it is aimed at influencing the growth and proportional development of the body.

ABNORMAL MOVEMENT

Problems with mobility include not only the difficulties of limited movement, but also those of abnormal movement such as in epilepsy or hyperactivity.

Epilepsy

Over two-thirds of seizures begin in childhood, and epilepsy has a direct influence on the quality of life for the child and family (Thiele et al 1999). It is estimated that 0.7–0.8% of school age children have epilepsy and in a significant number of cases the cause is idiopathic. An epileptic seizure is a paroxysmal disturbance of consciousness, motor function, sensation, perception, behaviour and emotion resulting from a cortical neuronal discharge (Swaiman 1989). Symptoms can occur singly or in any number of combinations. Seizures present in a number of forms, the most common type in children being grand mal seizures, the majority of which are idiopathic, and petit mal or absence seizures, in which the child loses consciousness for a few moments and may stare vacantly. In petit mal there is no muscle involvement and during the seizure the child remains upright. Simple and complex partial seizures may also occur.

Aromatherapy

Research undertaken by Betts (1996) at The Queen Elizabeth Hospital, Birmingham in relation to grand mal epilepsy has indicated that breathing the vapour of aromatic oil shortly before a seizure can reduce the severity of an attack. However, some oils are known to precipitate a seizure, so care must be taken. Unfortunately, Betts' list of suspect oils does not coincide with that of Tisserand (1994), who points out that reactions to essential oils by epileptics can be idiosyncratic. The system devised and refined by Betts involves patients selecting an aromatherapy oil, following which they have three full body massages with the chosen oil so that they experience feelings of relaxation, which many of them may not have enjoyed before. This is followed by auto-hypnosis training, with a post-hypnotic suggestion that they will feel very relaxed when they smell the oil.

They carry the oil with them and use it if they think they are going to have a seizure. This builds up a conditioned response, sometimes to the extent that the patient can develop a 'smell memory', so that they do not have to have the oil with them but can imagine it at will and so control their seizures. Betts also suggests that because patients gain some control over their seizures, they relax and become more confident, and this has a feedback effect on the seizures themselves. Betts was interested to note that the majority of his patients chose ylang ylang oil in preference to such favourites as lavender and chamomile, and suggests that it might have anti-convulsive properties. At the end of 1 year, 3 out of 25 patients had complete seizure control and were off medication, 7 had complete seizure control but were still on medication, 8 experienced at least a 50% reduction in seizures and an enhanced quality of life, 6 experienced no effect and 1 was worse.

Yamada et al (1994) subjected mice to a number of convulsions following inhalation of lavender essential oil. It was noted that inhaling lavender oil blocked nicotine-induced convulsions, and with electroconvulsive shock, the appearance of tonic extension and clonic convulsions gradually decreased, relative to the dose of lavender. Although the mechanism is not clear, this was thought to result from the augmentation of GABAnergic action (y-aminobutryic acid), a substance occurring mainly in the brain that transmits inhibitory impulses across synapses. Davis (1996) suggests that rosemary oil is anticonvulsive but very sensibly cautions against any aromatherapist treating epilepsy with aromatherapy unless medically trained.

TCM

TCM defines epilepsy as a problem of Phlegm blocking the Orifice of the Heart. As a result there is a functional disorder of Liver-Yin/ Kidney-Yin and this is the cause of most grand mal seizures in childhood, with febrile convulsions being a mild form of this imbalance. Children are particularly vulnerable as they are Yin deficient. Central nervous system (CNS) and congenital anomalies and lesions correlate with Kidney-Yin deficiency, whilst Liver-Yin deficiency is related to metabolic disorders. Babies and small children, who are in the Water stage of development, are particularly vulnerable to Kidney imbalances and neurological disorders.

The physiopathology of grand mal seizures is Liver-Yin deficiency leading to Liver-Yang excess which causes Wind. This Wind is further agitated by Heat and the combination of the two results in the tonic–clonic movements of the fit. Acupuncture is used to tonify Kidney-Yin and Liver-Yin. Prophylactic treatment includes clearing Heat and subduing Wind.

Absence seizures are caused by Liver-Yin/Heart-Yin deficiency. Since Shen or Mind resides in the Heart-Yin, a deficiency results in a brief loss of Mind or Shen. This is caused directly by Liver Wind carrying excess Phlegm which clouds the Heart and stops the Heart from housing the Shen (also a feature of insomnia), obstructing circulation to the eyes and resulting in an absence seizure. Treatment includes subduing internal Wind, dispelling Phlegm, tonifying Kidney and Heart-Yin and calming the Shen.

A number of studies have supported the use of acupuncture in the treatment of epilepsy. Using electro-acupuncture in a series of experiments, Oei et al (1992) demonstrated that high frequency electro-acupuncture will release a neuropeptide, cholecystokin-8, which has anticonvulsive activity. Shi (1987) gave acupuncture to 98 poorly controlled epileptics who were already on a variety of medications. When these patients had electro-acupuncture for 30 minutes in up to 15 treatments,

66% were reported to have had a marked reduction in the frequency of their attacks. In a review of the use of acupuncture in the treatment of epilepsy, Wu (1988) concedes that the use of anticonvulsive medication is indispensable. It is suggested that the concomitant use of acupuncture may be instrumental in reducing the dosage necessary to control the seizures. Encouraging evidence for this was given in a series of experiments on the effects of electro-needling on the actions of the neurotransmitters gamma-aminobutyric acid (GABA) and serotonin and of the hippocampus. Electro-needling reduced the subsidence of epiliform discharges by its direct restoration of attenuated cortical and hippocampal recurrent inhibition.

Herbalism

Mills (1989) suggests that the herb skullcap (*Scutellaria laterflora*) might help to reduce the severity and frequency of symptoms, since it is a central nervous system relaxant and an antispasmodic, although Barnes et al (2002) state that in spite of its traditional use as an anticonvulsant, there is no research at present to validate this claim.

Ayurvedic medicine

In Ayurvedic medicine, epilepsy is referred to as a condition characterised by entering into darkness and bewilderment, with aggravation of the doshas and loss of memory. It is characterised into four types:

1 Red or black auras, foaming at the mouth, biting and grinding teeth, deep breathing.
2 Yellow or red aura, yellow foaming at the mouth, thirst and feeling of heat.
3 White foaming at the mouth, feeling of cold and heaviness, white aura.
4 Mixture of one or more of the above.

It is treated with calamus root (*Acorus calamus*) which, according to Ayurveda, is anticonvulsive. Barnes et al (2002) have reviewed the use of this herb and support the use of the oil in particular as a spasmolytic and an anticonvulsant. Native Americans of the Cree tribe chewed the root for its hallucinogenic and stimulant effect and as an analgesic and anti-diabetic agent (Fetrow & Avila 2001). Shanmugasundaram et al (1991) describe the research into the use of a herbal formula (brahmighritham) for the control of epilepsy. The Ayurvedic formula includes the herbs *Herpestis monniera* (known as thyme leaved gratiola in English), *Cyperus rotundus* (nut grass) and *Saussurea lappa* (kut root). A compound of these herbs mixed with ghee (the dehydrated form of butter obtained from curd or fermented cows' milk) was administered to rats in whom epiliform seizures were induced. The rats were divided into three groups, a control group, an experimental group given brahmighritham, and a group given benzodiazepine for a period of 3 months. Results indicated that protection against induced epiliform seizures was afforded by brahmighritham to the same or better level than benzodiazepine.

Panjawani et al (1995) evaluated the use of Sahaja yoga meditation for stress management in patients with epilepsy. It was a small study of 32 patients who were randomly divided into three groups, one group practising Sahaja yoga, one group mimicking the Sahaja yoga postures and the third group acting as a control.

Baseline measurements were obtained and the patients monitored at 3 and 6 months. Results confirmed earlier reports that Sahaja yoga helped patients cope with the specific stresses associated with their condition. Specifically, measurements of galvanic skin response, blood lactate and urinary-vinyl mandelic acid were significantly improved in group one. These results indicated a reduction in stress in the patients and it is this that is thought to be responsible for the noted clinical improvement which has been reported in patients who practice Sahaja yoga.

Homeopathy and other therapies

Lockie (1990) suggests that epilepsy should be treated homeopathically by using constitutional remedies, although during a fit Cicuta (*Cicuta virosa*) should be given. Cicuta, common name water hemlock, is extremely poisonous in its natural state and causes symptoms similar to strychnine poisoning, with spasms, excessive salivation, sweating and hyperventilation. The constitutional remedy suggested by Herscu (1991) is *Calcarea carbonica* which is made from calcium carbonate derived from oyster shells. This remedy has a wide range of uses, acting mostly on the bones and teeth. In addition, Aconite might be useful after the fit is over and Bach Rescue Remedy can be of value. The calming and relaxing sequence from reflexology can also be helpful.

Attention deficit hyperactivity disorder

Hyperactivity or attention deficit disorder (ADD) and attention deficit hyperactivity disorder (ADHD) are chronic disorders of attention span and impulse control which can begin in infancy and may continue into adult life. A number of factors have been attributed to the development of the disorders, including heredity (parents or grandparents of children with ADD have been found to experience similar difficulties) and birth trauma. In some cases, metal toxicity has been implicated. The condition is characterised by a short attention span, poor impulse control and hyperactivity. Children who suffer from ADD may exhibit the following symptoms:

- Easily distracted
- Difficulty with listening and following directions
- Difficulty in focusing and sustaining attention
- Inconsistent performance in school work
- Difficulty in remaining seated
- General disorganisation in relation to everyday activities
- Poor study skills
- Excessive talking.

Children with ADHD also exhibit hyperactivity. In addition, some of these children may exhibit:

- Trouble with transitions and changes
- Aggressive behaviour
- Social immaturity
- Impulsivity and lack of control
- Low self-esteem and high frustration levels.

When the condition is left untreated it can give rise to school failure, peer rejection and family problems. The aetiology and treatment of the condition is extremely complex.

Conventional treatment

Conventional treatment includes behaviour modification and might include the use of the drug Ritalin (methylphenidate hydrochloride), which is a neurostimulant. The neurons in the regions of the brain that are implicated in executive control are rich in chatecholamines, i.e. dopamine, adrenaline and noradrenaline, in addition to other neurotransmitters such as serotonin, which may have a role in regulating dopamine transmission. The effect of Ritalin is to improve concentration and memory and it also helps to control frustration and anger. It works by raising the levels of resting dopamine, resulting in an increase in the availability of dopamine at dopamine receptor sites. With low dose drug treatment this results in a reduction in the relative rise in dopamine that is triggered by an impulse to move. As is to be expected with a powerful drug, there are side effects which include weight loss, appetite suppression, sleep disturbances and growth retardation.

Special diet

Investigations into hyperactivity in children have highlighted a number of potential causes, among which food intolerance is predominant. The increased use of processed food has led to more children ingesting additives such as food colouring, salicylates, sugars and sweeteners, and preservatives such as tartrazine (E102) and the benzoate preservatives (E210 and 219), all of which have been implicated in hyperactivity (Weiss 1986, Kaplan et al 1989, Kenyon 1993). Schauss (1984), who undertook studies in the USA, noted that simply reducing sugar and identifying and eliminating additives resulted in a marked reduction in antisocial behaviour, with the most aggressive individuals showing the best response. However, Wolraich et al (1985) failed to demonstrate that a sucrose challenge made hyperactive children worse and, taking other studies into account, concluded that the adverse effects associated with sucrose ingestion may be limited to a small subgroup of hyperactive children. In addition to sugars and additives, many hyperactive children can also be sensitive to cows' milk and dairy products (Kenyon 1993) and eliminating these foods can ameliorate many symptoms of hyperactivity.

Carter et al (1993) studied 78 children diagnosed as hyperactive, using a double blind crossover placebo controlled design. The study involved restricting children to a limited diet in order to eliminate possible triggers for ADHD. The results indicated that diet could contribute to behaviour disorders. The effects were not as large as in some trials, but the elimination of trigger foods would appear to work for some children. A further study by Boris and Mandel (1994) discussed the issue of single versus multiple food elimination trials and noted that single food elimination trials had failed to establish a clear link with hyperactivity.

Hyperactive children are frequently zinc deficient and benefit from supplementation. In addition, Davies and Stewart (1987) have suggested that these children may be magnesium deficient. Other supplements which have been suggested include B complex (Kenyon 1993). Part of the reason for zinc deficiency is these children's abnormal thirst, often coupled with ingestion of orange squash or coca cola which speed its excretion. Tartrazine reduces serum and uric zinc, and if a diet of junk food and sweet drinks is added to this, a deficiency in most minerals and vitamins will result.

The work of Dr Ben Feingold in the 1970s on the contributory role of additives on hyperactivity had a significant effect on the way in which hyperactivity was viewed. Although his work was criticised by the medical community, it is now recognised as pioneering in its approach. According to Dr Stephen Barrett, who writes on the Quackwatch web site, there have been no controlled trials to indicate that additives have contributed to the behaviours of the vast majority of children, but this does not prevent us from asking whether there are some children for whom this approach has worked. Success in using the additive exclusion diet is also dismissed with the suggestion that improvement is solely due to the fact that the child is receiving more attention. If only the treatment of ADHD was that easy. Exclusion diets can be trying on parents and children alike and, if not supervised properly, they can lead to serious dietary deficiencies. This is why work on hyposensitivities in children with food sensitivities is so valuable (Egger et al 1992). In Egger et al's trial, subjects followed an exclusion diet for 4 weeks and provoking foods were identified as they were re-introduced into the diet. Following this, patients received three doses of EPD (beta-glucuronidase) and small quantities of food antigens injected intradermally at 2-monthly intervals. Following this, the provoking foods were re-introduced into the diet. Results were encouraging and indicated that EPD permits children with food-induced hyperactivity to enjoy foods which had previously been denied them. However, Thompson (1998) is cautious about crediting many of these findings, stating that the link between hyperactivity and diet is 'very weak' and suggesting that much of the improvement from these studies is due to what she refers to as the more 'structured lifestyle associated with dietary restriction' and the 'encouragement of a daily routine'. Whilst the latter is indisputable, it would seem unnecessarily negative to refute any connection with diet. As paediatric nurses and health visitors are well aware, parenting styles are well established and often very resistant to change and it is highly unlikely that these styles would change suddenly over a 7-day period, which is often all the time needed to wash out the stimulant. Any change in parenting style is more likely to be due to the improved behaviour of the child, which is a response to the change in the diet. The study by Carter et al (1993) mentioned earlier included a measurement of family relationships as one of its outcome measures. They noted that a positive response to the diet was less likely where there was marital discord. However, this state of disharmony was also noted in 13% of the responders and 53% of the non-responders, which means that a large portion of the results were irrespective of family circumstance. The individuality of the child is paramount and most additive-free diets are healthy and inexpensive and may well work for a number of children.

Ayurvedic medicine

In the Ayurvedic framework, ADD and ADHD are seen as the result of vata and/or pitta imbalance. Specifically, they arise from a disturbance of prana vayu, the form of vata that is responsible for all higher cerebral functions. According to Ayurveda the condition may be congenital or acquired and may be the result of anything which provokes vata. Devi (1996) refers to our 'vata provoking society', citing the increased consumption of stimulants such as chocolate, white sugar, coca cola and various other soda type drinks as well as popcorn and chips. Douillard (1996) suggests that in vegetarian societies such as India, ADD is relatively unknown and recommends that a vegetarian diet should be examined as a potential treatment. He goes on to describe the cause of ADD and ADHD as a deficiency of prana or energy. This may seem an odd suggestion since the children appear to exhibit excessive amounts of energy, but this is due to a lack of the calming influence of the prana, which controls the vata system. Without sufficient prana, the nervous system will get out of control, and energy in the form of prana is necessary to calm down the nervous system. It is suggested that a sedative would further reduce the levels of prana. Douillard goes on to suggest that the nerve stimulant Ritalin paradoxically acts in the same way as prana. Devi (1996) notes that vata type hyperactivity will be worse in the autumn, on windy days and at dawn and dusk, and that the child tends to drink excess water and crave sweets and chocolate. Symptoms of vata type hyperactivity include:

- Restlessness
- Inattentiveness
- Wandering mind
- Poor memory
- Nervousness.

Children suffering from the pitta type of ADD more closely resemble children with ADHD in that they exhibit the following symptoms:

- Disordered understanding and comprehension
- Excess energy
- Tantrums
- Displays of anger and frustration.

Treatment of prana vayu disorder of vata includes regular massage with warm sesame oil, warm ginger baths and a vata pacifying diet which encourages the consumption of warm, heavy and oily foods, sweet food, dairy products, specific fruits and vegetables, chicken, turkey and seafood. This diet, which is rich in zinc, is discussed in greater detail in Section 3. Although ADD can be caused by vata or pitta imbalance, this diet can be used for all ADD imbalances because vata controls the nervous system and the diet will be generally calming and rejuvenating.

Of particular value for ADD is the herb Akar karabha (*Anacyclus pyrethrum*). Its active ingredient is anacycline, which acts on the brain improving cerebral perfusion and thus improving memory and understanding. It also works against tremor, and is anticonvulsant, antispasmodic and antidepressant.

Treatment of the pitta version of the disorder includes warm massage and a pitta pacifying diet, including the elimination of yellow and orange dyes, food additives and white sugar, which is in accordance with Western dietary advice. Just as Thompson (1998) attributes much of the success in treating ADD and ADHD to the more structured lifestyle and encouragement of daily routine resulting from dietary restriction, so Ayurveda recognises the importance of family input in treating these conditions. Devi (1996) refers to the vata provoked family that is characterised by fear, anxiety, restlessness, insecurity and disorganisation. The family may relocate frequently and life is unsettled. In a pitta provoked family system, the governing emotion may be anger with much judgemental criticism, and parents may drink heavily or use drugs.

Other general interventions which may be used include pranayama breathing exercises, which were discussed in Chapter 3, meditation, yoga, pancha karma and shirodhara. Pancha karma is a deep cleansing process allowing the body to release excess dosha from the cells and shirodhara is the flow of warm oil to the forehead to balance vata dosha and vata disorders, including insomnia, anxiety or worry. This procedure has been evaluated by Schneider et al (1990) and Waldschutz (1988), both reporting that the subjects had a significant reduction in stress, anxiety and depression. The value of yoga and transcendental meditation is discussed in greater detail in Section 3.

TCM

In TCM, ADD and ADHD are regarded as resulting from a deficiency in Kidney essence (Jing). This deficiency affects brain development, leading to delay in maturation and development. Specifically, there is a deficiency of Kidney-Yin leading to excessive expression of Kidney-Yang, which manifests itself as the hyperactivity of the wandering mind. Kidney-Yin precedes any activity and is the source of deepest tranquillity and the ultimate stillness.

The aim of treatment is to nourish the Kidney-Yin, opening the heart orifices and settling the agitated Yang. The essence or Jing which is housed in the Kidneys is the prenatal foundation of the body and is necessary for brain development and the development of power. The approach to treating this condition may vary from one physician to another, some prescribing a standard herbal preparation, others using different syndrome classifications (Dharmananda 1996, Kaptchuk 2000). The main substances used to treat ADD by Chinese doctors include dragon bone or dragon teeth, oyster shell or mother of pearl, succinum and cinnabar as well as herbs to clear the heart orifices and enhance mental function. These include acorus or sweet flag (*Acorus calamus*), polygala (*Polygalia tenuifolia*), curuma and alpinia (*Alpinia chinensis*).

A number of large scale clinical trials have demonstrated the value of these herbal formularies. In one trial, 66 children were administered the Chinese herbs normally used to treat ADD and ADHD, following TCM diagnosis, which was confirmed by DSM III R criteria (American Psychological Association 1987). The trial demonstrated an 84.8% effectiveness in ameliorating hyperactivity and improving attention span and school performance (Sun et al 1994). A further study using Chinese herbs showed that the results were comparable with Ritalin but there were fewer side effects. A number of clinical trials within the Chinese literature have yielded very positive results (Dharmananda 1996).

The role of acupuncture in the treatment of ADD and ADHD has been examined by Loo et al (1998) using TCM diagnostic criteria and DSM IV diagnostic criteria (American Psychological Association 1994). Laser acupuncture was used and six children in the treatment group showed a reduction in signs and symptoms of ADD.

Field et al (2000) evaluated the effect of t'ai chi on young people with ADD. Although the subjects in this study were adolescents, the technique could equally be applied to younger children. Thirteen adolescents of mixed ethnicity, each with a diagnosis of ADHD, following a baseline week without t'ai chi, then underwent 30 minutes of t'ai chi twice a week for 5 weeks. This was followed by 2 weeks without t'ai chi. At the end of each phase the subjects were assessed (blind) on the Conners Teacher Rating Scale. This rating score covers total hyperactivity with subcategories covering anxiety, antisocial behaviour, conduct, daydreaming and emotion. Results indicated that the subjects exhibited less anxiety, improved conduct, less daydreaming, fewer inappropriate emotions and less hyperactivity during the t'ai chi period compared with the pre-t'ai chi period. These improvements continued over the 2-week follow-up period when no t'ai chi was undertaken. These results echoed the results of other studies on adults, which have demonstrated the beneficial effect of t'ai chi on anxiety levels, showing reduced mental and emotional stress (Jin 1992) and improved mood (Jin 1989).

Other interventions

Research by Field (1998) on the role of massage in the treatment of ADD was carried out on adolescents and positive results were obtained. Scores on the Conners teacher rating scale indicated lower hyperactivity scores. Although Field notes that the mechanism is unclear, she suggests that raised serotonin levels noted in other massage studies may have a regulating effect on the elevated dopamine levels that have been noted in children with ADHD (Rogeness et al 1992).

Herbal and aromatherapy approaches to ADD and ADHD would include calming and relaxing the child, and the sedating effects of certain essential oils and herbs have already been discussed in Chapter 4 on sleep. Lockie (1990) suggests that homeopathic treatment for ADD and ADHD should be constitutional.

Olness and Kohen (1996) express reservation about the use of hypnosis for the treatment of ADD and ADHD but indicate that it can be helpful in lowering anxiety levels, enhancing the child's ability to recognise emotional lability, developing strategies for controlling emotional outbursts, managing associated problems such as sleep and interactions, and modifying attitudes towards school and learning. Research into the use of biofeedback in the treatment of ADD and ADHD has been very promising.

CHRONIC FATIGUE SYNDROME

One condition for which orthodox medicine has little to offer is ME or chronic fatigue syndrome (CFS), also known as post-viral fatigue syndrome, and many sufferers have turned to complementary medicine in order to try to obtain some relief from their symptoms. CFS is a devastating condition, the course of which is variable, but symptoms can include chronic fatigue, muscle and joint pains, muscle weakness, loss of concentration, depression and anxiety, poor sleep patterns and poor memory. Because it is poorly understood and, indeed, denied by some authorities, patients suffer greatly from a lack of support and sympathy. It is not a new disease, having been recorded during the 16th century, and outbreaks have been recorded in Coventry and at the Royal Free Hospital in London. The aetiology of the condition is unclear but certain viruses have been implicated, including the Epstein–Barr and Herpes viruses, since it commonly follows a viral infection. Feelings of tiredness and being 'washed out' are common after flu, but if the condition persists longer than 6 months then CFS is indicated. It has been suggested that some viruses alter the immune system, causing the body to become more vulnerable to external toxins.

Jordan et al (2000) reviewed the prevalence of the condition amongst children and adolescents and noted the difference between how children and adults display symptoms of fatigue: children present with irritability, distraction and fidgeting, whilst adults have difficulty in concentrating, lack energy and complain of tiredness. Adolescents present with adult-type symptoms and are frequently diagnosed as lazy. In the USA, the Center for Disease Control has attempted to estimate the prevalence rate for paediatric CFS. They estimate that the incidence of CFS amongst adolescents aged 12–17 years is 8.7 cases per 100 000. Gender differences indicate that pre-puberty, there are equal numbers of boys and girls with the condition, but in adolescence, the incidence amongst females increases. CFS does not seem to be confined to one social class (Gunn et al 1993, Hickie et al 1996).

In concordance with the notion that the condition presents differently in different people and that treatment should be tailored appropriately, Dowson (1993) reviewed a range of complementary therapies commonly used to treat this condition, including homeopathy, nutrition, acupuncture, healing and psychotherapy.

Nutritional strategies

Peters et al (1996) highlight the following factors which need to be addressed: optimise nutritional status, support the immune system, eliminate infections, eliminate food sensitivities, support the adrenals and reduce stress. However, it would appear that, individually, these interventions have little to offer, with no single treatment being universally effective. Peters et al (1996) suggest that the integrated approach provides more scope for optimism. Although it has been suggested by Truswell (1990) that nutritional supplementation is unnecessary in people who have a healthy diet, and the danger of vitamin toxicity has been highlighted by Evans and Lacey (1986), many CFS sufferers may well be poorly nourished and in a very debilitated state, in which case supplementation could be appropriate. Peters et al (1996) suggest nutritional supplements including B-complex, vitamins C and E, magnesium, zinc and selenium. Zinc is necessary for all cell function and loss of zinc gives rise to an increased susceptibility to oxidative damage, which has been highlighted as a possible contributing factor to CFS. It is necessary for good immune function, although excess doses can result in poor copper and iron absorption. Lack of selenium has been associated with muscle pain and tenderness, but the daily intake should not exceed 200 micrograms (Mason 1995). Of proven value in the treatment of CFS is intramuscular magnesium (Cox et al 1991). Deficiency of the mineral can result in lethargy and apathy, whilst coenzyme Q is reputed to be a free radical scavenger, an antioxidant and a membrane stabiliser. A review of nutritional strategies is offered by Werbach (2000).

Herbal remedies

Useful herbal remedies include St John's wort, hydrastis, which is antibacterial, and echinacea, which is immunity enhancing, with Siberian and Panax ginseng for the adrenals.

TCM

In TCM the exhaustion which is such a prominent feature of ME is said to be due to a weakness in Qi and to Blood deficiency and is also seen as a Damp/Heat problem. The TCM physician would use a combination of acupuncture and herbal medicine. TCM has reported some success with this condition and this is reviewed by Jiang and Franks (1994).

Massage

Field et al (1997) describe a study using massage to help to alleviate the symptoms of CFS. Two groups were established, one that received massage therapy and one that received sham TENS intervention. Both conditions were controlled for time and therapist intervention and pre- and post-session measurements were obtained using the profile of mood states, the state anxiety inventory and a visual analogue scale for pain. Pre- and post-test measurements indicated that depression and anxiety scores as well as pain scores were lower in both groups, but significantly lower in the massage group. Overall measurements taken on the first and last days of treatment in both groups showed reduction in depression and anxiety scores; in addition, the profile of fatigue symptoms score and the pain and sleep symptoms score were both improved. Although the mechanism for this is unclear, the authors suggest that reduced stress levels and enhanced sleep may account for the improvement in fatigue scores.

REFERENCES

American Psychological Association 1987 Diagnostic and statistical manual of mental disorders (DSM III R), revised 3rd edn. American Psychiatric Press, Washington

American Psychological Association 1994 Diagnostic and statistical manual of mental disorders (DSM IV), 4th edn. American Psychiatric Press, Washington

Barnes J, Anderson L, Phillipson J 2002 Herbal medicines: a guide for health care professionals, 2nd edn. Pharmaceutical Press, London

Betts T 1996 Fragrant breeze. Aromatherapy Quarterly 51: 25–27

Boris M, Mandel F 1994 Foods and additives are common causes of the attention deficit hyperactive disorder in children. Annals of Allergy 72(May): 462–468

Carter C, Urbanowicz R, Hemsley R et al 1993 Effects of a restricted food diet in attention deficit disorder. Archives of Diseases in Childhood 69: 564–568

Cox I, Campbell M, Dowson D 1991 Red blood cell magnesium and chronic fatigue syndrome. Lancet 337: 757–760

Davis P 1996 Aromatherapy: an A–Z. CW Daniel, Saffron Walden

Davies S, Stewart A 1987 Nutritional medicine. Pan Books, London

Dearmun A, Taylor A 1995 Nursing support and care: meeting the needs of the child and family with altered mobility. In: Carter B, Dearmun A (eds) Child health care nursing. Blackwell Science, Oxford

Devi A 1996 Ayurvedic specific condition review: attention deficit disorder/ hyperactivity. The Protocol Journal of Botanical Medicine 2(1): 32–39

Dharmananda S 1996 Traditional Chinese specific condition review: attention deficit disorder. The Protocol Journal of Botanical Medicine 2(1): 40–42

Douillard J 1996 Ayurvedic specific condition review: attention deficit disorder. The Protocol Journal of Botanical Medicine 2(1): 35–39

Dowson D 1993 The treatment of chronic fatigue syndrome by complementary medicine. Complementary Therapies in Medicine 1(1): 9–13

Edwards J 1999 Music therapy with children hospitalised for severe injury or illness. British Journal of Music Therapy 13(1): 21–27

Egger J, Stolla A, McEwen L 1992 Controlled trial of hyposensitisation in children with food-induced hyperkinetic syndrome. The Lancet 339(May 9): 1150–1153

Evans C, Lacey H 1986 Toxicity of vitamins: complications of a health movement. British Medical Journal 292(22 Feb): 509–510

Ewin D 1986 Emergency room hypnosis for the burned patient. American Journal of Clinical Hypnosis 26: 9–15

Ewin D 1999 Hypnosis in the emergency room. In: Remes R (ed) Medical hypnosis: an introduction and clinical guide. Churchill Livingstone, Edinburgh

Fetrow C, Avila J 2001 Professional's handbook of complementary and alternative medicines. Springhouse, Pennsylvania

Field T, Sunshine W, Hernandez-Reif M, Quintino O et al 1997 Massage therapy effects an depression and somatic symptoms in chronic fatigue syndrome. Journal of Chronic Fatigue Syndrome 3: 43–51

Field T, Quintino O, Hernandez-Reif M 1998 Adolescents with attention deficit hyperactivity disorder benefit from massage therapy. Adolescence 33: 103–108

Field T 2000 Touch therapy. Churchill Livingstone, Edinburgh

Glöckler M, Goebel W 1990 A guide to child health. Anthroposophical Press, Floris Books, Edinburgh

Gunn W, Connell D, Randall B 1993 Epidemiology of chronic fatigue syndrome: the Centers for Disease Control study. In: Bock G, Whelan J (eds) Chronic fatigue syndrome. Wiley, New York

Herscu P 1991 The homeopathic treatment of children. North Atlantic Books, Berkeley, California

Hickie I, Hooker A, Hadzi-Pavlovic 1996 Fatigue in selected primary settings: socio demographic and psychiatric correlates. Medical Journal of Australia 164: 585–588

Jiang D, Franks P 1994 Analysis of 50 cases of ME treated with Chinese herbs and acupuncture. Journal of Chinese Medicine 44: 13–20

Jin P 1989 Changes in heart rate, noradrenaline, cortisol and mood during t'ai chi. Journal of Psychosomatic Research 33(2): 197–206

Jin P 1992 Efficacy of t'ai chi, brisk walking, meditation and reading in reducing mental and emotional stress. Journal of Psychosomatic Research 36: 361–370

Jordan K, Ayers P, Jahn S et al 2000 Prevalence of fatigue and chronic fatigue syndrome like illness in children and adolescents. Journal of Chronic Fatigue Syndrome 6(1): 3–21

Kaplan BJ, McNicol J, Conter A, Maghadam HK 1989 Dietary replacement in pre-school aged hyperactive boys. Paediatrics 83: 7–17

Kaptchuk T 2000 Chinese Medicine: the web that has no weaver. Rider, London

Kelly K 1998 Integrating holistic nursing care in the treatment of asthma: a case study. Journal of Emergency Nursing 24(6): 489–491

Kenyon J 1993 Hyperactivity: a consideration of the alternatives. Complementary Therapies in Medicine 1: 78–80

Lee C-T, Lei T 1999 Qigong. In: Jones W, Levin J (eds) Essentials of complementary and alternative medicine. Lippincott, Williams & Wilkins, Philadelphia

Lockie A 1990 The family guide to homeopathy. Penguin Books, Middlesex

Loo M, Naeser M, Hinshaw S Laser acupuncture and treatment for ADHD. NIH grant # IR03 MH 56009-01

Mason P 1995 Handbook of dietary supplements. Blackwell Science, Oxford

May L, Carter B 1995 Nursing support and care: meeting the needs of the child and family with altered cerebral function. In: Carter B, Dearmun A (eds) Child health care nursing. Blackwell Science, Oxford

Meadows R, Newell S 2000 Lecture notes in paediatrics. Blackwell Science, Oxford

Miller R 1996 An investigation into the management of spasticity experienced by some patients with multiple sclerosis using acupuncture based on Traditional Chinese Medicine. Complementary Therapies in Medicine 4(1): 58–62

Mills S 1989 The complete guide to modern herbalism. Thorsons, London

Milton D 1998 Using alternative and complementary therapies in the emergency setting. Journal of Emergency Nursing 24(6): 500–508

Mokone S 2000 Qigong and t'ai chi in physical therapy. In: Charman R (ed) Complementary therapies for physical therapists. Butterworth-Heinemann, Oxford

Oei L, Chen X, Van Ree J 1992 Potentiation of electro acupuncture-induced analgesia by CCK-8 antagonist L-365, 260 in Wistar rats but not in acoustically evoked epileptic rats. Acupuncture in Medicine 10: 47–52

Olness K, Kohen D 1996 Hypnosis and hypnotherapy with children. The Guildford Press, London

Panjawani U, Gupta H, Singh S et al 1995 Effect of sahaja yoga practice on stress management in patients with epilepsy. Indian Journal of Physiological Pharmacology 39(2): 111–116

Peters D, Lewis P, Chaitow L 1996 Chronic fatigue. Complementary Therapies in Medicine 4(1): 31–36

Rogeness G, Javors M, Pliszka S 1992 Neurochemistry and child adolescent psychiatry. Journal of the American Academy of Child and Adolescent Psychiatry 31: 765–781

Sancier K 1996 Medical applications of Qigong. Alternative Therapies 2(1): 40–46

Schauss A 1984 Nutrition and behaviour: complex interdisciplinary research. Nutrition and Health 3(1–2): 9–37

Schneider R, Cavanaugh K, Kasture H 1990 Health promotion within a traditional system of natural health care: Maharishi Yurveda. Journal of Social Behaviour and Personality 5(3): 1–27

Shanmugasundaram E, Mohammed Akbar G, Radha Shanmugasundaram K 1991 Brahmighritham, an Ayurvedic herbal formula for the control of epilepsy. Journal of Ethnopharmacology 33: 269–276

Shi Z et al 1987 The efficacy of electro acupuncture on 98 cases of epilepsy. Journal of Traditional Chinese Medicine 7(1): 21

Sun Y, Wang Y, Qu X et al 1994 Clinical observation and treatment of hyperkinesias in children by Traditional Chinese Medicine. Journal of Traditional Chinese Medicine 14(2): 105–109

Swaiman K 1989 Pediatric neurology, principles and practice. Mosby, St. Louis

Taylor A, Lin Y, Snyder A, Eggleston K 1998 ED staff members' personal use of complementary therapies and recommendations to ED patients: a southeastern US regional survey. Journal of Emergency Nursing 24(6): 495–498

Thiele E, Gonzalez-Heydrich J, Riviello J 1999 Epilepsy in children and adolescents.

Child and Adolescent Psychiatric Clinics of North America 8(4): 671–694

Thompson J 1998 Nutritional requirements of infants and young children. Blackwell Science, Oxford

Tisserand R 1994 The art of aromatherapy. CW Daniel, Saffron Walden

Truswell S 1990 who should take vitamin supplements? British Medical Journal 301 (21 July): 135

Tse S, Bailey D 1992 T'ai chi and postural control in the elderly. American Journal of Occupational Therapy 46: 295–300

Vickers A 1993 Complementary medicine and disability: alternatives for people with disabling conditions. Chapman & Hall, London

Waldschutz R 1988 Influence of Maharishi Ayurveda purification treatment on physiological and psychological health. Erfahrungsheilkunde Acta Medica Empirica 11: 720–729

Weiss B 1986 Food additives as a source of behavioural disturbances in children. Neurotoxicology 7: 197–208

Werbach M 2000 Nutritional strategies for treating chronic fatigue syndrome. Alternative Medical Review 5(2): 93–108

Wolf S, Barnhart H, Ellison G 1997 The effect of t'ai chi chuan and computerised balance training on postural stability in older subjects. Physical Therapy 77(4): 371–381

Wolraich M, Milich R, Stumbo P et al 1985 Effects of sucrose ingestion on the behaviour of hyperactive boys. The Journal of Pediatrics 106(4): 675–682

Wu D 1988 Suppression of epileptic seizures with acupuncture: efficacy, mechanism and perspective. American Journal of Acupuncture 16(2): 113–117

Yamanda K, Mimaki Y, Sashida Y 1994 Anticonvulsive effects of inhaling lavender oil vapour. Biological Pharmaceutical Bulletin 17(2): 359–360

9 **Problems related to washing and dressing**

CHAPTER CONTENTS

- **Introduction   134**
- **Eczema   135**
  Aromatherapy   135
  Anthroposophical medicine   136
  Homeopathy   137
  TCM   137
  Herbalism   138
  Hypnosis   139
  Reflexology and Bach flower remedies   139
- **Wound care   140**
  Aromatherapy   140

Herbalism   140
Ayurvedic medicine   142
Anthroposophical medicine   143
Homeopathy   143
- **Burns   143**
  Hypnosis   143
  Massage and music therapy   144
- **Other issues relevant to wound care and burns   144**
- **References   144**

INTRODUCTION

Problems with washing and dressing can be exacerbated by any problem which compromises the integrity of the skin. However, a number of skin conditions will respond well to adjunctive treatment with CAM, frequently resulting in the reduced use of topical steroids, aggravating creams and the long-term use of antibiotics.

Not only is the skin the largest organ of the body, it also has a vital social function and often, even minor skin complaints can cause more anguish than more serious conditions, possibly leading to a negative self-image (Williams 1997).

Price (1999) describes the development of a normal body image as taking place over time and suggests that children begin to map their body, learning about its boundaries and capabilities during their preschool years and later, at school, using their peers to ascertain how acceptable their appearance is to other people. He suggests that altered body image can be defined as a 'state of personal distress defined by the patient which indicates that the body no longer supports self esteem and which is dysfunctional to individuals' (Price 1995).

Two conditions which affect body image are considered here. First eczema, which is debilitating to both the child and the family, is discussed. Secondly, since accidents are the commonest cause of mortality and morbidity in childhood, the role of CAM in wound care, including the treatment of burns, is discussed.

ECZEMA

Eczema is an inflammatory condition presenting as patches of dry skin that become red, scaly and itchy, leading to extensive scratching, which results in lichenification, excoriation and superimposed infections. It has a wide spectrum of clinical manifestation, from small areas of dry skin to a severe, remitting generalised dermatitis requiring hospital treatment. The UK diagnostic criteria (Williams et al 1994a) include six key features distinguishing atopic dermatitis from other inflammatory conditions. Although it can be difficult to provide an accurate estimation of the incidence of atopic eczema in children, recent studies indicate a frequency of between 5% and 10% (Williams 1995) and it appears to be a condition of the more affluent (Williams et al 1994b). In 90% of cases, eczema starts before the age of 5 years and often within the first 3 months of age (Yates et al 1983). There is evidence that the incidence of the condition is increasing, which suggests that there might be an environmental as well as a genetic element to the condition (Williams 1995).

As children start to attend playgroups, and later school, there is a dramatic increase in the size of their immediate peer group. As the child socialises and interacts with others, there is a resulting development of self image and social competence. Children who have physical and psychological problems will be inhibited in this process (Perrin et al 1984). Specifically, children who suffer from eczema have been noted to exhibit emotional disturbances which have been indicated as a precursor to behavioural problems (Daud et al 1993). In one study (Absolon et al 1997), the extent of psychological disturbance in the eczema group was twice that of the comparison group, the degree of disturbance correlating with the severity of the eczema. Of the children with eczema, 80% were noted to have an emotional disorder associated with excessive worries, fears, stomach aches and sleep disorders, although whether these were a result or a precursor of the development of eczema is not clear. The effect of eczema on family life has been documented by Elliott and Luker (1997), and Daud et al (1993) noted that family life suffered increased strain owing to parents' perceptions of having little support and few friends, resulting in their social life becoming very restricted. This was echoed by Lawson et al (1995) who noted that parental stress was related to the parents' perception of the ability of the child to cope with the condition.

Conventional treatments for eczema include the use of emollients, the avoidance of identified allergens, the application of topical steroids, possibly some dietary manipulation and, in severe cases, wet wrapping.

Aromatherapy

Aromatherapy can have an important function as a supportive therapy in the treatment of eczema both at a physical level, as a topical application, and at a psychological level, for its calming and soothing properties. The potential for the use of aromatherapy is supported by a number of studies. Monges et al (1994) investigated the moisturising properties of three gels containing essential oils of mandarin, German chamomile and orange (the botanical origins were not indicated). Subjects acted as their own control and 1 mL of the oils at 5% concentration in identical aqueous gels was applied to four areas on the inner surfaces of the arms of six volunteers. Measurements were taken regularly from each zone for 2 hours after the application of the gels. Results, measured by IRFT spectroscopy and the electrical capacitance of the skin, indicated an immediate effect of the three preparations compared with the control zone. All three gels produced an immediate hydrating effect; however, with the German chamomile gel, the hydration was more intense and had a longer lasting effect compared with the other two gels, and it is thought that the presence of hydrocarbons in the German chamomile may be instrumental in the moisturising process.

Aertgeets et al (1985) compared the use of Kamillosan (chamomile) cream with steroidal (0.25% hydrocortisone, 0.75% fluorcortin butyl ester) and non-steroidal (5% bufexamac) dermatological agents as a maintenance therapy for eczema. The study was carried out over a period of 3–4 weeks and results indicated that the Kamillosan cream was as effective as the 0.25% hydrocortisone but superior to the non-steroidal anti-inflammatory agent (5% bufexamac) as well as to the 0.75% fluorcortin butyl ester.

Anderson et al (2000) investigated the use of essential oils and massage on childhood atopic eczema in children who had not been responsive to conventional therapy. Sixteen children aged between 3 and 7 years were randomly assigned either to a control group, who had a massage without essential oils, or to the experimental group who had a massage with a blend of three essential oils chosen by their mothers. The oils were chosen from marjoram, frankincense, German chamomile, myrrh, thyme, benzoin and spike lavender and, following standard aromatherapy practice, each blend was diluted with almond oil. The children in each group were given a 30-minute massage once a week by a therapist who visited them at home and, in addition, a massage was given each day by their mothers over a period of 8 weeks. Day time irritation and night time disturbances were noted by the mothers, who had been trained in the recording technique. The results showed that there was no difference in improvement scores between the essential oil group and the massage alone group; however, day time irritation scores and night time disturbance rates were reduced in both groups. Unfortunately, this improvement was reversed during two subsequent 8-week treatment periods during which there was a slight exacerbation of the eczema in the essential oil group. The authors suggest that this might be due to two factors: either the reduction of the placebo effect of increased mother–child interaction, or an allergic reaction to the oils. However, looking at the oils chosen by the mothers, better long-term results might have been obtained by using one oil at a time, chosen for its anti-inflammatory activity and calming effect (e.g. chamomile or lavender), since the role of stress and emotional factors in the development and exacerbation of eczema has been identified (Brown 1972, Koblenzer 1988).

Anthroposophical medicine

Within Anthroposophical medicine, the skin is seen to reflect the three-fold nature of humankind, i.e. the nerve–sense pole (because it is a sense organ), the metabolic pole (because it is an organ of excretion) and the rhythmic aspect (because the skin is also an organ of respiration), and many disturbances of the skin are seen as a result of disturbances of the liver. Treatment of eczema will, therefore, include a basic treatment of the liver consisting of Hepatodoron (Fragaria vesca fol. 20%/Vitis vivifera fol. 20%), which is wild strawberry and grape vine and is useful for all liver conditions (Bott 1996). Externally applied remedies might include calendula baths and the use of Balsamicum ointment, which is made up of marigold (*Calendula officinalis*), dog's mercury (*Mercurialis perennis*) Peru balsam tree (*Myroxylon peruiferum*) and antimony (*Stibium*). Calendula, which is antiseptic, anti-inflammatory and immunostimulant, has been in use as a skin healer since ancient times. Research supports its traditional use as a wound healer, its anti-inflammatory effects and its value in dermatological conditions (Boucard-Maitre et al 1988, Akihisa 1996), and its stimulation of physiological regeneration and epithelisation (Kioucek-Popova et al 1982).

Homeopathy

In the homeopathic approach to care, eczema is not regarded as one but a range of presentations, which are treated individually. Graphites is the key remedy for skin conditions and the treatment of choice for the eczema that presents as weepy, particularly behind the ears. It is known to be excellent for skin complaints and was proved by Hahnemann after he noted that workmen who worked in a mirror factory were using graphite to heal cold sores. For dry, itchy skin Alumia (*aluminium oxide*, the base for gems such as ruby, emerald and sapphire) is prescribed, whilst dry, sensitive skin which is prone to infection will respond to Psorinium. Psorinium, which was 'proved' by Hahnemann in 1833, is one of the nosodes, which means it is prepared from attenuated disease matter, in this case the scabies vesicle. Sulphur is recommended for dry, red, rough itchy skin made worse by washing or heat.

TCM

In Traditional Chinese Medicine, as in Anthroposophical medicine, the link between the skin and lungs is acknowledged. In addition, it is the function of the Kidneys to nourish and moisten the skin. Eczema is the result of the accumulation of Heat and Damp combined with Blood and Yin deficiency. Other internal organs which can be involved include Lung, Spleen, Kidney and Liver. There are two basic types of eczema in children, Wind/Heat and Damp/Heat eczema, and both are due to a deficiency of Lung and Kidney Defensive Qi, the Wind/Heat type being more related to the Lungs, and the Damp/Heat type to the Kidneys. Eczema due to Damp/Heat is moist, oozing fluid, and red and itchy, whilst Wind/Heat eczema is very dry, red and itchy.

Itching, which is such a distressing aspect of eczema and the cause of so much damage to the skin, is seen in TCM as the result of Lung imbalance. The Lung houses the Corporeal Soul which is responsible for the child experiencing excessive physical sensations such as intense itching. Treatment is aimed at dispersing Heat and Damp and tonifying chronic deficiencies in chronic eczema. Herbs may be applied externally and acupuncture would also be part of the treatment. Loo (2002) points out that acupuncture has been found to be successful for itching in eczema, as do Lun and Rong (2000) and Sun and Wang (1996).

Scott (1994) describes the use of acupuncture in the treatment of infantile eczema, indicates the acupuncture points which would be used, and recommends the topical use of the Western herb heartsease (pansy) to reduce irritation.

Atherton et al (1992) describe the effective use of Chinese herbs in the treatment of eczema in children. It came to the notice of a number of clinicians in the dermatology department of Great Ormond Street Hospital that some of the children attending the clinic, who had not hitherto responded to Western medicine, were suddenly getting better. It transpired that the childrens' parents were taking them to a Chinese doctor who was prescribing a collation of individually prescribed TCM herbs for the treatment of their eczema. The Western clinicians were so impressed with the results of this treatment that they subsequently undertook a clinical trial using a protocol of symptoms and one of four pre-prepared tea bags of the herbs. Following TCM tradition, the herbs represented a hierarchy of effect, as described in Chapter 1. Although TCM treatments are normally prescribed individually, it was agreed that for the purpose of the clinical trial, four standard prescriptions would be used, the Chinese doctor indicating which type of patients should have which prescription. A placebo controlled double blind trial of a specific prescription of ten Chinese herbs was undertaken with 47 selected children who had non-exudating atopic eczema. Preparation of the medicine involved boiling the herbs for 90 minutes and taking the decoction orally. The patients were assessed and scored on erythema and surface damage. It was found that two-thirds of the treated children had a 60% reduction in eczema activity scores, although this was smaller than the reduction obtained by the Chinese doctor using individual prescriptions. It was shown that Chinese herbs were effective as a treatment for atopic eczema in children. Research by Latchman et al (1996) indicated that the herbal prescriptions have the ability to target various immunological parameters which may be involved in the pathogenesis of eczema.

Herbalism

The anti-allergic and anti-inflammatory activities of the herbs German and Roman chamomile, through the inhibition of histamine release, have been well documented (Issac 1979, Tubaro 1984, Mann & Staba 1986). Chamomile can be used both internally, where it exerts a calming effect, and externally as a topical application. Using the croton oil test (a local skin irritant) and comparing German chamomile in a cream base, hydrocortisone ointment and a simple cream base, the chamomile cream exhibited 70% of the activity of the hydrocortisone ointment. In a similar experiment an experimentally produced toxic contact dermatitis was induced in volunteers and was treated with chamomile ointment which was compared with an ointment base and a 1% hydrocortisone acetate. The chamomile ointment demonstrated a superior soothing effect in comparison with the hydrocortisone acetate (Albring et al 1983). In a large-scale survey of general practitioners, it was reported that good therapeutic effect was obtained from a chamomile cream containing 2% standardised herbal extract, and the use of this cream allowed for a reduction in the level of topical steroids used. In addition to using a topical application, a medical herbalist would address all aspects of the person's life and might suggest a calming prescription addressed specifically to the person's eliminative system, since the functioning of this system is considered to be relevant to the treatment of eczema and other skin disorders.

Hypnosis

Shenefelt (2000) has reviewed the use of hypnosis in dermatology and has identified a range of conditions for which it is of value, including warts, urticaria and verrucas. Unfortunately, there have been few large-scale clinical trails on the role of hypnosis in dermatology (Sokel et al 1993, Stewart & Thomas 1995), although it has been demonstrated to be useful in controlling physiological processes (Dikel & Olness 1980, Olness 1986). This facility can be applied appropriately in clinical settings (Olness 1986). The use of hypnosis in the treatment of eczema might include using images of coolness, water, snow or wind, as well as post-hypnotic suggestions as an adjunct to habit reversal techniques, to reduce and interrupt the itch/scratch/itch cycle, or the use of glove anaesthesia (mentioned in Chapter 5 on pain relief). Hypnosis is also of great value in addressing the psychological issues relating to eczema, such as self-confidence, learning to ignore other peoples' comments on the state of the child's skin, improving sleep patterns and the general reduction of stress and anxiety, which can contribute to the exacerbation of the problem. In a very detailed study Laidlaw et al (1996) demonstrated that subjects could reduce the size of an experimentally generated histamine-induced weal in response to self-hypnotic suggestion, following a histamine titration series. A variety of suggestions were used to effect the change, including the suggestion that the histamine solution was just water, or imagining that there was a protective layer over the skin. Some subjects created their own visualisations. The majority of the participants were able to decrease the size of the weals, even the larger, more itchy weals produced by the high concentrations of histamine.

Sokel et al (1993) described the treatment of atopic eczema in children with hypnosis and biofeedback, specifically to reduce the subjective experience of itching (and, therefore, scratching). Forty-four children aged between 5 and 15 years took part in a controlled trial using either hypnosis or biofeedback based on galvanic skin resistance as relaxation techniques, whilst a third control group took part in group discussions about eczema. Results showed no improvement in the percentage of the body covered by eczema, but the amount of lichenification and surface damage was significantly reduced, compared with its original severity, by visit three in the hypnosis and biofeedback groups, compared with the discussion group. There was no difference in reduction between the hypnosis and biofeedback groups. There would seem to be a case for using biofeedback or hypnosis to reduce scratching and interrupt the scratching/itching/scratching cycle.

Reflexology and Bach flower remedies

Chronic conditions such as eczema may respond well to interventions such as reflexology, where treatment would include calming and relaxing sequences, leading to increased feelings of calm and wellbeing (Thomas 1989), as well as the active massaging of the specific reflex zones related to the areas afflicted with the eczema. Since the skin is an organ of elimination, additional reflex areas that would be massaged include those related to the excretory organs and the lungs. Children who are taking the Bach flower remedies may have a prescription containing Crab apple for feelings of self-hatred and uncleanliness, common in many children who suffer from eczema, Gentian for discouragement and despondency, which occur when the condition repeatedly flares up after periods of acquiescence, and Agrimony for putting on a brave face in a depressing situation. As previously stated, all Bach flower remedies can be taken alongside conventional medication.

WOUND CARE

Gelbart (1998) reviews the history of wound care from ancient times, when the main treatment was the application of mud and leaves. Sesame oil was used in Babylon around 2250 BC and is thought to inhibit the action of staphylococcus. Honey and sugar were staple agents and wounds might be irrigated with sea water (advocated by Hippocrates 460–370 BC) or vinegar (advocated by Celsius, 25 BC–50 AD). The Romans treated wounds with myrrh, which has been shown to be bacteriostatic against *Staphylococcus aureus*. The physician Galen advocated the use of wine as a wound cleanser. Wound sepsis was a continuing problem and it was poorly understood. Before the advent of antibiotics, wound infection was mainly due to haemolytic streptococcus; now, however, since the development of methicillin-resistant staphylococcus aureus (MRSA), *Staphylococcus aureus* is the predominant pathogen isolated from wounds, followed by *E. coli.*, *Streptococcus faecalis* and *Pseudomonas aeruginosa*.

Aromatherapy

As we have seen in Chapter 3, essential oils have bacteriostatic properties although their role in wound care has yet to be firmly established. In an excellent review of the use of essential oils in wound care, Baker (1998) raises the issue of the lack of consensus on oil use between aromatherapists. In particular, there is no definition of what constitutes a small wound, there is some discrepancy in views on how the oils should be applied to the wounds, and no references are given. Of particular concern to Baker is the advice given on the use and management of dressings which is at variance with current wound care practice. Bearing in mind that aromatherapy books are available to the general public who may not be aware of current practices in wound care, nurses may need to modify the patients' application and use of essential oils. One good example of this is the use of lavender oil on burns. Tiran (2000) tells the story of Gattefoss, the originator of modern aromatherapy, who burned himself in his laboratory, plunged his hand into a bowl of lavender oil and reported that his hand healed up very quickly and without any scarring. However, practitioners need to be aware that the St John's Ambulance and the British Red Cross Society do not recommend the use of any oils or ointments on a burn as a first aid measure.

Herbalism

The use of honey as a wound cleanser and a promoter of healing has been known for 4000 years. It promotes granulation and tissue formation, is antimicrobial and reduces oedema (Efem 1988, in Bone 1994). The key ingredient has been identified as hydrogen peroxide which is formed as a result of glucose oxidase from the bee with glucose in diluted honey (White & Stubers 1963). Allen et al (1991) noted that New Zealand honey from one specific source, Manuka, was superior to 26 other types of honey against *Staphylococcus aureus*. Comparing the honey with another monofloral honey (*Knightia excela*) against a number of wound pathogens, Manuka honey showed superior results against *E. coli* and *Staphylococcus aureus*, whilst *Knightia excela* was more responsive to *Streptococcus pyogene* and *Salmonella typhus*. However, neither was particularly active against *Pseudomonas aeruginosa* and *Proteus mirabilis*, which are common contaminants of Superficial wounds. However, as Postmes et al (1993, in Bone 1994) point out, the composition of honey is not always constant and it may contain traces of pesticides or drugs used in bee keeping. They suggest that the highest possible standards must be maintained if honey is to be used for medicinal purposes: it must be sterile and free of any contaminants, and more research is needed into its use.

Another bee product, already mentioned in Chapter 3, that has a key role in the treatment of wounds is propolis, which has been used since ancient times to heal sores and ulcers. Today, it is still used regularly in Eastern Europe. Propolis has been shown to be effective against *Staphylococcus aureus*, although less effective when compared with standard antibiotics (Scheller 1977, in Bone 1994). However, in vitro tests have demonstrated that propolis can potentiate the action of other antibiotics (Kivalkina & Gorshunova 1973, in Bone 1994) and antibiotic resistant strains of *Staphylococcus aureus* have become sensitive to the antibiotics erythromycin, tetracycline and penicillin when the drugs were combined with propolis (Shub et al 1981, in Bone 1994).

One trial of propolis on patients with infected wounds found that external treatment with propolis accelerated wound healing, with half of the invading organisms disappearing within 4 days (Damyanliev et al 1982, in Bone 1994). (Scheller et al 1980, in Bone 1994) in demonstrated that topical use of propolis on surgical wounds, burns and ulcers achieved up to 80% faster healing rate when compared with conventional healing methods.

Other wound care treatments include the herb St John's wort which will be discussed again in Section 3. Paracelsus describes it in the treatment of wounds as follows: 'Its virtue is beyond all description, how great it truly is and what can be achieved by it … it is not possible that any better remedy for wounds will be found in any country.' One of the reasons it was used as a remedy was the ancient doctrine of signatures, based on the concept that the therapeutic properties were reflected in the herb's shape and colour. When the leaves of the St John's Wort are crushed they stain the fingers red, thus giving the idea that they are good for stopping bleeding and, according to Culpeper, 'it is a singular wound herb … it heals inward hurts and bruises … and as an ointment closes up the lips of wounds' (Culpeper 1653). Hahn (1992) reviews its use against *Staphylococcus aureus* in the form of hyperforin, and it is anti-inflammatory and anti-ulceric (Berghofer & Holzl 1989).

Comfrey (*Symphytum officinale*) is an impressive local healing agent for wounds and slow healing ulcers. Also known as bone knit, its claim to be a miracle worker is pre-eminent. Its leaf structure contains more protein than any other member of the vegetable family (Bremness 1995). The leaf and roots contain allantoin, which encourages cell division, and mucilage, which promotes the reconstruction of tissue (Bremness 1995). Wound healing and analgesic activities have been shown in animal studies (Goldman 1985). The toxicity of comfrey has been under debate for some time. Two incidents of hepatotoxicity have been reported following ingestion of comfrey. In both incidents, the ingestion was chronic and resulted in veno-occlusive disease, whilst acute toxicity can result in hepatic necrosis. Liver damage is by no means inevitable, as demonstrated by Anderson and McLean (1989) who examined 29 chronic users of comfrey who showed no signs of hepatotoxicity. However, it is now recommended that comfrey be used only on intact skin (Barnes et al 2002), although Mills (1993) points out that some species of comfrey are lower in alkaloids than others and suggests that drying and metabolising the herb further reduces their availability. He further points out that the leaf has always been shown to have negligible quantities of the alkaloid.

In animal studies, aloe vera (*Aloe barbadenis*) in a gel preparation it has been shown to be effective against radiation burns, skin ulcers and peptic ulcers (Parmar 1986). Clithra et al (1998) demonstrated the use of aloe vera in healing dermal wounds on diabetic rats. Following serial examination of the wounds, results indicated that aloe vera enhanced the healing process by influencing each of the healing phases, i.e. inflammation, fibroplasias, collagen synthesis and maturation and wound contraction. It was thought that the effect of the gel was due to its hypoglycaemic properties. The role of aloe vera as an anti-inflammatory agent was demonstrated by Vazquez et al (1996) using the classic induced oedema in a rat's paw. In the treatment of pressure sores to assist healing, aloe vera exhibited an anaesthetic reaction, antibiotic reaction and increased local microcirculation (Cuzzell 1986). The action of the aloe vera gel is said to be related to the high water content of the gel (Grindlay & Reynolds 1986) and the sugars within the gel are thought to inhibit bacterial growth. It has been suggested that the gel mimics modern polysaccharide hydrogel and hydrocolloid dressings. In vivo studies have reported activity against *Pseudomonas aeruginosa*, *Staphylococcus aureus*, *E. coli* and *Klebsiella pneumoniae* (Grindlay & Reynolds 1986). Marshall (1990) summarised some of the problems in evaluating aloe vera, stating that few of the studies are precise enough in identifying the exact species of aloe vera or the plant part from which the gel is extracted, and that more good research is needed. In a review of the research since 1986 into the action of aloe vera, Reynolds and Dweck (1999) state that research has largely upheld the therapeutic claims for the plant.

Ayurvedic medicine

In Ayurveda, aloe vera is regarded as a general tonic for the liver. Its effects are anti-vata, anti-pitta and anti-kapha so it is generally rebalancing. It is seen to have cooling properties and is used with the herb turmeric for the treatment of burns and traumatic wounds. Turmeric has anti-inflammatory properties, and is a general tonic and a natural antibiotic. Traditionally, ghee is said to pacify all three doshas, and imbalances of the three doshas affects the body's natural resistance or agni, which leaves the body vulnerable to infection. Ghee promotes the healing of wounds and is used locally on burns. Honey is recognised for its healing properties and is seen as a warming substance, acting to reduce vata and kapha. A ghee made from licorice is also used on septic wounds.

Anthroposophical medicine

Anthroposophical medicine suggests that wounds are washed with calendula 20% and that burns are treated with compresses of combudoron, which is later used as an ointment. Combudoron consists of a blend of leopard's bane (*Arnica montana*) and nettle (*Urtica urens*). Wound healing in Anthroposophical medicine is related to the polarity principle. The original wound, exhibiting signs of inflammation and pain, indicates increased activity of the astral body and ego (heat). As the wound starts to heal, the etheric body regenerates the destroyed tissues. When the wound heals, the etheric body partly withdraws and the astral body resumes its actions.

Homeopathy

The homeopathic approaches to wound care and pain (Ch. 5) should be considered in conjunction with one another, and the specific types of wounds and their presenting symptoms indicate specific remedies. Gemmell (1997) cautions against leaving infected wounds too long and recommends hospital or medical referral if the patient is feeling feverish and unwell, or if the wound is exuding any pus. However, for minor, clean wounds a homeopath may recommend bathing the area with Calendula lotion and taking Calendula to stimulate healing, Aconite for shock and Arnica to reduce bruising. Since some parents who use homeopathic remedies may not have had their children inoculated, they should be appraised of the dangers of tetanus and urged to have the anti-tetanus vaccine. Puncture wounds, for example animal bites, would be treated with *Ledum palustre*, however all animal bites must be referred for medical attention, although homeopathic remedies may be given at the same time.

BURNS

Hypnosis

An American doctor, Dabney Ewin, who is also a professor of psychiatry and surgery has pioneered the use of hypnosis in the emergency department, specifically in the early treatment of burns. He contends that suggestions to patients that they are feeling cool and comfortable, and that the burn is already beginning to heal, should be made as early as possible after the incident and that paramedics should be trained to use hypnosis in this way. Ewin points out that patients coming into the emergency department following a trauma are in a 'trance equivalent state' and are particularly responsive to suggestion. The use of entonox will also induce this condition. Although a review of the evidence for the effectiveness of hypnosis specifically for wound care has suggested that the evidence is slim, Olness and Kohen (1996) suggest that because hypnosis is successfully used on children in the treatment of other dermatological conditions, its use in this way is quite reasonable. As has already been seen, hypnosis can induce and enhance sleep as well as helping with stress and anxiety, encouraging a more healing environment, and many of the hypnosis techniques suggested in Chapter 5 on pain may be utilised during dressing changes or burn debridement. A pilot study was undertaken by van der Does et al (1988) with a group of burns patients including two adolescents, both of whom used self-hypnosis successfully for pain control. Betcher (1960) describes the successful use of hypnosis for dressing changes with a 10-year-old girl who suffered third degree burns. Later, further surgery was needed for which a general anaesthetic was unsuitable and hypnosis was used as the main anaesthetic agent.

Massage and music therapy

Field et al (1998) conducted a study on the use of massage therapy prior to burn debridement, to reduce anxiety and to alleviate pain during the procedure. Pain from burns treatment, i.e. cleansing and debridement, is described as short but intense and may be more painful and distressing than the burn itself (Andreasen et al 1972). Subjects were offered a 5 day course of massage therapy lasting for 30 minutes prior to burn debridement. Results indicated that these patients had lower levels of depression and anxiety, lower cortisol levels and reduced pain. Prenser et al (2001) describe the use of music in reducing pain and anxiety in the management of burn treatment in a number of case studies, using music as an aid to relaxation and as a diversionary tactic.

OTHER ISSUES RELEVANT TO WOUND CARE AND BURNS

CAM techniques and interventions described in earlier chapters of this book may also be useful in wound care. For example, effective wound healing requires good nutrition, which is impossible if patients are suffering from loss of appetite or nausea and vomiting (Ch. 6). Chapters 4 and 5 on sleep and pain control will be relevant, as well as some aspects of Chapter 7 on elimination related to constipation, often a problem if the child is seriously injured or burned and confined to bed. During recovery, normal physiotherapy might be augmented by the use of massage, yoga and t'ai chi, affecting the body's 'vitality' (Mokone 2000), which underpins the body's ability to regenerate and grow. It has been noted in earlier chapters that Qigong has been shown to increase feelings of wellbeing and to enhance balance and body and spatial awareness. This is particularly valuable if medical treatment has resulted in a change of body image, since it is also a force by which children can re-map their new body.

REFERENCES

Absolon C, Cotterell S, Elmridge S, Glovers M 1997 Psychological disturbance in atopic eczema: the extent of the problem in school age children. British Journal of Dermatology 137: 241–245

Aertgeerts P, Albring M, Klaschka F 1985 Comparative testing of Kamillosan cream and steroidal (0.25% hydrocortisone, 0.75% fluorcortin butyl ester) and non steroidal (5% bufexamac) dermatological agents maintenance therapy of eczematous diseases. Zeitsher Hautkrankh 60: 270–277

Akihisa T 1996 Triterpene alcohols from the flowers of compositae and their anti-inflammatory effects. Phytochemistry 43: 1255–1260

Albring M, Albrecht H, Alcorn G et al 1983 Methods and Findings in Experimental and Clinical Pharmacology 5(8): 575–577

Allen K 1991 A survey of antibacterial activity of some New Zealand honeys. Journal of Pharmacy and Pharmacology 43: 817–822

Anderson P, McLean A 1989 Comfrey and liver damage. Human Toxicology 8: 55–74

Anderson C, Lis-Balchin M, Kirk-Smith M 2000 Evaluation of massage with essential oils on childhood atopic eczema. Phytotherapy Research 14: 452–456

Andreasen N, Noyes R, Hartford C 1972 Factors influencing adjustment of burn patients during hospitalisation. Psychosomatic Medicine 34: 517–526

Atherton D, Sheehan M, Rustin M et al 1992 Treatment of atopic eczema with traditional Chinese medicinal plants. Pediatric Dermatology 9(4): 373–375

Baker J 1998 Essential oils: a complementary therapy in wound management. Journal of Wound Care 7(7): 355–357

Barnes J, Anderson L, Phillipson J 2002 Herbal medicines: a guide for health care professionals, 2nd edn. Pharmaceutical Press, London

Berghofer R, Holzl J 1989 Isolation of 13', 118-biapigenin (amentoflavone) from Hypericum perforatum. Planta Medica 55: 91

Betcher A 1960 Hypnosis as an adjunct to anaesthesiology. New York State Journal of Medicine 60: 816–822

Bone K 1994 Propolis: a natural antibiotic. Australian Journal of Medical Herbalism 6(3): 61–65

Bott V 1996 Spiritual science and the art of healing: Rudolf Steiner's anthroposophical medicine. Healing Arts Press, Vermont

Boucard-Maitre Y 1988 Cytotoxic and anti tumoral activity of Calendula officinalis extracts. Pharmazie 43: 220

Bremness L 1995 Herbs. Dorling Kindersley, London

Brown D 1972 Stress as a precipitant factor of eczema. Journal of Psychosomatic Research 16: 321–327

Clithra P, Sajithlal G, Chandrakasan G 1998 Influence of aloe vera on the healing of dermal wounds in diabetic rats. Journal of Ethnopharmacology 59(3): 195–201

Cuzzell R 1986 Readers' remedies for pressure sores. American Journal of Nursing 86: 923–924

Daud L, Garralda M, David T 1993 Psychosocial adjustment in pre-school children with atopic eczema. Archives of Disease in Childhood 69: 670–676

Dikel W, Olness K 1980 Self-hypnosis, biofeedback and voluntary peripheral temperature control in children. Pediatrics 66(3): 335–340

Efem S 1988 Clinical observations on the wound healing properties of honey. British Journal of Surgery 75 (July): 679–681

Elliott B, Luker K 1997 The experiences of mothers caring for a child with severe atopic eczema. Journal of Clinical Nursing 6: 241–247

Field T, Peck M, Burman I, Krugman S 1998 Massage therapy effects on burn patients. Journal of Burn Care and Rehabilitation 19: 241–244

Gelbart M 1998 Time's great healers. Nursing Times 94(34): 65–68

Gemmell D 1997 Everyday homoeopathy. Beaconsfield Publishers, Beaconsfield, UK

Goldman R 1985 Wound healing and analgesic effect of crude extracts of Symphytum officinale. Fitoterapia 6: 323–329

Grindlay D, Reynolds T 1986 The aloe vera phenomenon: a review of the properties and modern uses of the leaf parenchyma gel. Journal of Ethnopharmacology 16: 117–151

Hahn G 1992 Hypericum perforatum (St John's Wort): a medicinal herb used in antiquity and still of interest today. Journal of Naturopathic Medicine 3(1): 94–96

Isaac O 1979 Pharmacological investigations with compounds of chamomile. Planta Medica 35: 118–124

Kioucek-Popova E 1982 Influence of the physiological regeneration and epithelization using fractions isolated from Calendula officinalis. Acta Physiologica et Pharmacologica Bulgarica 8: 63–67

Koblenzer C 1988 Stress and the skin: significance of emotional factors in dermatology. Stress Medicine 4: 21–26

Laidlaw T, Booth R, Large R 1996 Reduction of skin reactions to histamine after a hypnotic procedure. Psychosomatic Medicine 58(3): 242–248

Latchman Y, Banerjee P, Poulter L et al 1996 Association of immunological changes with clinical efficacy in atopic eczema patients treated with traditional Chinese herbal therapy. (Zemaphyte) International Archives of Allergy and Immunology 109(3): 234–239

Lawson V, Lewis-Jones M, Reid P 1995 Family impact of childhood atopic eczema. British Journal of Dermatology 133(suppl 45): 19

Loo M 2002 Pediatric acupuncture. Churchill Livingstone, Edinburgh

Lun X, Rong L 2000 Twenty-five cases of intractable cutaneous pruritus treated by auricular acupuncture. Journal of Traditional Chinese Medicine 20(4): 287–288

Mann C, Staba E 1986 The chemistry, pharmacology and commercial formulations of chamomile. In: Mann C, Staba E (eds) Herbs, spices and medicinal plants: recent advances in botany, horticulture and pharmacology, vol 1. Oryx Press, Arizona

Marshall J 1990 Aloe vera gel: what is the evidence? Pharmaceutical Journal 244: 360–362

Mills S 1993 The essential guide to herbal medicine. Penguin Books, Harmondsworth

Mokone S 2000 Qigong and t'ai chi in physical therapy. In: Charman R (ed) Complementary therapies for physical therapists. Butterworth-Heinemann, Oxford

Monges P, Joachim G, Bohor M et al 1994 Comparative in vivo study of the moisturising properties of three gels containing essential oil: mandarin, German chamomile and orange. Nouvelle Dermatologie 13(6): 470–475

Olness K 1986 Hypnotherapy with children: new approach to solving common paediatric problems. Postgraduate Medicine 79: 95–105

Olness K, Kohen D 1996 Hypnosis and hypnotherapy with children. Guildford Press, London

Parmar N 1986 Evaluation of aloe vera leaf exudate and gel for gastric and duodenal anti ulcer activity. Fitoterapia 57: 380–381

Perrin E, Gerrity S 1984 Development of children with chronic illness. Pediatric Clinics of North America 31(1): 19–31

Postmes T, van den Bogaard S, Hazen M 1993 Honey for wounds, ulcers and skin graft preservation. Lancet 341(8847): 756–757

Prenser D, Yowler C, Smith L et al 2001 Music therapy for assistance with pain and anxiety management in burn treatment. Journal of Burn Care and Rehabilitation 22(1): 83–88

Price B 1995 Assessing altered body image. Journal of Psychiatric and Mental Health Nursing 2(3): 169–175

Price B 1999 Altered body image. Nursing Times Clinical Monograph no 29. Emap Healthcare, London

Reynolds T, Dweck A 1999 Aloe vera leaf gel: a review update. Journal of Ethnopharmacology 15(68): 3–37

Scott J 1994 Treatment by acupuncture: infantile eczema. Journal of Chinese Medicine 45(May): 9–13

Shenefelt P 2000 Hypnosis in dermatology. Archives of Dermatology 136(3): 393–399

Sokel B, Kent C, Lansdown R et al 1993 A comparison of hypnotherapy and biofeedback in the treatment of childhood atopic eczema. Contemporary Hypnosis 10(3): 145–154

Stewart A, Thomas S 1995 Hypnotherapy as a treatment for atopic dermatitis in adults and children. British Journal of Dermatology 132: 778–783

Sun Y, Wang D 1996 Acupuncture treatment of dermopathies and pediatric diseases. Journal of Traditional Chinese Medicine 16(3): 214–217

Thomas M 1989 Fancy footwork. Nursing Times 85(41): 42–44

Tiran D 2000 Complementary therapies for pregnancy and childbirth, 2nd edn. Baillière Tindall, Edinburgh

Tubaro A 1984 Evaluation of anti inflammatory activity of a chamomile extract after topical application. Planta Medica 50: 359

Van der Does A, Van Dyke R, Spijker R 1988 Hypnosis and pain in patients with severe burns: a pilot study. Burns 14(5): 399–404

Vazquez B, Avila G, Escalante B 1996 Anti-inflammatory activity of extracts from aloe vera gel. Journal of Ethnopharmacology 55(1): 69–75

White J, Stubers M 1963 Studies in honey inhibine. 2. A chemical assay. Journal of Apicultural Research 2: 93–100

Williams H 1995 On the definition and epidemiology of atopic dermatitis. Dermatological Clinics 13(3): 649–657

Williams H 1997 Dermatology health care needs assessment. In: Stevens A, Rafferty J (eds) The epidemiology based needs assessment review. Radcliffe Medical Press, Oxford

Williams H, Burney P, Hay R et al 1994a The UK Working Party's diagnostic criteria for atopic dermatitis. 1. Derivation of a minimum set of discriminators for atopic dermatitis. British Journal of Dermatology 131: 383–396

Williams H, Strachan D, Hay R 1994b Childhood eczema: disease of the advantaged? British Medical Journal 308: 1132–1135

Yates V, Kerr R, MacKie R 1983 Early diagnosis of infantile seborrhoeic dermatitis and atopic dermatitis clinical features. British Journal of Dermatology 108: 633–638

SECTION CONTENTS

Chapter 10 Problems with communication 151
Chapter 11 Problems related to sleep 162
Chapter 12 Problems related to expressing sexuality 167
Chapter 13 Problems related to washing and dressing 177
Chapter 14 Problems with eating and drinking 185
Chapter 15 Problems with elimination 192
Chapter 16 Problems related to working and playing 196

INTRODUCTION

Section 2 has laid the foundation for the use of CAM with children in a range of clinical situations, and many of the problems and treatments that have been addressed in the previous chapters are just as relevant to adolescents. However, Section 3 will concentrate on the problems specific to adolescence, and will upgrade the interventions suggested in Section 2, as appropriate, although there may be some repetition of material. Again, Roper's categories have been adopted as a framework.

ADOLESCENCE

The developmental stage of adolescence, generally regarded as between 12 years and 18 years, has been described by Piaget as the years of formal operational thinking and the development of abstract thought, while Erikson sees adolescence as the stage of identity versus role confusion. The successful completion of this stage leads to the emergence of a psychosocial identity and the attainment of a durable set of values.

In Chinese culture adolescence corresponds to the Fire Element and key organs at this stage of development are the Heart (seat of passion) and the House of Shen (Spirit and Mind), the development of which enables the adolescent to deal with abstract thought since the Mind is able to go beyond concrete operations into formal operations and encompass a far wider view of the world and the universe. An unbalanced Fire in adolescence can lead to dangerous behaviour and reckless passion, with serious consequences. Such young people present as rebellious, trying to establish themselves as separate in identity from their parents (Loo 2002).

Anthroposophical medicine sees adolescence as starting at around 14 years, at the beginning of the third 7-year cycle of development. At this stage the astral body frees up new forces, which adolescents need to learn how to use. This allows the young people to test themselves, their peers and particularly their parents. It is thought that the freed astral body affects boys and girls in different ways. Boys become shy and embarrassed, turning inwards on themselves, whilst girls are more outward directed, testing out their social strengths (Bott 1996).

Adolescence is a time of great emotional, social and physical upheaval and whilst a good number of young people weather this with little disturbance, others have a more problematic time. It is a time of changing relationships, exploring new values and preparing for major life choices, for example deciding on a career or leaving home for the first time. In Eriksonian terms, this is described as finding an identity and, inherent in this, is the challenging of orthodox rules and regulations whether in behaviour, dress or language. For adolescents with a medical condition, some of this rebellion may be directed against their condition, making compliance with treatment more difficult. Because of this reluctance to accept the 'orthodox', adolescents may well be motivated to use CAM.

Gardiner and Wornham (2000) have reviewed the use of CAM in adolescence and have identified a number of reasons why adolescents and their parents choose to use CAM:

- Personal recommendation of either the therapy or the therapist
- Concern about the side effects of conventional medicine
- A solution to a chronic health problem
- Dissatisfaction with conventional care.

In this section we discuss a wide range of conditions, medical and psychological, which affect adolescents and for which CAM may be able to offer an extra dimension of treatment. Nurses working with adolescents are well aware of the developing and challenging intellect of young people, and that their interests are wide-ranging, making them open to new ideas and suggestions. For this reason it is important that nurses are aware of which complementary therapies are suitable for which conditions, and are able to counsel their patients appropriately. One danger is that in their desire to establish their identity as separate from that of their parents and their desire to rebel against authority, young people may elect to adopt CAM interventions which would adversely affect their wellbeing and future health. Of particular importance for nurses is the understanding of alternative methods of treating diabetes and cancer, and awareness of the dangers of dietary manipulation, which is addressed in Section 2.

In his paper on the need for specialist nurses for adolescents, Needham (2000) describes the recent rise in the profile of adolescent health care, noting that adolescents are at a distinctive and significant developmental stage that requires special health care provision. He goes on to note, however, that a national strategy for adolescent health care provision under the NHS is still lacking. The fifth report of the House of Commons Select Committee on Health (1997) stated that 'Adolescent health needs, in regard to both health promotion and treatment of sickness are given insufficient priority and lack of focus, with poorly developed services. Services for adolescents should be given greater focus and priority.' Needham (2000) states that adolescence may be seen as 'a discrete and significantly different stage from that of childhood or adulthood. It is a period of physical, emotional and social changes and there is also an immense psychological change'.

Wheatley (1998) suggests that nurses who work with adolescents should have additional nursing skills, including health promotion, confirming Sparocino's (1993) suggestion that part of the specialist nurse's role in adolescent care is to assist the young person to recognise or to avoid health damaging behaviour. Needham (2000) expands the role further by pointing out that part of the role of the specialist nurse for adolescents is the development of patient autonomy as a legal and ethical right, an ethos supported by the philosophy of CAM. For a discussion of the link between CAM and health promotion see Whitehead (1999) and for a review of the role of CAM in health promotion see Mantle (2002). In response to these approaches, much of this section centres around interventions for lifestyle behaviours which contribute to ill health.

REFERENCES

Bott V 1996 Spiritual science and the art of healing: Rudolf Steiner's anthroposophical medicine. Healing Arts Press, Vermont

Gardiner P, Wornham W 2000 Recent review of complementary and alternative medicine used by adolescents. Current Opinion in Pediatrics 12(4): 298–302

House of Commons Select Committee on Health 1997

Loo M 2002 Pediatric acupuncture. Churchill Livingstone, Edinburgh

Mantle F 2002 Complementary therapies and health promotion. British Journal of Community Nursing 7(2): 102–107

Needham J 2000 The nurse specialist role in adolescent health. Paediatric Nursing (Oct) 12(8): 28–30

Sparocino P 1993 The CNS influence on patient autonomy. Clinical Nurse Specialist 7(3): 110

Wheatley M 1998 Running a teenage drop in clinic in school. Primary Health Care 8(3): 26–29

Whitehead D 1999 The relationship between health promotion and complementary therapies. Complementary Therapies in Nursing and Midwifery 5(6): 171–175

10 Problems with communication

CHAPTER CONTENTS

- **Introduction   151**
- **Depression   151**
  Herbalism   151
  Homeopathy   152
  Bach flower remedies   153
  Aromatherapy   153
  Cultural differences   154
  TCM   155
  Anthroposophical medicine   156
  Ayurvedic medicine   156

- **Stress and anxiety   157**
  Herbalism   158
  Massage   158
  Reflexology   158
  Ayurvedic medicine   158
  TCM   159
- **References   159**

INTRODUCTION

The stereotype of the moody, 'misunderstood' adolescent who is unable to communicate in anything more linguistic than grunts is a good standby for situation comedies. However, for some young people this period of their lives can be one of crippling emotional distress and with all that is going on in their lives it is not surprising that many young people experience high levels of stress, anxiety and depression.

DEPRESSION

Classic symptoms of depression include withdrawal of contact, flattened affect and reduced speech, as well as anxiety, agitation and loss of self-confidence. Symptoms of anxiety include agitation, insomnia and disturbed eating patterns. Ambrosini (2000) has reviewed the literature on the use of pharmacological interventions in childhood and adolescent depression and noted that, in general, tricyclic antidepressants were of little value. However, significantly better effects were obtained with fluoxetine and paroxetine. He suggests that this specific response is due to the changing hormone status of children and the differing rates of maturation of the noradrenergic versus serotonergic neurotransmitter systems.

Herbalism

Although not suggested as a treatment for severe depression, St John's wort (*Hypericum perforatum*) has a well-validated research base to support its value in the treatment of mild to moderate depression. St John's wort has a long history of use, from the herbal scholars of the Greek and Roman Empires, and it was well known for its efficacy as a wound healer. It obtained its name during the advent of Christianity. Previously, it had been associated with Balder, the Norse god of light, and the herb was supposed to have properties to ward off evil spirits (Sumner 2000). Culpeper (1653) stated that it is a 'singular wound herb ... it heals inward hurts and bruises ... and closes up the lips of wounds'. Strangely, he does not suggest its use for anxiety and depression, although it had been observed from early times to have a calming and sedative effect (Linde et al 1996, Kim 1999). Its action resembles that of a monoamine oxidase inhibitor (MAOI) and serotonin re-uptake inhibitor, although the mode of action is not at all clear (Rasmussen 1998, Miller 1998). The MAOI action is very weak and does not require any of the usual adjustment in diet that is needed in MAOI treatment, although this assertion has been challenged by the Irish Medical Board who sought to ban St John's wort as an over-the-counter preparation. McIntyre (2000) points out that a search of the literature failed to identify a single case of MAOI type adverse reaction. For a full and balanced review of the issues and benefits of St John's wort see McIntyre (2000). Overall, patients tolerated the herb better than conventional antidepressants, specifically the tricyclics. This reflects the observations of Paracelsus, the German-Swiss alchemist and physician (1493–1541), who extolled the herb's virtue and many uses, specifically noting its safety and lack of side effects. However, a modern interaction which needs to be noted is the potential for St John's wort to reduce the therapeutic effect of certain prescribed medications such as cardiac medications, anticoagulation therapy and the contraceptive pill. It should not be taken concurrently with other antidepressant medication.

Homeopathy

For adolescents who choose to use homeopathy in the treatment of depression, the prescription might include Ignatia for excitability and depression, Sepia and Nat. mur for irritability and Lycopodium for stress and depression. Ignatia is particularly good if part of the patient's mental set is to want to be well thought of, with a tendency to self-pity accompanied by frequent changes of mood. Boyd (1989) lists the traits of Ignatia as paradoxical, unexpected and perverse, whilst Gibson (1996) notes the key features as being instability with a tendency to resent contradiction, being sensitive to blame and generally feeling misunderstood. Ignatia is made from the seed pods of the *Ignatia amara*, which contain strychnine which acts on the nervous system (Lockie 1990). Sepia is made from the ink of the cuttle fish and reflects the action of the cuttle fish which, in adversity, hurriedly scuttles away to hide, so it is particularly suited to those who want to hide themselves away and who resent intrusion, with a loss of interest in and indifference to life (Boyd 1989), and those who Gibson (1996) refers to as sad, silent individuals, apathetic and solitary, with undifferentiated fear. Nat. mur is especially relevant to the adolescent since it addresses emotional stress relating to broken love affairs and unrequited love, rejection and vulnerability to emotional injury while putting on a hard front to hide one's feelings. These adolescents tend to harbour resentments and imagined or real injuries. Boyd (1989) describes them as 'Nice to know but difficult to live with'. Lycopodium is used if the depression is secondary to severe anxiety about the possibility of failure and the young person is trying to escape responsibility with illness. There are a number of advantages of using homeopathy for depressed patients, including its safety in the event of overdose. Homeopathic medicines are also safe from abuse or addiction.

Bach flower remedies

The Bach flower remedies are aimed at addressing negative emotional states (see Ch. 1) and three types of depression are recognised:

- Depression that descends suddenly and for no apparent reason, for which the remedy Mustard is prescribed
- Despair and utter hopelessness, for which Gorse is suggested
- Deep mental anguish and emotional pain, for which Sweet Chestnut is recommended.

Mustard, first potentised in 1935 after Dr Bach had settled in the village of Sotwell in Oxfordshire, is prepared by the boiling method whilst Gorse was first potentised in 1933 and is prepared by the sun method. White chestnut, which is used for what might be called reactive depression, is prepared by the sun method and was potentised at Sotwell in 1935. As ever, Rescue Remedy is a good all-round remedy for adolescents, as is Walnut, to help them to cope with all the physical and emotional changes which can cause distress, whilst Crab apple is also of value.

Aromatherapy

Tiran (2000) suggests that there are number of essential oils in a range of combinations which can be used for depression, depending on the presenting symptoms. Amongst them are bergamot (*Citrus bergamia*), ylang ylang (*Cananga odorata*), rose (*Rosa damascena*), neroli (*Citrus aurantium*), chamomile (*Matricaria chamomilla*) and lavender. Unfortunately, there is a variation of opinion amongst practitioners regarding the therapeutic qualities of some essential oils. For example, Davis (1996) suggests bergamot for depression but Price (1993) and Ryman (1989) do not confirm this, whilst Tisserand (1994) suggests ylang ylang and bergamot for anxiety and chamomile, neroli or rose for depression. However, there is good research to support the therapeutic effects of a number of these oils, particularly their muscle relaxing and sedative effects; for example, rosemary (*Rosmarinus officinalis*) (Aquel 1992), *Geranius pelargonium* (*Gervaniaceae*) (Lis-Balchin et al 1998), and other essential oils (Buchbauer et al 1993). Good evidence for the use of lavender (*Lavandula augustifolia*) for insomnia is offered by Buchbauer et al (1991) and for the use of neroli (*Citrus aurantium*) for insomnia by Jager et al (1992). There is some evidence for the effect of citrus fragrances in treating depression (Kormani et al 1995). For this research the researchers created a new citrus fragrance consisting of lemon oil mixed with orange and bergamot. A constant concentration of a volatile gel of the oil was put in a room in which the depressed subjects spent most of the day and night. The concentration of the oil was measured continually during the experiment. The dosages of antidepressants were reduced gradually over a period of a few weeks, as the subjects felt was appropriate, and all the subjects in the experimental group were exposed to the citrus fragrance until their depression remitted. Measurements were taken using the Hamilton rating scale for depression and the self rating depression scale. Results showed that it took 4–11 weeks of treatment with the citrus fragrance before remission occurred. Although there was no statistical difference between the groups in the HRSD scores or number of days of hospital treatment, in the experimental group the dosages of antidepressants were markedly reduced and by the end of treatment, 9 of the 12 patients did not need antidepressants. In the control group, all the subjects retained and needed their normal dosage of antidepressants. Measurement of cortisol and dopamine levels before treatment started showed no difference between the two groups; however, whilst these levels were reduced in both groups during the experiment, the levels in the citrus fragrance group were significantly lower than in the control group. Although the authors agreed that it could be open to question whether the citrus fragrance had a direct antidepressant effect, it did, in this study, contribute to a better clinical outcome.

Warren and Warrenburg (1993) conducted a series of studies using a range of clinical outcomes to investigate the mood-altering attributes of a range of flower fragrances. In the first series of studies, changes in blood pressure were used as a measure of stress levels. The researchers combined a flower fragrance with the essential oil of nutmeg (*Myristica fragrans*), which has a traditional role of reducing stress. Results showed that the addition of nutmeg to the fragrance induced a lowering of blood pressure compared with the same fragrance without the nutmeg oil. In further studies they used a mood profiling procedure in order to detect mood changes evoked by flower fragrances. Mood profiling is a self-administered psychological assessment tool for measuring subjective changes evoked by the fragrances. It measures eight dimensions of mood which are affected by fragrance: four positive and four negative categories. The tool was tried out on five fragrances. Results showed that muguet decreased depression, apathy and irritation but not stress, and increased happiness, relaxation and stimulation. Douglas fir decreased apathy, stress, depression and irritation and increased relaxation and happiness. Tuberose decreased apathy, depression, stress and irritation and increased relaxation, sensuality and happiness; however, it was not recorded as being stimulating. Osmanthus increased happiness and was stimulating, decreasing irritation, stress, depression and apathy, whilst hyacinth decreased irritation, stress, depression and apathy, thus increasing happiness, sensuality and relaxation, and was also regarded as stimulating.

Cultural differences

Because adolescents from minority cultures may find it easier to talk about their feelings and emotions in the language of their own medical system, the charity MIND has recommended that we revise our Western medical orientated diagnostic approach and try to speak the language of the specific cultures (MIND 1993). In her paper on post-natal depression, for example, Gerrard (2000) points out that some cultures do not have a word for depression. Laungani (2000) expands on this, stating that the word depression is not an easy one to understand in many cultures and noting that there is, for example, no equivalent word for it in any of the 38 languages currently spoken in India.

TCM

In Traditional Chinese Medicine, emotional problems are related to the principles of Qi, Blood and Yin and treatment would be aimed at correcting the imbalance between these elements. As Fruehauf (1995) points out, the main characteristic of Eastern thought is the inseparable mind/body continuum. The mind/body dyad is in constant interaction, one affecting the other, and Chinese practitioners would always recognise that emotional factors play a part in health and illness. The Seven Emotions are considered to be most important and it is recognised that the difference between them may be small or that a mixture of emotions may be present at any one time. Each emotion is related to a specific organ.

- Joy is related to the Heart
- Anger relates to the Liver
- Sadness and grief relate to the Lungs
- Fear and fright relate to the Kidneys
- Pensiveness relates to the Spleen.

A pulse reading would indicate the patient's state of mind, depending on which organ pulse is affected. The two organs that are most susceptible to emotional disturbance are the Heart and the Liver. As noted in Chapter 4 on sleep, the Heart stores the Shen which is the Spirit of the body. When the Shen is disturbed it can result in insomnia, crying, muddled thinking and inappropriate behaviour. The Liver regulates the emotions, since the Liver network is responsible for the harmonious distribution of Qi and disturbance of Liver-Qi will result in emotional distress. In general, TCM would classify depression as a problem relating to stagnation of (predominantly) Liver-Qi, and treatment is aimed at the restoration of the Qi flow. In his review of the treatment of mental and emotional problems in TCM, Maciocia (1994) discusses the pathology of these problems in terms of their effects on Qi, Blood and Yin. The mind and body are one, and just as emotional problems have an effect on Qi, Blood and Yin, so disorders of Qi, Blood and Yin will have an effect on the Mind. Maciocia classifies these effects into three categories: mind obstructed, mind unsettled and mind weakened. In particular, the condition 'mind unsettled' includes many of the symptoms that adolescents might experience. This condition can be caused by an imbalance within a number of subsystems, such as deficiency of Blood-Yin, stagnation of Qi, or stasis of Blood, Fire, Phlegm-Fire or Empty-Heart. This particular condition is manifested in anxiety, mental restlessness, insomnia and agitation. In addition, patients may experience depression and an inability to plan their lives, as well as suffering from nightmares and irritability (Maciocia 1994). The approach to treatment would involve nourishing Blood or Yin and calming the Mind; other interventions would include the use of acupuncture and herbal remedies. These have been described by Fruehauf (1995), who suggests formulas for problems such as anxiety, involving 'quietening the spirit', and depression, involving a range of decoctions addressing the Liver network, which is in charge of the harmonious distribution of Qi. Most unhappy emotions in TCM are attributed to stagnant Qi. 'In a patient full of sadness the Qi becomes depressed and does not move' (from an unspecified classic Chinese text, cited in Fruehauf 1995).

As has been pointed out earlier, acupuncture should not be viewed in isolation but as part of a TCM package of care. It has been used since ancient times as a treatment for mental disturbances and a number of studies have been undertaken to assess the effectiveness of acupuncture in the treatment of depression. Luo et al (1985), for example, conducted a study with two groups, one in which the 27 participants received electro-acupuncture and one with 20 participants who received 100–200 mg per day of amitriptyline over a 5-week period. Independent assessors, using the Hamilton Depression Rating Scale, assessed the participants before and after the interventions. Both groups achieved a statistically significant improvement, but with fewer side effects reported by the acupuncture group. The results were attributed to increased serotonin output and noradrenaline turnover and the rebalancing of Yin and Yang. Similar results were noted in a study by Yang (1994), who again compared acupuncture with amitriptyline over a period of 6 weeks. There was no significant difference between the groups except that participants in the acupuncture group reported that they were feeling much more stable by 4 weeks. Tao's (1993) single blind study using the Hospital Anxiety and Depression Score (HADS) pre- and post-treatment with acupuncture, noted a highly significant reduction in the levels of anxiety and depression 1 month after treatment. This study showed that in 42 out of 60 patients, the levels of anxiety were reduced to within the normal range as measured by the HADS scale, i.e. 0–7. Of the depressed patients, a score within the normal range was obtained in 45 out of 50 patients, showing that acupuncture can induce a reduction in anxiety and depression without the use and side effects of medication. It is suggested in the paper that it is the release of endorphins by the use of acupuncture which results in the decrease in anxiety levels and that the use of acupuncture in the treatment of depression has a similar effect to the use of pyrasidol-type antidepressants. Low serotonin levels are associated with depression and, in one study, the use of electro-acupuncture was noted to raise levels of serotonin significantly (Mao et al 1980).

The philosophy of TCM lies firmly in the preventative sphere and the use of acupuncture may help many suffering from stress or depression, as a preventative measure and to protect health. Allen et al (1998) investigated the use of acupuncture in the treatment of major depression in women. In his paper he endorsed this health promotion approach, suggesting that alternative therapies might well be accepted by patients as adjuncts or substitutes for existing treatments. He also points out the need for maintenance treatments.

Anthroposophical medicine

In Anthroposophical medicine the liver is seen as the organ of life and if it ceases to function properly it can give rise to a fear of life and an increasingly anxious state. If this situation continues it can lead to feelings of depression with developing inertia and loss of spirit. It can be seen that this is a very similar ethos to that of TCM. Treatment would involve the use of homeopathic remedies, which have already been discussed, as well as massage.

Ayurvedic medicine

In Ayurvedic medicine the treatment of affective disorders is a process of rebalancing the prevailing dosha. Some affective disorders such as anxiety are linked specifically with one dosha, in this case the vata dosha, whilst depression can be related to any of the three doshas. An imbalance in the vata dosha will give rise to symptoms such as difficulty in concentration, flight of ideas, insomnia, increased sensitivity and depression. Preceding this imbalance there is often a history of emotional injury or traumatic event or a history of parental neglect. An imbalance of the kapha dosha will demonstrate symptoms of inertia, denial and a general slowing down of the whole body and mind. These are the sort of symptoms normally associated with seasonal affective disorder. Pitta disorders manifest themselves in a high level of aggression and in deception and jealousy. They can involve destructiveness and violence, and may include compulsive–obsessive disorders. This type of disorder is often the result of chronic stress before exams or of prolonged social or personal injustices. It may also be the result of an ambition being thwarted with possible loss of face; for example, failure to gain a part in the school play, a place on a sports team, or selection at a chosen university or college. It is considered to be the most dangerous form of depression because of the potential for violence either against other people or against oneself. Treatment in Ayurvedic medicine is achieved by the use of herbs, diet and yoga to pacify and reduce the excess dosha. For depression, Lad (1984) suggests the plough, corpse, palm tree and lotus positions. One herbal treatment is the preparation triphala, described earlier, which is a regulator for all the doshas. Other treatments include pancha karma, which is a deep cleansing process allowing the body to release excess dosha from the cells, and shirodhara, which is the flow of warm oil to the forehead to balance vata dosha and vata disorders, including insomnia, anxiety or worry. This procedure has been evaluated by Schneider et al (1990) and Waldschutz (1988) and both reported that the subjects had a significant reduction in stress, anxiety and depression.

Diet can be used to reduce vata energy. Lad (1984) suggests that encouraging the client to eat fish, seafood, beef, bananas, turkey, chicken, oats and wheat will calm excess in the vata doshas. Buhrmann (1996) states that protein is important and advises eating cheese, milk, eggs and yoghurt, since low protein can lead to reduced serotonin levels, affecting mood. Low levels of serotonin can cause depression but this can be raised by increasing tryptophan, which is present in foods such as chicken, turkey, bananas and yeast extract and has been implicated in the treatment of insomnia and depression (Kitahara 1987, Delgardo 1990). Seafood and beef are both rich in zinc, a lack of which can lead to mental lethargy and impaired taste (Mason 1995), whilst avocado, sweet potatoes, fish and wheat cereals are excellent sources of pyridoxine (vitamin B6). Davies and Stewart (1987) note that dietary deficiencies can affect mental function. The lack of B vitamins has been linked to irritability and depression, and lack of zinc can cause depression or mood swings, whilst low levels of potassium cause depression and apathy. The use of diet in the treatment of depression has been reviewed by Spencer and Jacobs (1999).

STRESS AND ANXIETY

Although not perhaps as serious as overt depression, stress and anxiety can exert a crippling effect on a young person struggling with new experiences, new expectations and an uncertain future.

Herbalism

In addition to remedies discussed in Section 2, adolescents might find the following interventions of use. Herbs which can be of value include chamomile, both Roman and German, which has been noted in Section 2 as a gastro-intestinal relaxant and sedative. Over-the-counter remedies which adolescents may access include products containing valerian (*Valerian officinalis*) and passiflora (*Passiflora incarnata*). Valerian has a long history of use as a sedative, for example by the 19th century Shakers, and is routinely prescribed in Germany. Similarly to chamomile, it is thought to act like the benzodiazepines (Sumner 2000). Wong et al (1998) give an excellent review of the use of herbs in psychiatric care.

Massage

In Section 2 the value of massage for anxiety in small children was noted. Field (1998, 2000) provided an extensive overview of the value and effectiveness of massage therapy in alleviating stress, depression and anxiety in adolescent mothers when she compared massage with relaxation therapy, including yoga exercises followed by progressive muscular relaxation. Using self-report, observation and urinary cortisol levels as outcome measurements, her results showed that the massage group reported less anxiety and depression and exhibited lower cortisol levels during the study. This confirmed Field's earlier (1992) study on infants, discussed in Chapter 6. Watson and Watson (1997) note the therapeutic effects of touch and its effects on muscle relaxation.

Reflexology

Evidence for the role of reflexology in reducing stress and anxiety is offered by Thomas (1989) who, in a well-designed study, demonstrated a reduction in anxiety levels of psychiatric hospital patients, whilst Trousdell (1996) indicated that reflexology had a marked effect on clients' feelings of wellbeing.

Ayurvedic medicine

Bera et al (1998) have described a trial of the use of yoga to reduce stress, but of particular value to adolescents is the research undertaken by Malathi et al (1998) on the use of yoga to reduce exam stress in medical students. The research was conducted on 50 students aged 18–19 who were not familiar with yoga as a therapy. They undertook a 1 hour session of yoga asanas three times a week for a period of 3 months, whilst a control group continued with normal reading and studying activities for the hour. Pre- and post-assessment measures, using the Spillberger's anxiety score, were taken to determine the anxiety scores of both groups. Two measurements were taken, one before and one after practice, 1 month before the exam as a baseline and pre- and post-practice on the day of the exam. On both occasions there was a significant reduction in stress levels compared with scores prior to yoga practice. Specifically the students reported that they noticed improved concentration, self-confidence, wellbeing and relaxation.

In addition, they recommended that yoga should be an ongoing activity and should be included in the undergraduate curriculum. Similarly, Malathi et al (2000) using the subjective wellbeing inventory reported that results showed that participants had improvement in general wellbeing and confidence at the significance levels.

TCM

Lewis (2000) has provided an excellent introduction to t'ai chi and Qigong, tracing their development from an ancient martial art to their present use as therapeutic exercise. The aim of the t'ai chi movements, known as the Form, is to even out and balance the Qi. The principles behind this include relaxation, evenness of movement, balance and focus. As has been stated earlier, in TCM the mind and body are seen as one, so the relaxing, balancing and focusing of the physical movements have a similar effect on the mind, increasing relaxation and reducing anxiety. The general treatment of anxiety in TCM has been addressed in Section 2.

The effects of exercise on mental functioning have been well documented. Chen and Snyder (1999) have reviewed the role of t'ai chi as a nursing intervention. They point out that the potential benefits of t'ai chi have been investigated since the 1980s, primarily for cardiovascular or chronic conditions. Jin (1992) investigated the role of t'ai chi in stress reduction, comparing it with brisk walking, reading or meditation. Results indicated that all four interventions improved the subjects' moods and that the effect of t'ai chi was similar to walking briskly. It was also noted that t'ai chi was more effective than reading in reducing anxiety and increasing the vigour of the subjects.

REFERENCES

Allen J, Schnyer R, Hill S 1998 The efficacy of acupuncture in the treatment of major depression in women. Psychological Science 9(5): 397–401

Ambrosini, P 2000 A review of pharmacotherapy of major depression in children and adolescents. Psychiatric Services 51(5): 627–633

Aqel, M. 1992 A vascular smooth muscle relaxant effect of Rosmarinus officinalis. International Journal of Pharmacology 30(4): 281–288

Bera T, Gore M, Oak J 1998 Indian Journal of Physiological Pharmacology 42(4): 473–478

Boyd H 1989 Introduction to homeopathic medicine, 2nd edn. Beaconsfield Publishers, Beaconsfield

Buchbauer G, Jirovetz L, Jager W 1991 Aromatherapy: evidence for sedative effects of the essential oil of lavender after inhalation. Zeitschrift der Naturforschung 4(c): 1067–1072

Buchbauer G, Jirovetz L, Jager W 1993 Fragrance compounds and essential oils with sedative effects upon inhalation. Journal of Pharmaceutical Sciences 82(6): 660–664

Buhrmann S 1996 Ayurvedic psychology and psychiatric approaches to the treatment of common affective disorders. The Protocol Journal of Botanical Medicine 2(1): 1–8

Chen K-M, Snyder M 1999 A research based use of t'ai chi movement therapy as a nursing intervention. Journal of Holistic Nursing 17(3): 267–279

Culpeper N 1653 Complete herbal: a book of natural remedies for ancient ills. Wordsworth Editions, Hertfordshire

Davies S, Stewart A 1987 Nutritional medicine. Pan Books, London

Davis P 1996 Aromatherapy: an A–Z. CW Daniel, Saffron Walden

Delgardo P 1990 Seratonin function and the mechanism of antidepressant action. Archives of General Psychiatry 47: 411–418

Field T 1992 Infants of depressed mothers. Development and Psychopathology 4: 49–66

Field T 1998 Massage therapy effects. American Psychologist 53(12): 1270–1281

Field T 2000 Touch therapy. Churchill Livingstone, Edinburgh

Fruehauf H 1995 Commonly used Chinese herbal formulas for the treatment of mental disorders. Journal of Chinese Medicine 48(May): 21–34

Gerrard J 2000 Postnatal depression. NT Books, Emap Healthcare, London

Gibson D 1996 Studies of homeopathic remedies. Beaconsfield Publishers, Beaconsfield

Jager W, Buchbauer G, Jirovetz L 1992 Evidence of the sedative effect of neroli oil, citronella and phenylethyl acetate on mice. Journal of Essential Oil Research 4: 387–394

Jin P 1992 Efficacy of t'ai chi, brisk walking, meditation and reading in reducing mental and emotional stress. Journal of Psychosomatic Research 36: 361–370

Kim H 1999 St John's wort for depression. A meta analysis of well defined clinical trials. Journal of Nervous and Mental Disorders 187: 532–539

Kitahara M 1987 Dietary ratio tryptophan and suicide in the United Kingdom, Ireland and States, Canada, Australia and New Zealand. Omega Journal of Death and Dying 18n(7): 1–6

Kormani T, Fujiwara R, Tanida M et al 1995 Effects of citrus fragrance on immune function and depressive states. Neuroimmunomodulation 2: 174–180

Lad V 1984 Ayurveda, the science of self healing: a practical guide. Lotus Press, Wisconsin

Laungani P 2000 Postnatal depression across cultures: conceptual and methodological considerations. International Journal of Health Promotion and Education 38(3): 86–94

Lewis D 2000 T'ai chi ch'uan. Complementary Therapies in Nursing and Midwifery 6(4): 204–206

Linde K, Ramirez G, Mulrow C 1996 St John's wort for depression: an overview and meta analysis of randomised clinical trials. British Medical Journal 313: 253–258

Lis-Balchin M, Patel J, Hart S 1998 Studies on the mode of action of essential oils of scented leaf Pelargonium (Geraniaceae). Phyto-therapy Research 12: 215–217

Lockie A 1990 The family guide to homeopathy. Penguin Books, Middlesex

Luo H, Jia Y, Li Z 1985 Electro acupuncture vs amitryptiline in the treatment of depressive states. Journal of Traditional Chinese Medicine 5: 3–8

McIntyre M 2000 A review of the benefits, adverse events, drug interactions and safety of St John's wort. The implications with regard to the regulation of herbal medicines. The Journal of Alternative and Complementary Medicine 6(2): 115–124

Maciocia G 1994 The treatment of mental and emotional problems with acupuncture and Chinese herbs, pt 11. American Journal of Acupuncture 22(4): 305–334

Malathi A, Damodaran A, Shah N 1998 Psychophysiological changes at the time of examination in medical students before and after practice of yoga and relaxation. Indian Journal of Psychiatry 40(1): 35–40

Malathi A, Damodaran A, Shah N et al 2000 Effect of yogic practices on subjective well being. Indian Journal of Physiological Pharmacology 44(2): 202–206

Mason P 1995 Handbook of dietary supplements. Blackwell Science, Oxford

Mao W, Ghia J, Scott D et al 1980 High versus low intensity acupuncture analgesia for treatment of chronic pain: effects on platelet serotonin. Pain 8: 331–342

Miller A 1998 St John's wort (Hypericum perforatum) clinical effects on depression and other conditions. Alternative Medicine Review 3(1): 18–26

MIND 1993 MIND's policy on black and minority ethnic people and mental health. MIND, London

Price NS 1993 Aromatherapy workbook. Thorson's, London

Rasmussen P 1998 St John's wort: a review of its use in depression. Australian Journal of Medical Herbalism 10(1): 8–13

Ryman D 1989 The aromatherapy handbook. CW Daniel, Saffron Walden

Schneider R, Cavanaugh K, Kasture H 1990 Health promotion within a traditional system of natural health care: Maharishi Yurveda. Journal of Social Behaviour and Personality 5(3): 1–27

Spencer J, Jacobs J 1999 Complementary/ alternative medicine: an evidence based approach. Mosby, London

Sumner J 2000 The natural history of medicinal plants. Timber Press, Oregon

Tao DJ 1993 Research on the reduction of anxiety and depression with acupuncture. American Journal of Acupuncture 21(4): 327–329

Thomas M 1989 Fancy footwork. Nursing Times 85(41): 42–44

Tiran D 2000 Complementary therapies for pregnancy and childbirth, 2nd edn. Baillière Tindall, Edinburgh

Tisserand R 1994 The art of aromatherapy. CW Daniel, Saffron Walden

Trousdell P 1996 Reflexology meets emotional needs. Journal of the Association of Complementary Medicine 14(11): 9–12

Waldschutz R 1988 Influence of Maharishi Ayurveda purification treatment on physiological and psychological health. Erfahrungsheilkunde Acta Medica Empirica 11: 720–729

Warren C, Warrenburg S 1993 Mood benefits of fragrance. Perfumer and Flavorist 18: 9–18

Watson S, Watson S 1997 The effects of massage: an holistic approach to care. Nursing Standard 11(47): 45–47

Wong A, Smith M, Boon H 1998 Herbal remedies in psychiatric practice. Archives of General Psychiatry 55(11): 1033–1044

Yang X 1994 Clinical observations on needling extra channel points in treating mental depression. Journal of Traditional Chinese Medicine 14: 14–18

11 Problems related to sleep

CHAPTER CONTENTS

- ■ **Introduction** 162
  - *General approaches* 162
- ■ **Therapeutic interventions** 163
  - *Hypnosis* 163
  - *Herbal remedies* 163
  - *Homeopathy* 164

- *Bach flower remedies* 165
- *Ayurvedic medicine* 165
- *Aromatherapy* 165
- *Anthroposophical medicine* 166
- *TCM* 166
- ■ **References** 166

INTRODUCTION

Stress, anxiety and depression can lead to problems in sleeping and, with adolescents as with younger children, lack of sleep can result in hypersomnia during the day and can be due to a range of sleep disorders. For adolescents, lack of sleep due to work load and socialising, and sleep problems resulting from an erratic schedule are key problems. However, there are two conditions that need to be excluded in adolescence. One is narcolepsy, which typically develops during the adolescent period; the other is Kleine–Levin syndrome, which starts in adolescence. Ryan et al (1987) noted that 25% of depressed adolescents complained of hypersomnia.

General approaches

Building on previously mentioned remedies such as essential oil of lavender, the herb chamomile and isocones, there are a number of remedies which can be of particular value in addressing adolescents' erratic lifestyles. A review of a number of non-pharmacological treatment modalities and meta-analyses of treatment outcomes (Morin et al 1994) has shown that sleep restriction (curtailing the amount of time spent in bed to that actually spent asleep), stimulus control (regulating the time of retiring and getting up, reducing stimulants such as caffeine and alcohol and ensuring a period of quiet before going to bed) and cognitive relaxation (imagery, meditation, thought stopping) produced the best reduction of sleep latency, to less than 30 minutes. Generally, patients suffering from sleep-onset insomnia responded better to treatment than patients with mixed insomnia or sleep-maintenance insomnia. Overall, stimulus control was the most effective single therapy for either sleep-onset or sleep-maintenance insomnia and procedures aimed at reducing cognitive arousal were slightly more effective than those aimed at reducing physiological arousal, e.g. muscle relaxation. However, it was suggested that general recommendations about caffeine, exercise and diet are unlikely to be sufficient on their own for treating chronic insomnia.

THERAPEUTIC INTERVENTIONS

Hypnosis

Hypnosis can be particularly useful in the treatment of insomnia, especially for very anxious adolescents who are often able to keep their anxiety at bay during the day by distracting themselves with daily tasks, but whose anxiety begins to surface as evening draws on, specifically focusing on fears that they may not get off to sleep and concerns that they will not get enough sleep. Other approaches to insomnia would involve addressing the underlying medical or psychological problems. Exploratory techniques may need to be employed to discover any underlying reasons for the insomnia, such as childhood incidents, nightmares or phobias. As with younger children, suggestions which emphasise warmth, safety and security whilst lying in bed, along with general suggestions evoking a calm and peaceful state are helpful. The removal of any anxiety about not sleeping, with positive suggestions about going off to sleep, staying asleep and awaking refreshed in the morning is central to this approach.

Herbal remedies

Herbal preparations which are traditionally used to induce sleep include nervous restoratives such as St John's wort, vervain (*Verbena officinalis*), rosemary (*Rosmarinus officinalis*), wild lettuce (*Lactuca virosa*), skullcap (*Scutellaria laterifolia*) and lavender (*Lavandula officinalis*) (Mills 1994). The overall approach of a medical herbalist would be to use calming and relaxing agents rather than heavy sedatives. St John's wort, mentioned in relation to depression, has a calming effect but can also act as a restorative tonic for the nervous system. For relaxation, gentle calming agents such as chamomile should be tried first, whilst lime flowers (*Tilia cordata*) or lemon balm (*Melissa officinalis*) have a traditional use in the treatment of anxiety states and tension, although no scientific evidence is available to support this. However, lime flowers should not be used in people with cardiac problems. Herbs with a stronger sedative effect include hops (*Humulus lupulus*), skullcap (*Scutellaria laterifolia*), valerian (*Valeriana officinalis*), or passion flower (*Passiflora incarnata*). Barnes et al (2002) offer evidence for the antispasmodic and sedative effects of hops but caution that this herb should not be taken by anyone suffering from depression as the sedative effect may exacerbate the symptoms of depression. In addition, alcohol and orthodox sedative therapy will enhance the therapeutic action. In spite of the traditional use of skullcap as a relaxant and anticonvulsant, there are no documented scientific data to support these claims. Animal research into the action of passion flower indicates evidence of central nervous system depression and anticonvulsive properties. There were no reported side effects to passion flower, but excessive doses may give rise to heavy sedation and may potentiate MAOI therapy (Barnes et al 2002).

Valerian is an ancient medicinal herb (the name derives from *valere* which means 'to be in health') used in Galen's time for epilepsy (Bremness 1995), and is particularly good as an additive in very stressful circumstances. It is for this reason that it was issued to the civilian population during World War II to help them sleep through the blitz. Research using a double blind repeated measures random order design supported the hypothesis that extract of valerian would shorten sleep latency times in people having problems getting off to sleep, as well as shortening the time taken in settling down to sleep. According to the authors, the design was chosen to mimic the 'occasional' sedative consumption typical of poor sleepers; secondly, it is more complex than the straightforward crossover design and reduces the risk that volunteers might detect the different treatments by other means than sensing their effects on sleep; and thirdly, the design allowed the researchers to detect any carry-over effects as they occurred. Although the valerian did not increase the total sleep time, it did produce more stable sleep during the first quarter of the night and, overall, did not diminish or disrupt the normal levels of movement during the night. In addition, subjects reported improved sleep with no side effects such as nightmares or feeling 'hung over' the next morning. Sleep latency times were reduced by an average of 7 minutes. The researchers concluded that valerian was as effective as small doses of benzodiazepines and barbiturates (Leathwood & Chauffard 1985). They also noted that valerian improved the quality of sleep.

Good results were also obtained using valerian with subjects who had all suffered sleep difficulties and fatigue. Half of them regularly or periodically took conventional sedatives. The subjects were randomised into two groups with regard to which tablet should be taken the first night. Twenty-one out of twenty-seven subjects rated the valerian better than the control and again reported that they slept very well, with no side effects and with the disappearance of the nightmares and disturbed sleep that they had reported as occurring with conventional medication (Lindahl & Lindwall 1989).

Research on the use of St John's wort on sleep patterns noted that it produced an increase in deep sleep during the total sleep period; however, sleep latency, sleep maintenance and total sleep time were not affected (Schultz & Jobert 1994). Again, these sedative herbs should not be taken alongside conventional sedatives.

Homeopathy

Building on the homeopathic remedies for insomnia discussed in previous chapters, remedies which are particularly relevant to adolescents who have problems with sleeping might include Coffea cruda, particularly for those who have an overactive mind, with general feelings of agitation, possibly as a result of study for exams or anticipation of an interview. For those who have been overworking, are unable to switch off and are feeling irritable, angry and very stressed, Nux. vomica is recommended. These two remedies are very similar and it may be necessary to try both before the correct remedy is found. Both are useful if the young person is having difficulties in sleeping whilst in the midst of a series of exams and finds it difficult to switch from thinking about one exam (and the statutory post-mortem on the paper) to thinking about the next. Of the remedies mentioned, readers may recognise Coffea, which has been used medicinally throughout the Middle East as a remedy to address problems that resemble the ingestion of too much coffee; just as too much coffee can stimulate symptoms of over excitement, so homeopathic doses of Coffea have the opposite effect.

Bach flower remedies

Two of the Bach flower remedies are of particular value since they address the sort of problems common to those who cannot get off to sleep. White Chestnut is helpful specifically for the times when the mind is full of problems, ideas, thoughts and recurrent anxieties or mental arguments, and Red Chestnut is helpful for those who worry incessantly about other people and those who strongly identify with the sufferings of others. Both these remedies were first potentised in 1935.

Ayurvedic medicine

Suggested yoga positions for help in dealing with insomnia include the cobra, corpse and backward bend (Lad 1984). The erratic lifestyle of the adolescent militates against the routine of Ayurvedic medicine, but for insomnia, which is usually caused by excess vata, the interventions outlined under depression should be used.

Aromatherapy

In addition to the research discussed in earlier chapters on the efficacy of lavender essential oil, research has also been conducted using essential oils of passiflora (*Passiflora incanarta*) and lime blossoms (*Tilia cordata*). Mobility in mice was reduced by 55% by the inhalation of lime blossoms, whilst there was no reduction in mobility for passiflora. However, when caffeine overactivity was induced, motility was reduced by inhalation of both lime blossoms and passion flower (Buchbauer et al 1992).

Research into the activity of essential oil of neroli (*Citrus aurantium*) (Jager et al 1992) demonstrated the sedative effects of the oil and the effect was noted to be greatest during the first 30 minutes of exposure to the vapours. This was confirmed by an interesting study which was conducted on the effect of oils on sleep latency, using EEG and psychological scoring. The aim of the study was to test the effect of oils on sleep latency under stress conditions. The oils used included spike lavender, sweet fennel, bitter orange (neroli), linden, valerian and marjoram (the botanical sources were not stated). The odour of bitter orange shortened the time it took to go to sleep significantly compared with no odours, suggesting that the odour of bitter orange affected the cortex and inhibited the excitement of the central nervous system, thus encouraging sedation. The subjects reported that they found it easy to sleep even under conditions of mental stress (Miyake et al 1991).

A further review of the data by Buchbauer et al (1993), investigating the traditional uses of essential oils, confirmed the sedative properties of sandalwood, neroli and lavender essential oils and showed that lavender oil exhibited a superior sedative effect, but found that the traditional use of rose oil as a sedative was not confirmed (the botanical sources were not stated). The fact that lavender proved to be sedative, even after hyperactivity was induced by caffeine, might be useful to adolescents who have difficulty in getting off to sleep after drinking too much coffee or too many caffeine drinks.

Anthroposophical medicine

In Anthroposophical medicine, Steiner advocated meditation exercises to facilitate connection with the spirit world, as well as Anthroposophical remedies such as Coffea tosta or Belladonna. Attention would also be addressed to living patterns, such as times of eating. Anthroposophical medicine recognises a number of causes for insomnia, e.g. psychological shock, for which silver is the remedy of choice, or insomnia as a result of nervous restlessness, which is treated with Avena Sativa comp, a mixture of valerian, passion flower, hops, oats and a high homeopathic potency of Coffea, or Malvae comp. tea, which contains mallow, lavender flowers and valerian root.

TCM

The use of isocones, which were referred to in Section 2, could be of value for adolescents since they may help to adjust the erratic sleep patterns that occur when adolescents are out of synchronisation with circadian rhythm.

REFERENCES

Barnes J, Anderson L, Phillipson J 2002 Herbal medicines: a guide for health care professionals, 2nd edn. Pharmaceutical Press, London

Bremness L 1995 Herbs. Dorling Kindersley, London

Buchbauer G, Jirovetz L, Jager W 1992 Passiflora and lime blossoms: motility effects after inhalation of the essential oils and of some of the main constituents in animal experimentation. Archive of Pharmacology 325: 247–248

Buchbauer G, Jirovetz L, Jager W 1993 Fragrance compounds and essential oils with sedative effects upon inhalation. Journal of Pharmaceutical Sciences 82(6): 660–664

Jager W, Buchbauer G, Jirovetz L 1992 Evidence of the sedative effect of neroli oil, citronella and phenylethyl acetate on mice. Journal of Essential Oil Research 4: 387–394

Lad V 1984 Ayurveda, the science of self healing: a practical guide. Lotus Press, Wisconsin

Leathwood P, Chauffard F 1985 Aqueous extract of valerian reduces latency to fall asleep in man. Planta Medica 51: 144–148

Lindahl O, Lindwall L 1989 Double blind study of a valerian preparation. Pharmacology Biochemistry and Behaviour 32: 1065–1066

Mills S 1994 A complete guide to modern herbalism. Thorsons, London

Miyake Y, Nakagawa M, Asakura Y 1991 Effects of odors on humans (1) effects on sleep latency. Chemical Senses 16(2): 183

Morin C, Culbert J, Schwartz M 1994 Non-pharmacological interventions for insomnia: a meta analysis of treatment efficacy. American Journal of Psychiatry 151(8): 1172–1180

Ryan N, Puig-Antich J, Rabinovich H et al 1987 The clinical picture of major depression in children and adolescents. Archives of General Psychiatry 44: 854

Schultz H, Jobert M 1994 Effects of hypericum extract on the sleep EEG in older volunteers. Journal of Geriatric Psychiatry and Neurology suppl 1: S39–43

12 Problems related to expressing sexuality

CHAPTER CONTENTS

- **Introduction 167**
- **Premenstrual syndrome 167**
  Bach flower remedies 168
  Aromatherapy 168
  Massage 168
  Homeopathy 168
  TCM 169
  Herbal remedies 169
  Ayurvedic medicine 170
  Reflexology 171
  Nutritional intervention 171

- **Dysmenorrhea 172**
  Approaches to treatment 172
  TCM 172
  Homeopathy and aromatherapy 173
  Ayurvedic medicine 173
  Herbal remedies 174
- **Gynaecological infections 174**
- **References 174**

INTRODUCTION

Depression, stress and anxiety can have a negative effect on the adolescent's self-image which is an integral part of being able to express their developing sexuality. For adolescents, physical and emotional changes can leave them feeling awkward and selfconscious leading to a lack of confidence, particularly if they experience gynaecological problems, which can inhibit social life.

PREMENSTRUAL SYNDROME (PMS)

Premenstrual syndrome often starts in adolescence, and presents as a collection of well-recognised physical and emotional symptoms which classically affect women 7–10 days before a period starts. Abraham (1980) proposed four sub-categories of PMS according to the presenting symptoms:

- PMS-A which is the commonest type, affecting 66–80% of PMS sufferers. Predominant symptoms include anxiety, irritability, insomnia and nervous tension caused by raised oestrogen in relation to progesterone.
- PMS-H occurs in 60–66% of sufferers and includes weight gain, bloatedness, breast tenderness and oedema of the face, hands and feet.
- PMS-C presents as increased appetite, craving for sweets, headaches, fainting, fatigue, dizziness, palpitations and trembling.
- PMS-D is characterised by depression and suicidal tendencies.

Although there is a classification of symptoms, each woman's experience is individual and symptoms can fluctuate over a number of cycles, making research into the condition problematic. Conventional therapy includes the use of diuretics, antidepressants and hormone therapy, although no one single treatment has been identified as superior. Of particular concern is the fact that PMS has been linked with poor academic performance in adolescents.

Bach flower remedies

Bach flower remedies which are of help include Mustard for depression, Crab apple for feelings of dissatisfaction with the body and mind, Impatiens for irritability and Beech for annoyance and intolerance, with Holly for bad temper. In addition, Cherry plum is helpful for fear of losing control. Cherry plum, which is prepared by the sun method, was first potentised in Sotwell in 1935.

Aromatherapy

Davis (1996) suggests that PMS can be helped by lymphatic drainage massage using essential oils of geranium (*Pelargonium graveolens*) to restore hormonal balance and rosemary (*Rosmarinus officinalis*), a diuretic, for fluid retention, with bergamot (*Citrus bergamia*), chamomile and rose oils (*Rosa centifolia* and *Rosa damascena*) for depression and irritability. She also points out that rose is the best oil for any disorders of the female reproductive system and suggests that it be used specifically for women who lack confidence in their own desirability or for sexual insecurity, although there is no evidence for this claim.

Massage

Field (2000) compared massage therapy (which has been noted to be of value in the treatment of depression) and relaxation in their effect on PMS. The massage therapy group received a 30 minute massage twice a week for 5 weeks, starting at the beginning of the premenstrual week and ending on the last day of the premenstrual week of the next cycle. Meanwhile, the relaxation group had progressive muscle relaxation training. Following initial training, this group received written instructions in the technique and were encouraged to practise for 30 minutes twice a week. Results were recorded using the State Trait Anxiety Inventory and the menstrual distress questionnaire and Profile of Mood States. Results indicated an immediate decrease in anxiety and improvement in mood following the first relaxation and massage sessions. Anxiety was also decreased after the last day session, but only in the massage group. The women in the massage group also reported a reduction in water retention.

Homeopathy

Homeopathic remedies for PMS include Nat. mur for tender breasts, bloated body and a tendency towards depression and introversion. This remedy is also appropriate for those suffering from premenstrual migraines, particularly those involving visual disturbances, and for those who break out in acne at this time. Pulsatilla is recommended for the oversensitive who have changeable moods with physical symptoms of vertigo, cystitis and mastitis, and Sepia for the sad and depressed, particularly if displaying symptoms of irritability and anger. Physically they may suffer from left sided headache, nausea or loss of appetite, they may feel generally sluggish and may have an exacerbation or outbreak of acne.

TCM

TCM defines four stages of menstruation:

1 Post menstruation: at this stage, following the blood loss, there is a relative deficiency of Blood and Yin.
2 Mid-cycle: this marks the transition from Yin to Yang, and this transition ensures proper ovulation.
3 Pre-menstruation: this period sees the growth of Yang-Qi. Since Kidneys are the root of Yin and Yang in the body and dominate sexual development, healthy transition from Yin to Yang is dependent on the Kidneys. In addition, the growth of Liver-Qi is necessary to move the Blood, which gives rise to menstruation.
4 Menstruation: during menstruation emphasis is on the free flow of blood and problems with this caused by stagnant Liver-Qi give rise to PMS.

Flaws (1985) notes that PMS categories are all variations of a basic Liver-Qi stagnation, since the Liver-Qi meridian passes through the uterus and ovaries and, as we have noted earlier in Chapter 10 on depression, disturbances of Liver-Qi affect the emotional state. The commonest symptoms are represented by Liver-Qi stagnation and symptoms include premenstrual breast tenderness and abdominal distension, irritability, clumsiness, moodiness and depression.

PMS can also be caused by a deficiency syndrome, particularly Liver-Blood deficiency which presents as weepiness and depression premenstrually with poor memory, tiredness and slight breast distension. PMS occurs when the Liver-Blood is deficient because Blood is being diverted towards the uterus.

Deadman (1995) gives a complete overview of TCM's ten patterns of pre-menstrual syndrome. General principles of treatment include addressing the presenting symptoms and rebalancing the Liver-Qi. Acupuncture treatment would start just after ovulation and would be given every other day, and treatment would need to be given over three menstrual cycles to have any effect. Flaws (1985) describes the range of herbal remedies used in the treatment of PMS.

Herbal remedies

Western herbal remedies for treating PMS would include those already mentioned under stress and anxiety (Ch. 10) and, in addition, there is excellent evidence for the value of agnus castus (*Vitex agnus castus*) in treating PMS. Agnus castus has a long history of efficacy as a 'woman's herb' and recent studies indicate that it works by correcting the oestrogen/progesterone balance. It acts at the level of the anterior pituitary, causing a decrease in the production of follicle stimulating hormone and an increase in the secretion of luteinizing hormone. The overall effect is the increase in the production of progesterone. It is of value in the treatment of all cases of PMS with the exception of type C (Mills & Bone 2000). Turner and Mills (1993) undertook a double blind clinical trial of agnus castus in the treatment of PMS. 217 women completed the full 3 months of treatment, 105 taking the herb and 112 on placebo. Only one symptom showed a statistical difference between the placebo and treatment groups, and that was the "feel jittery or restless" symptom at the 5% level; however, subjective reporting by 25 of the women on agnus castus showed they felt that their symptoms had improved. Four stated that their water retention had improved, five had fewer headaches, while eight said their breast tenderness had improved. The researchers concluded that the research design did not reflect all the differences between the placebo and the herb and that more research should be carried out, particularly in relation to symptoms of water retention.

More recent research by Schellenberg (2001) compared agnus castus with placebo. The study was a randomised, double blind placebo controlled trial over three menstrual cycles. 170 women who had PMS according to the DSM III criteria (American Psychological Association 1987) took agnus castus or a placebo daily for three consecutive menstrual cycles. Outcome measurement was the women's self-assessment of irritability, anger, headache, bloating and breast fullness. Improvement was greater in the active group than the placebo group ($p < 0.001$) with high tolerance level. The group reported a 50% reduction in symptoms.

Another herb, discussed earlier in relation to depression (Ch. 10), that has been evaluated recently for PMS is St John's wort (Stevinson & Ernst 2000). This was an uncontrolled observational study of 19 women with PMS who took the St John's wort for the duration of two menstrual cycles, leading to a significant reduction in all outcome measurements on the anxiety and depression scale and social adjustment scale. The participants reported that the degree of improvement was 51% (similar to agnus castus). This was not a controlled trial and the researchers agree that more work needs to be done.

Ayurvedic medicine

In Ayurveda, all three doshas are implicated in the menstrual cycle and symptoms are related to the respective dosha. Vata symptoms include bloated belly, low backache, insecurity, anxiety and fear, irregular menses and painful joints. Pitta symptoms are hot flushes, sensitive nipples, migraine headache, and anger resulting in argumentativeness. Fluid retention, tender breasts, weight gain, tiredness with excess sleep, and craving for sweets and chocolate are kapha symptoms. The predominant dosha is vata and, as has been explained previously, the main aim of Ayurvedic treatment is the pacification of the dominant dosha. Throughout the menstrual period the woman is encouraged to rest for 3 days or to reduce her work schedule, avoiding heavy work. A light, vata-reducing diet is suggested, including avoiding red meat, carbonated drinks, fried food and chocolate (Sharma & Clark 1998). In Ayurveda the menses are seen as a purifying activity and therefore internal tampons are not recommended. PMS is the result of two sub-doshas: ranjaka pitta, which is responsible for blood formation, and apana vata, which moves waste matter downwards. Additional treatment includes pancha karma, the relief of constipation and the reduction of stress. If one of the presenting symptoms is anger, then treatment would also be aimed at reducing pitta. It was pointed out in the previous section that the pitta type of depression was particularly serious in terms of self-harm and harming others.

Reflexology

Oleson and Flocco (1993) undertook a randomised controlled study to determine the effects of reflexology on PMS symptoms. Thirty-five women were randomly assigned to be treated by ear, hand and foot reflexology or to receive placebo reflexology. Subjects were carefully screened prior to the study for pregnancy, prior experience of reflexology or psychiatric illness. In addition, all subjects were screened by a clinical psychologist for psychological disturbance. During the study, each subject kept a daily diary which monitored 38 premenstrual symptoms on a four point scale and recorded them for 2 months prior to the study, for 2 months during the reflexology and for 2 months afterwards. Treatments were administered for 30 minutes once a week for 8 weeks. Unfortunately, the study suffered from a high attrition rate, which the researchers put down to the length of the study and the intensive input from the participants. In the true reflexology group appropriate reflex points for the treatment of PMS were stimulated, whilst the placebo group were given non-specific, uneven stimulation to points unrelated to the treatment of PMS. Baseline measurements of the two groups were similar before the treatments started.

Results showed that the participants in the true reflexology group reported a 46% reduction in symptoms from baseline during the treatment phase and 41% during the post treatment phase, which compares well with the results of the other studies of CAM treatments and PMS in this chapter. In addition, the 19% reduction in symptoms in the placebo group was less than half the amount of reduction in the true reflexology group.

In her review of the evidence for the effectiveness of CAM in the treatment of PMS, Stevinson (2000) intimates that there is no convincing evidence for its effectiveness, citing, rather strangely, that in some instances only one trial is available and noting particularly that there is a sizable placebo response in PMS, making comparison problematic. However, Oleson and Flocco (1993) pre-empt this somewhat dismissive approach, indicating in their study that PMS does indeed respond to placebo intervention, but pointing out that a number of other researchers had put the reduction in PMS symptoms in response to placebo intervention at less than 20%. As seen in the last three studies discussed in this chapter, response rates to treatment rather than placebo have consistently been at least twice this figure.

Nutritional intervention

A double blind trial of a nutritional programme for PMS had a positive outcome. Of the two groups engaged in the study, one received dietary advice and a nutritional supplement, Optivite, whilst the other received dietary advice and a placebo. The dietary advice suggested a low fat diet, vegetable proteins and fresh fruit, along with encouragement to reduce intake of coffee, tea, alcohol, salt, sugar and refined carbohydrates. The results were encouraging. All the participants showed a substantial reduction in symptoms which appeared to be due to the dietary improvement rather than to the supplement (Stewart et al 1993).

In her review of nutritional interventions, Head (1997) noted that the multi-factorial aetiology of PMS precludes any definitive dietary intervention but suggests that, where appropriate, the administration of specific dietary interventions may help. This is echoed by Dr Christiane Northrup, an obstetrician and gynaecologist with many years of experience in treating PMS with both orthodox and alternative approaches, in her excellent book *Women's Bodies Women's Wisdom* (Northrup 1995). She suggests that a reductionist approach, looking for a cause or magic bullet cure, will not work since the causes of the condition are multifactorial and treatment must be approached holistically. Therefore a number of treatments might work for a variety of women and nurses should be able to discuss these options and help adolescents make their own health choice.

DYSMENORRHOEA

Primary dysmenorrhoea starts 6–12 months after menarche. It is characterised by intense localised pain in the lower abdomen which may accompany other symptoms such as nausea and vomiting, diarrhoea, headache and irritability.

Approaches to treatment

Research undertaken by Balbi et al (2000) reviewed the dietary habits of 356 female students who suffered from primary dysmenorrhoea. They noted that, in keeping with the fact that eggs and fruit have a high magnesium and calcium content, girls who did not eat fruit or eggs experienced more severe symptoms of dysmenorrhoea. Calcium is able to regulate the ability of the muscular cells to respond to nervous stimuli, whilst a reduction in magnesium causes muscular hyperexcitability. The research suggests that attention to the diet of adolescents who suffer from primary dysmenorrhoea may prove to be of value in reducing the pain of menstruation. The potential of complementary therapies in the treatment of menstrual pain was highlighted by Campbell and McGrath (1999) when they reviewed the use of analgesia by adolescents. They noted that approximately 30% of adolescents did not use over the counter analgesics and approximately 15% of women did not respond to or were not able to tolerate the medications typically given for menstrual discomfort, and that medication may only provide limited relief. Of their sample of 299 female students, 31% said they used alternative methods of pain control because they worked, 28% said that the methods were convenient and 27% said they did not like using drugs, while 21% said that drugs did not have any therapeutic effect.

TCM

In TCM, dysmenorrhoea is seen as the result of Kidney and Spleen deficiency, with pain before and after the period indicating stagnant Blood and Qi deficiency. In TCM the foot is regarded as the root of the tree (body), and to nourish the root will heal the tree, thus a foot massage is often given for dysmenorrhoea.

In addition there are a number of herbs which are used routinely for gynaecological conditions, aimed predominantly at treating Qi weakness and Blood. Although these are known as Women's Precious Pills, because their action is good for anaemia and general lassitude, paradoxically they can be used by men.

Wang Xiaoma (1987) reviewed the effect of acupuncture and moxibustion in 100 cases of dysmenorrhoea. The patients presented with three syndromes: 46 were suffering from stagnation of Qi and Blood, 27 related to Cold and 17 had deficiency of Qi and Blood. The emphasis of the treatment was on the promotion of the smooth circulation of Blood and Qi. Treatment was given daily starting 8 days before the period and each course consisted of 12 treatments. Results showed that 54 patients were cured (complete relief of dysmenorrhoea and accompanying signs and symptoms), 27 had marked improvement (marked relief of dysmenorrhoea), and there was some improvement in 13 cases and failure in 6, making the total effective rate 94%. This therapeutic intervention proved to be simple, effective and economical.

Zhang (1984) reviewed 49 cases of dysmenorrhoea caused by Cold and Blood stasis. Acupuncture treatment was started 7–10 days before the onset of the period and was administered every other day until the period started. Results indicated that 42 patients had a complete cure and 6 had a marked improvement. Helms (1987) did a randomised controlled clinical trial using four groups of patients. One group was given acupuncture treatment, one was given sham acupuncture, one group had non-acupuncture visits with the project physician and one group acted as the control group. Results showed that there was a 41% reduction in analgesia used by women in the real acupuncture group. Thomas et al (1995) used a placebo controlled trial of four different modes of acupuncture and three different modes of TENS. Twenty-nine patients were treated 7 and 3 days before their expected periods. Results indicated that all the acupuncture methods showed improvements in outcome measures that reached significance level for pain. However, with the exception of low frequency electro-acupuncture, this did not result in a decrease in analgesia consumption. Low frequency TENS also gave significant reduction in pain and in analgesia consumption. High frequency TENS and placebo TENS did not result in significant improvement. At 3-month follow-up the improvement was maintained at significant levels, indicating that pre-emptive use of acupuncture and low frequency TENS resulted in reduced pain during menstruation.

Homeopathy and aromatherapy

Homeopathic treatments which might be indicated in treating dysmenorrhoea include Pulsatilla for pain in the lower back and abdomen, Calc. phos which is particularly good for adolescents with lower back ache and Belladonna for cramp-like pain before the period starts.

The antispasmodic oils of lavender, marjoram or chamomile, used as a hot compress on the abdomen, are said to bring relief.

Ayurvedic medicine

In Ayurvedic medicine the cause of dysmenorrhoea is the same as in PMS, i.e. excess of apana vata, and much of the advice is the same for both, with the added intervention of abdominal massage, working clock-wise and using sesame oil and pancha karma for dysmenorrhoea. This helps reduce symptoms, and a vata-reducing diet will also help. Lad (1983) suggests taking aloe vera for menstrual cramps.

Herbal remedies

Because of its normalising effect on the menstrual cycle, agnus castus is of value in the treatment of painful periods; however, it should be noted that because of its normalising action it can interfere with the effectiveness of the contraceptive pill.

GYNAECOLOGICAL INFECTIONS

Gynaecological infections such as thrush can be debilitating and depressing. A number of studies have indicated the use of tea tree oil as a useful treatment (Carson & Riley 1994, Belaiche 1985, Hammer et al 1998, Cox et al 2000). The bee product propolis, which is active against *Candida albicans* and is shown to act synergistically with antimycrotic drugs, lowering the resistance of the yeast to the drug (Bone 1994), is also useful. Propolis is also highly active against *Trichomonas vaginalis* (Bone 1994) and it has also been seen to be effective against *Herpes genitalis*. In the results of two unpublished studies described by Ring (1995), patients reported that symptoms began to be alleviated within 12 hours of initiation of treatment, with complete healing of the lesions occurring within 4 days of starting treatment.

REFERENCES

Abraham G 1980 Premenstrual tension. Problems in Obstetrics and Gynaecology 3(12): 1–39

American Psychological Association 1987 Diagnostic and statistical manual of mental disorders (DSM-III-R), 3rd edn. American Psychiatric Press, Washington

Balbi C, Musone R, Menditto A et al 2000 Influence of menstrual factors and dietary habits on menstrual pain in adolescence age. European Journal of Obstetrics and Gynaecology and Reproductive Biology 91(2): 143–148

Belaiche P 1985 Treatment of skin infections with essential oil of Melaleuca alternifolia. Phytotherapy 15: 15–17

Bone K 1994 Propolis: a natural antibiotic. Australian Journal of Medical Herbalism 6(3): 61–65

Campbell M, McGrath P 1999 Non pharmacological strategies used by adolescents for the management of menstrual discomfort. The Clinical Journal of Pain 15(4): 313–320

Carson C, Riley T 1994 The antimicrobial effect of tea tree oil. Medical Journal of Australia 160: 236

Cox S, Mann C, Markham J et al 2000 The mode of action of antimicrobial action of the essential oil of Melaleuca alternifolia (tea tree oil). Journal of Applied Microbiology 88: 170–175

Davis P 1996 Aromatherapy: an A–Z. CW Daniel, Saffron Walden

Deadman P 1995 Acupuncture in the treatment of premenstrual syndrome. Journal of Chinese Medicine 48(May): 5–14

Field T 2000 Touch therapy. Churchill Livingstone, Edinburgh

Flaws B 1985 Premenstrual syndrome (PMS): its differential diagnosis and treatment. American Journal of Acupuncture 13(3): 205–222

Hammer K, Carson C, Riley T 1998 In vitro activity of essential oils, in particular Melaleuca alternifolia (tea tree) and tea tree oil products against Candida spp. Journal of Antimicrobial Chemotherapy 42(5): 591–595

Head K 1997 Premenstrual syndrome: nutritional and alternative approaches. Alternative Medical Review 2(1): 12–25

Helms J M 1987 Acupuncture for the treatment of primary dysmenorrhea. Obstetrics and Gynecology (Jan) 69(1): 51–56

Lad V 1983 Ayurveda, the science of self healing: a practical guide. Lotus Press, Wisconsin

Mills S, Bone K 2000 Principles and practice of phytotherapy: modern herbal medicine. Churchill Livingstone, Edinburgh

Northrup C 1995 Women's bodies, women's wisdom. The complete guide to women's health and wellbeing. Piatkus, London

Oleson T, Flocco W 1993 Randomised controlled study of premenstrual symptoms treated with ear, hand and foot reflexology. Obstetrics and Gynaecology 82(6): 906–911

Ring S A 1995 Antiviral complex of flavonoids from propolis in the treatment of herpes infections. Journal of Alternative and Complementary Medicine Jan: 9–10

Schellenberg R 2001 Treatment of premenstrual syndrome with agnus castus fruit extract: prospective, randomised, placebo controlled study. British Medical Journal 322: 134–137

Sharma H, Clark C 1998 Contemporary Ayurveda. Churchill Livingstone, Edinburgh

Stevinson C 2000 Evidence for complementary therapies in premenstrual syndrome. Focus on Alternative and Complementary Therapies 5(3): 185–188

Stevinson C, Ernst E 2000 Hypericum perforatum for the treatment of premenstrual syndrome. British Journal of Obstetrics and Gynaecology 107: 870–876

Stewart SC, Tooley SH, Paterson-Jones J, Tooke J, Stewart M 1993 Effect of a nutritional programme on premenstrual syndrome and work efficiency. Complementary Therapies in Medicine 1(2): 68–72

Thomas M, Lundeberg T, Bjork G 1995 Pain and discomfort in primary dysmenorrhea is reduced by pre-emptive acupuncture of low frequency TENS. European Journal of Physical Medicine and Rehabilitation 5: 71–76

Turner S, Mills S 1993 A double-blind clinical trial on a herbal remedy for pre-menstrual syndrome: a case study. Complementary Therapies in Medicine 1(2): 73–77

Wang X 1987 Observations of the therapeutic effects of acupuncture and moxibustion in 100 cases of dysmenorrhoea. Journal of Traditional Chinese Medicine 7(1): 15–17

Zhang Y 1984 A report of 49 cases of dysmenorrhoea treated by acupuncture. Journal of Traditional Chinese Medicine 4(2): 191–102

13 Problems related to washing and dressing

CHAPTER CONTENTS

- **Acne   177**
  Aromatherapy   178
  Nicotinamide   178
  Ayurvedic medicine   179
  Anthroposophical medicine   179
  Herbalism   179
  TCM   179
  Homeopathy   180
  Bach flower remedies   180

- **Psoriasis   181**
  Herbal remedies   181
  TCM   181
  Anthroposophical medicine   182
  Homeopathy   182
  Ayurvedic medicine   182
  Psychological interventions   182
  Other interventions   183
- **References   183**

ACNE

One condition which is a blight on the young person's life is acne. Acne vulgaris is a chronic inflammatory disease characterised by the development of comedones, ethrythematous papules and pustules on the face, chest and back. Acne is common during adolescence, predominantly between the ages of 14 and 18 years, and it is triggered by the activity of the sebaceous glands and by androgenic stimulants at puberty. As with other skin conditions, it fluctuates in its severity, and flare-ups have been associated with stress, which is particularly high during adolescence. Causes of stress include taking national exams, coping with interpersonal relationships and making career choices. The fact that most adolescents grow out of acne is of no consolation to the young person who is suffering from it and does nothing to help their self confidence. Koo (1995) quotes Sulzberger and Zaidems (1948) who say that: 'There is no single disease which causes more psychic trauma, more maladjustment between parent and children, more general insecurity and feelings of inferiority and greater sums of psychic suffering than does acne vulgaris.'

It is the social and psychological effects of acne which prompt young adults to seek help. Koo (1995) suggests, and this has been confirmed by other dermatologists, e.g. Williams (1995), that skin problems and acne in particular are regarded as purely cosmetic problems and that the psychosocial effects are seriously underestimated. Attempts to evaluate the impact of acne using standard psychometric instruments normally used in mental health on adolescents have had mixed results. Koo's research, using interviews with acne sufferers, produced a number of consistently mentioned issues, including lack of self-esteem and self-confidence, poor body image, embarrassment, social withdrawal, limitations on lifestyle, and anger. Many sufferers reported feeling ugly and one refused to use mirrors (Koo 1995). Jowett and Ryand (1985) noted that adolescents with acne had poorer academic functioning when compared with others. Cunningham (1998), a nurse specialist who runs an acne support group, calls acne the 'forgotten disease' and highlights the need for early intervention to avoid scarring. Conventional treatments using benzoyl peroxide and systemic antibiotics usually provide good results but can cause unacceptable side effects. It has been noted that good results can also be obtained by using the less aggressive tea tree oil, which is antifungal and antibacterial (Lis-Balchin et al 1996) as well as being an immunostimulant.

Aromatherapy

Bassett et al (1990) conducted a single, blind randomised clinical trial on 124 patients with mild to moderate acne, using a 5% tea tree gel versus a 5% benzoyl peroxide preparation. The severity of each patient's acne was defined using the counting technique of Burke and Cunliffe (1984) as well as an assessment of skin tolerance related to dryness and erythema. The benzoyl peroxide caused more dryness and scaling but no difference in erythema. Both treatments were effective in reducing the number of infectious lesions throughout the trial and the reduction between baseline and final assessment was significant in both groups. Although effects from the tea tree oil took longer to become apparent than did the effects from the benzoyl peroxide, the tea tree oil was better tolerated by facial skin since it did not cause the dryness and skin scaling of the benzoyl peroxide preparation. Tea tree oil was considered an effective topical treatment for acne, with fewer side effects, but the authors suggest that a 100% tea tree oil would have had a quicker result.

Nicotinamide

A study was made by Shalita et al (1995) of the comparative merits of nicotinamide versus clindamycin gel in the treatment of inflammatory acne vulgaris. The study was stimulated by the problem of using systemic and topical antimicrobials, which are associated with the emergence of resistant pathogens and an increase in microorganism resistance. Nicotinamide gel is a potent anti-inflammatory agent, but without the risk of inducing bacterial resistance. A comparison was made between a 4% nicotinamide gel and a 1% clindamycin gel in a treatment population of 76 patients randomly assigned to the groups and who applied the gels twice daily for 8 weeks. Evaluation was carried out using the physician's global evaluation, acne lesion counts and an acne severity rating. Results were very encouraging, with the nicotinamide gel giving an 82% improvement and the clindamycin 1% giving a 68% improvement, with statistically similar reductions in acne lesions. The researchers suggest that nicotinamide gel is a useful and desirable alternative to antimicrobials for the treatment of acne vulgaris. Lis-Balchin et al (1996) noted that the antimicrobial and antifungal effects are most effective against *Staphylococcus aureus* and less active against *E. coli* and pseudomonas, but not effective against *propione bacterium acnes,* which is specific to acne.

Ayurvedic medicine

Ayurvedic medicine describes acne as Tarunya Peetika, which means a disease of adolescence. It is caused by excess of pitta dosha in the lymph tissue. In a very well controlled clinical trial, four Ayurvedic formulations in the treatment of acne vulgaris were compared with a placebo. Subjects were controlled for sex, age, diet, smoking and types of complexion and a 2 week wash out period was instigated at the beginning of the trial to eliminate the effects of existing medication. The skin care regimen was standardised for all the young people and the medication, which was taken in tablet form, was to be taken three times a day. Observer bias was controlled for and assessment of the treatment was done blind. On evaluation, the group taking the medication called Sunder vati was associated with a significant reduction in the total number of inflammatory lesions within 2 weeks and a further reduction at 6 weeks, whilst the other treatment groups showed no significant difference when compared with baseline values. This particular medication consisted of the herbs Kutaj (*Holarrhena antidysenterica*, Apocynaceae), Amalaki *(Emblica officinalis)*, Vidanga *(Embelia ribes*, Myrsinaceae) and Sunth (*Zingiber officinale,* Zingiberaceae). The mechanism is not clear but the authors (Chopra et al 1982) suggest that Amerlaki, a fruit, is rich in vitamin C. Vidanga is a common Indian medicine and may have antibiotic action against *Staphylococcus aureus* and *E. coli*. Kutaj bark has astringent activity and Sunth is reported to have an anti-inflammatory action.

Anthroposophical medicine

In Anthroposophical medicine, acne is seen as a deficiency of excretion. A special diet is advocated, consisting of a 1 week apple diet followed by 3 months on a vegetarian diet, along with a general treatment of Quartz D30 alternately with Sulphur D3, with Erysidoron 1 and 2 for severe cases. Local applications of hot water with Calendula 20% are added.

Herbalism

Again, the traditional role of herbalism is to restore the proper function of the body and increase health and vitality, thus herbs are widely used as supportive remedies, particularly in chronic, degenerative and inflammatory conditions, as was noted in Chapter 3 in relation to eczema. A more validated treatment of acne is the use of agnus castus, which can also be used by men.

TCM

TCM regards acne as a problem of Phlegm and Heat that can be aggravated if the patient has been eating too much Hot, Damp food or if the digestive tract is unbalanced, resulting in the malfunction of Stomach channels, or if the Lungs have been invaded by Wind/Heat. As with Western herbal treatment, Traditional

Chinese Medicine concentrates on ridding the system of toxins, and a diet avoiding foods containing Heat and Phlegm is advised. Lui (1995) describes the use of auricular acupuncture in the treatment of acne. The patients were diagnosed as having Wind/Heat invading the Lung channel or an accumulation of Heat in Spleen and Stomach. The acupuncture points were punctured with thumb tack needles and the course of treatment involved the needles being manipulated 3–5 times per day up to a total of 15 manipulations. 46 patients were treated and results showed that 28 were deemed to be cured, the criteria being the disappearance of skin lesions. For 10 subjects, the treatment was markedly effective (evaluated as the disappearance of 90% of the skin lesions) and 3 had a marked improvement, in total an effective rate of 93%. All the cured cases were followed-up for 6 months and none of them suffered any relapse. In his review of clinical studies on the treatment of skin disease using acupuncture, Rosted (1994) noted that methods varied considerably between therapists, although the intervention had a high level of effectiveness overall.

Homeopathy

Homeopathic remedies for acne include Pulsatilla, which is recommended for teenage acne, particularly if too much rich food has been consumed, and Hepar. sulph, where there are a large number of infected spots. Long-standing acne responds to Sulphur, whilst Kali. brom is recommended for chronic acne and Antimonium crudum for infected spots.

Bach flower remedies

As was pointed out in the introduction to this chapter, skin conditions not only cause a great deal of psychological damage but can themselves be triggered or aggravated by emotion, stress or trauma. Since the Bach flower remedies act solely on the emotions to facilitate the return of equilibrium, some adolescents may find them helpful. Relevant remedies for acne, which is normally age-related, include Walnut for the changes experienced during adolescence, Scleranthus for the accompanying mood swings that aggravate the condition, Wild oat to help determine a path in life and Mustard for depression, notably for the type which descends out of the blue and is part and parcel of the mood swings. Since skin conditions fluctuate in their intensity and in response to different treatments, Gentian should be recommended for the discouragement that this can cause.

A key remedy for all skin conditions is Crab apple for the lack of self-esteem and sometimes almost revulsion at the state of the skin. Howard suggests putting drops of the remedy Crab apple into clear water to rinse the face, as well as the application of Rescue Remedy cream, which contains honey for healing. Larch is indicated for lack of self-confidence and Willow for self-pity and resentment. Gentian was first potentised by Dr Bach in Kent in 1931 and is prepared by the sun method. It was one of the original twelve healers described in his book of that name (Bach 1933). Larch, along with Mustard, are among the last remedies identified by Dr Bach after he had settled in Sotwell, and these are prepared by the boiling method.

PSORIASIS

Perhaps one of the most distressing skin conditions is psoriasis. Psoriasis is a chronic inflammatory condition which is characterised by raised plaques of thickened, scaly epidermis and affects about 2% of the population. It tends to be familial and, as with other skin conditions, tends to relapse and remit spontaneously, and it can start at any age. It is characterised by multiple, discrete red patches with silvery white scales, most frequently occurring on the knees and elbows. The cause is unknown but is thought to be related to metabolic or immunological events. Orthodox treatment includes anti-inflammatory drugs or immunosuppressive therapy such as methotrexate.

Herbal remedies

Herbal medicine applies the same principles of treatment as outlined in Chapter 9 with the addition of a topical application of chrysarobin of which dithranol is the cheaper synthetic analogue.

Traditionally, oatmeal has been used as a bath additive, being particularly good for irritating conditions. Aloe vera has been known and used medicinally since the 4th century BC and was used by Alfred the Great and revered by the Mohammedans (Hollis 1994). It is also thought to have been one of Cleopatra's beauty secrets (Hollis 1994, Bremness 1995). Barnes et al (2002) have pointed out that aloe vera is the mucilaginous tissue located in the leaf parenchyma of *aloe vera* and other related aloe species. They suggest that some documented studies have not used pure aloe vera but have used other extracts of aloes rather than the pure aloe vera. Syed et al (1996) investigated the use of aloe vera (*Aloe barbadensis*) in the treatment of psoriasis with good results. In this study, aloe vera was dispensed at 0.5% in a hydrophilic cream and applied to the areas of psoriasis three times a day for 5 consecutive days per week for 4 weeks. A control group used a placebo. Patients were examined on a weekly basis for 16 weeks and those who showed a progressive reduction in lesions, desquamation followed by decreased erythema, infiltration and reduced PASI score were deemed to be cured. The subjects were subsequently followed up for a further 8 months. The aloe vera group had a significantly larger number of cures than the placebo group, 83.3% compared with 6.6% in the placebo group, and the active group also had the largest number of healed chronic lesions. Biopsy analysis showed that the aloe vera group had a decrease in the levels of epidermal acanthosis, parakeratosis, thinning and inflammatory infiltration. No side effects were recorded.

TCM

Psoriasis has been shown to respond well to acupuncture. 61 cases of psoriasis were treated, many having quite extensive involvement of the body, and each patient received an average of 9 acupuncture sessions. Half of the patients had complete or almost complete clearance of the condition, 14 patients had two-thirds clearance and 8 had a clearance of one-third, while 9 patients had minimal or no improvement. The authors suggest that there was a possible involvement of the cutaneous reticuloendothelial system in the clearance of the skin lesions (Liao et al 1992).

Fujiwaki and Furusho (1992) described the use of rice bran broth bathing in the treatment of atopic dermatitis. 16 outpatients undertook the rice broth bathing for 2–5 months and their skin condition was checked every month. None of the 16 experienced negative effects and the efficacy of the treatment was excellent in 4 of the subjects, good in 7, slightly effective in 4 and ineffective in 1. The authors concluded that the treatment of psoriasis by this method is safe and clinically useful.

Anthroposophical medicine

Anthroposophical treatments for psoriasis include using the apple and vegetarian diet already described in the treatment of acne. In addition, Betula cortex, Quartz, Gallae halepenses D2–D3 and Agaricus muscarius D10 in a decoction of Species anti-psoriases are recommended.

Homeopathy

A locally applied homeopathic cream has been evaluated by Gieler et al (1995). *Mahonia aquifolium* (Rubisan) was tested on a sample of 375 patients over a period of 12 weeks. Results showed that symptoms improved or disappeared completely. The preparation was well tolerated by the subjects and the researchers suggest that the ointment offers an alternative to conventional treatments for psoriasis. Further research has been done on this preparation by Augustin et al (1999), who examined the effects of *Mahonia aquifolium* as a topical application in the treatment of psoriasis, comparing it with dithranol. The ointment was applied daily for 4 weeks. Biopsies of the lesions were taken prior to and on completion of the study and results demonstrated the efficacy of both *Mahonia aquifolium* and dithranol as treatments for psoriasis, having effects on both the cellular cutaneous immune mechanisms and on the hyperproliferation of keratinocytes. The effect of dithranol was more pronounced than that of *Mahonia aquifolium*.

Ayurvedic medicine

In Ayurvedic medicine, psoriasis is seen as excess pitta in the blood as well as an imbalance between perspiration and urination, and in both cases blood purification and the rebalancing of the excess dosha is seen as the correct treatment. Diet would be adjusted to rebalance the dosha.

Psychological interventions

A number of studies have examined the role of psychological interventions in the treatment of psoriasis. Zachariae et al (1996) looked at the effects of psychotherapy, and Gaston et al (1988) looked at meditation and imagery. Gaston's research compared meditation and imagery with routine treatment and waiting list groups. Although there was a significant difference between treatment and control group, it was noted that imagery offered no additional benefit to meditation. Although the sample size was small, the results do offer an additional intervention in the treatment of psoriasis. In a further study by Gaston et al (1991), a larger sample size showed again that the practice of meditation may be clinically effective for some patients in reducing their psoriasis symptoms. For one of the control groups the relationship between psychological stress and psoriasis was examined prospectively over a period of 20 weeks using standardised measures. Results indicated a positive correlation between the severity of psoriasis symptoms and psychological stress and the impact of adverse life events, although the authors point out that within this there were important individual differences. They suggest that stress reduction techniques should be regarded as part of the treatment for psoriasis.

Other interventions

One interesting review of results in the treatment of psoriasis comes from a clinic on the Dead Sea. Whilst in no sense of the term is the report a research trial, a review of 1448 patients treated at the clinic was undertaken by Abels et al (1995). Treatment at the clinic involved an increasing exposure to the sun for up to 6 hours per day and bathing in the Dead Sea for up to 1 hour per day, as well as the application of topical emollient creams. Recommended treatment time was 28 days. Results indicated that over 99% of patients improved at least 50%, and 58% had a complete clearing of their condition. The Dead Sea has been credited with unique therapeutic benefits for over 2000 years. The authors suggest that this is due to its unusual geographical situation, 390 metres below sea level, engendering a unique, natural ultra-violet spectrum of light, combined with the fact that the sea is rich in salts and minerals. There was, however, a difference in response between Israeli patients and those from overseas. One reason for this might be that the Israelis stayed for only 2 weeks whilst overseas patients stayed for the full 28 days. Dead sea salt can be obtained by mail order, although how effective it is without the accompanying holiday and ultra-violet light is not clear. In a previous study, Gruner et al (1990) compared treatment of psoriasis with salt from the Dead Sea, plus ultra-violet light, with baths containing sodium chloride in comparable concentrations, and demonstrated a reduced amount of Langerhan's cells in the epidermis of subjects in the Dead Sea group, the sodium chloride treatment having no effect at all.

REFERENCES

Abels D, Rose T, Bearman J 1995 Treatment of psoriasis at a Dead Sea dermatology clinic. International Journal of Dermatology 2: 134–137

Augustin M, Andrees U, Grimme H et al 1999 Effects of Mahonia aquifolium ointment on the expression of adhesion, proliferation and activation markers in the skin of patients with psoriasis. Forsch Komplementarmed Apr 6 (Supp 2): 19–21

Bach E 1933 The twelve healers and other remedies. CW Daniel, Saffron Walden

Barnes J, Anderson L, Phillipson J 2002 Herbal medicines: a guide for health care professionals, 2nd edn. Pharmaceutical Press, London

Bassett I, Pannowitz D, Barnetson St C 1990 A comparative study of tea tree oil versus benzoyl peroxide in the treatment of acne. Medical Journal of Australia 153: 455–458

Bremness L 1995 Herbs. Dorling Kindersley, London

Burke B, Cunliffe W 1984 The assessment of acne vulgaris – the Leeds technique. British Journal of Dermatology 111: 83–92

Chopra R, Chopra I, Handa K 1982 Indigenous drugs of India. Academic Publishers, Calcutta, p 673–684

Cunningham M 1998 Spot check. Nursing Times 94(50): 61–63

Fujiwaki T, Furusho K 1992 The effects of rice bran bathing on patients with atopic dermatitis. Acta Paediatrica Japanica 34: 505–510

Gaston L, Crombez J, Joly J et al 1988 Efficacy of imagery and meditation techniques in treating psoriasis. Imagination, Cognition and Personality 898(1): 25–38

Gaston L, Crombez J, Lassonde M et al 1991 Psychological stress and psoriasis: experimental and prospective studies. Acta Mermo-Veneriologica 156 (suppl): 37–43

Gieler U, Von der Weht A, Heger M 1995 Mahonia aquifolium. A new type of topical treatment for psoriasis. Journal of Dermatological Treatment 6(1): 31–34

Gruner S, Zwirner A, Boonen H 1990 Effect of treatment with salt from the Dead Sea (Tomesa therapy) on epidermal Langerhans cells – a clinical study. Zeitschrift fur Hautkrankheiten 65(12): 1146–1151

Hollis S 1994 The country diary herbal. Bloomsbury Books, London

Jowett S, Ryand T 1985 Skin disease and handicap: an analysis of the impact of skin conditions. Social Science Medicine 20(4): 425–429

Koo J 1995 The psychosocial impact of acne: patients' perceptions. Journal of the American Academy of Dermatology 32(5) part 3: s26–s28

Liao S 1992 Acupuncture treatment for psoriasis. Acupuncture and Electro-therapeutics Research 17: 195–208

Lis-Balchin M, Hart S, Deans S 1996 Comparison of the pharmacological and antimicrobial action of commercial plant essential oils. Journal of Herbs, Spices and Medicinal Plants 4(2): 69–86

Lui Z-H 1995 Ear point embedding in the treatment of acne vulgaris. International Journal of Clinical Acupuncture 6(1): 113–115

Rosted P 1994 Survey of recent clinical studies on the treatment of skin diseases with acupuncture. American Journal of Acupuncture 22(4): 357–361

Shalita A, Smith J, Parish L et al 1995 Topical nicotinamide compared with clindamycin gel in the treatment of inflammatory acne vulgaris. International Journal of Dermatology 34(6): 434–437

Sulzberger M, Zaidems S 1948 Psychogenic factors in dermatological disorders. Medical Clinics of North America 32: 669

Syed T, Ahmad A, Holt A et al 1996 Management of psoriasis with aloe vera in a hydrophilic cream: placebo controlled, double blind study. Tropical Medicine and International Health 1(4): 505–509

Williams H 1995 On the definition and epidemiology of atopic dermatitis. Dermatological Clinics 13(3): 649–657

Zachariae R, Oster H, Bjerring P et al 1996 Effects of psychological intervention on psoriasis: a preliminary report. Journal of the American Academy of Dermatology 34(6): 1008–1015

14 Problems with eating and drinking

CHAPTER CONTENTS

- **Introduction** 185
- **Anorexia nervosa** 185
  Massage 186
  Music therapy 187
  Hypnosis 187
  Other useful interventions 187
- **Bulimia nervosa** 188
  Hypnosis 188

- **Obesity** 188
  Hypnosis 189
  TCM 189
  Other interventions 190
- **Conclusion** 190
- **References** 190

INTRODUCTION

Adolescents have a great need to be socially accepted and considered attractive by their peers, which is dependant on having a good self image. Unfortunately, the pressures resulting from this may lead to problems with eating and drinking. Eating disorders stem from a psychological illness in which the patient's emotional distress presents as various problems with eating. Young people with these disorders have been known to present with a number of personality disorders, and there can be a high incidence of coexisting psychiatric conditions, such as mood disturbances, major depression and obsessive/compulsive disorders. In addition, they suffer from feelings of inadequacy, lack self-confidence, and have poor self-esteem and poor coping mechanisms.

ANOREXIA NERVOSA

Coman and Evans (1995) note that anorexia nervosa develops from a number of causes, including personality characteristics, perceptual disturbances, feelings of personal inadequacy and family interaction factors. They suggest that family dysfunction is a factor in most cases of anorexia. Fornari et al (2001) highlight the role of parental neglect (in terms of failure to cooperate with treatment) in anorexia nervosa, and state that parental non-compliance exposes the young person to a wide variety of long-term and short-term health risks, including death.

The serious and complex condition of anorexia nervosa requires skilled medical and nursing intervention, but patients can also benefit from supportive therapies, particularly in the recovery phase. Anorexia nervosa has been described as a condition commonly affecting middle to upper class families, but as Kohn and

Golden (2001) point out, this stereotype is no longer applicable and there appears to be no cultural immunity for anorexia. In fact, the incidence of the condition is increasing in countries such as China and Japan as well as among Native Americans and Hispanics (Crago et al 1996). Rural areas are affected as much as urban ones and Kreipe (1995) reports a bimodal diagnostic peak at ages 14 and 18 years.

Most eating disorders are triggered by a desire to lose weight and involve a fear of fullness or loss of control around food. Presenting symptoms of anorexia include:

- A refusal to maintain normal body weight
- An intense fear of weight gain and fatness
- A dysmorphic body image (Kohn & Golden 2001).

This can result in changes of mood and inability to think coherently, as well as a preoccupation with food. This leads to a diet low in fat and carbohydrate, leading to a loss of water, body fat and eventually loss of essential body tissue. Treatment of this condition is far from simple and requires a long-term commitment from the patient and the family, but it is suggested that any complementary therapy which helps to address the underlying depression, anxiety and stress may be of help. Clearly, not all the interventions explored in this book would be appropriate and treatment would depend on the skilled practitioner's assessment of which therapies might be of value at any one stage of the patient's illness.

Massage

Any therapy which enables patients to develop realistic perceptions of their own bodies and to feel positive about themselves will be beneficial. Field (2000) described the role of massage as a supportive treatment for this very complex condition and investigated the effect of massage in relieving the anxiety and depression often associated with anorexia.

Nineteen females undergoing treatment for anorexia nervosa were randomly assigned to either a massage therapy group or a group undergoing conventional treatment and normal activity. The two groups were assessed using the State Trait Anxiety Inventory (STAI) and the Profile of Mood States (POMS), and samples were taken for saliva cortisol. In addition, on the first and last days of the trial the following assessments were performed: the center for epidemiological studies depression scale, the eating disorder inventory (EDI) and a urine analysis. The massage therapy group received a 30 minute full body massage twice a week for 5 weeks. Following the study the assessment scores on the STAI and the POMS for the massage group decreased and the saliva cortisol levels reduced, suggesting an immediate reduction in anxiety and stress hormone levels, and improved mood following the massage. Long-term measures indicated that the massage group had reduced EDI scores. Overall, the subjects reported decreases in anxiety and improvement in mood following the massage sessions. By the end of the study the women in the massage group were reporting less body dissatisfaction on the EDI, with the scores for the control group being unchanged. Field suggested that the success of the massage therapy may have been due to the desire for tactile nurturing described by Gupta et al (1995). Field also suggested that the massage might be helping the women to feel more comfortable with their bodies and may also have facilitated an increase in close physical contacts and a more intimate relationship.

Music therapy

Two interesting papers by Smeijsters (1996) and Robarts and Sloboda (1994) describe the use of music therapy in the treatment of anorexia nervosa. Both sets of authors confirm the role of music as a form of non-verbal communication in patients who are unable to express their feelings, or who may not understand their feelings in any other way. Smeijsters (1996) writes that music therapy, whether vocal or instrumental, encourages the patient to develop a better sense of body awareness and can include the use of relaxation exercises. Robarts and Sloboda (1994) describe two case studies in which music therapy was used as an adjunct to other treatments. They noted that anorectics display a number of common musical symptoms which reflect their distorted sense of self. These symptoms include lack of musical structure, rapid playing, avoidance of phrasing, i.e. no pauses between sections, preference for high notes over lower tones, lack of expression of any emotion and lack of flexibility. The two case studies illustrate how music therapy encourages the patients to develop a sense of self and of self in relation to another and can help towards the emergence of individuality and autonomy.

Hypnosis

Coman and Evans (1995) reviewed the role of hypnosis in the treatment of anorexia. Whilst it has been shown that hypnosis can be effective in treating lack of self-confidence, low self-esteem and stress, Coman and Evans suggested that the restrictive nature of anorexia would make the patient a poor subject for hypnosis. The role of hypnosis is discussed further in the next section on bulimia.

Other useful interventions

T'ai chi and yoga, with their slow, controlled movements, are a means of increasing body awareness, by increasing chi and prana and inducing a calm and peaceful state of mind, while at the same time maintaining body tone and suppleness.

Anorexics frequently have strong feelings of self-loathing and adolescents who use the Bach flower remedies may be using formulas that include the following: Crab apple as a cleansing agent for the mind and body, especially for those who are unhappy with their image; Rock water for the rigid self-denial of the anorexic; Mimulus for the fear of putting on weight; and Elm and Walnut for fear of not being able to cope with the increasing adult responsibilities and the mental and physical changes of adolescence.

Homeopathic remedies which patients might be using for this condition include Nat. mur (which is particularly effective), Pulsatilla or Argentum nit, which is recommended where a phobic element is present.

A search of the Ayurvedic medicine literature did not reveal any studies on the treatment of anorexia nervosa but a review of the symptoms of anorexia nervosa indicates a strong concordance with the symptoms of excess vata and treatment would be to redress this.

BULIMIA NERVOSA

Bulimia nervosa is characterised by binge eating followed by purging on a regular basis, i.e. more than twice a week. It tends to present in later adolescence and is associated with poor impulse control. Patients may be underweight, of normal weight or overweight. Bulimia and anorexia represent the spectrum of eating disorders, and 10–30% of patients cross over from one disorder to the other during their illness (Strober et al 1997), with 40% of anorexic patients having symptoms of bulimia (Golden & Sacker 1984). Features of bulimia include:

- Self-induced vomiting
- Abuse of laxatives or diuretics
- Fasting
- Excessive exercise
- And a feeling of loss of control when bingeing.

Coman (1992) highlighted the personal characteristics of bulimic patients: feelings of shame, self-criticism, a need for immediate gratification, a strong need for approval and heightened interpersonal sensitivity (Groth-Marnat & Schumaker 1989). Johnson and Larson (1982) suggest the condition is an addictive disorder, with the food being used for tension release.

Hypnosis

In Coman's (1992) review of the role of hypnosis in the treatment of bulimia, he notes that some psychiatric disorders, including phobic disorders and eating disorders, are characterised by high levels of hypnotisability. Patients with bulimia nervosa have been noted to score at higher hypnotisability levels than patients with anorexia or patients in a control group. Groth-Marnat and Schumaker (1990) argue that extreme weight control behaviours may be similar to hypnotic-like states such as dissociation, which is a reported characteristic of bulimics during binge eating. They further argue that this dissociation might be related to cognitive and perceptual distortions reported by many patients with eating disorders. However, this view has been challenged by Frasquilho and Oakley (1997), who point out that hypnosis and dissociation are only loosely correlated and that few studies have linked this with bulimic behaviour. Coman (1992) suggest that a contributory factor for patients in controlling their eating is their phobic absorption in their eating behaviour and their levels of generalised anxiety. Treatment of bulimics with hypnosis would include supportive intervention during cognitive and behavioural change, dealing with underlying triggers to the condition, and long-term maintenance therapy.

OBESITY

In the health survey of 1991 (White et al 1993), 15% of the English population were classified as being obese, a problem which has been on the increase over the last 30 years. The causes of obesity are many and embrace such factors as genetic predisposition, family eating patterns, availability of food, culture, chaotic lifestyle and, increasingly in our technological age, lack of exercise. Food habits are notoriously difficult to alter. They are formed early in childhood and are long-lasting (Fieldhouse 1996). Hill and Peters (1998) have highlighted the environmental factors that currently promote overeating and thus compound the potential for obesity. Specifically, they cite the 'super sizing' of fast food portions and the high fat content of many ready meals. They also note changes in lifestyle, such as increased technology and transportation, reducing the need for physical activity, and the increased tendency for more sedentary pursuits amongst children.

The growing problem of childhood and adolescent obesity (defined as a body mass index over the ninety-seventh centile relative to age or gender) has been noted by the health care industry as a serious economic factor, leading as it does to increased morbidity and mortality. The therapeutic input for addressing this problem is psychological and family therapy, exercise programmes, behaviour modification and nutritional education. In general, the aim is to control the child's calorie input and allow weight redistribution to occur naturally as the child grows. However, during adolescence (allowing for some individual variations) young people have attained most of their adult height and, following the growth spurt at 12 years for girls and 14 years for boys, the potential for weight adjustment by normal growth is diminished. 60–85% of obese children and adolescents will remain obese as adults.

Hypnosis

Coman and Evans (1995) have reviewed the efficacy of hypnosis in the treatment of obesity. Hypnosis is particularly valuable for clients who need to lose weight in that it can address a number of underlying psychological barriers to successful weight loss. Specifically, it can address faulty cognition around food, identify antecedents to eating, and help with stimulus control difficulties and other lifestyle issues on an individual basis (Coman and Evans 1995). Schaumberg et al (1995) addressed the issue of the link between self-esteem and weight. In a well-designed control trial they found that, in general, hypnosis was an effective clinical intervention for weight reduction in young women.

TCM

In Traditional Chinese Medicine, obesity is thought to be caused primarily by dysfunctions of Stomach, Spleen, Liver and Kidney. Loo (2002) describes the differentiation of obesity and its aetiology in TCM. Causes of obesity are age-related, the most common syndrome being Spleen and Stomach-Qi deficiency leading to Dampness in the Middle Energiser. Children who have a constitutionally weak Spleen are prone to developing Spleen and Stomach deficiency. The result is the inefficient transformation of food into Qi and its transportation round the body. These children tend to be sedentary, not just because of their weight gain but because muscle weakness due to Spleen deficiency makes them feel easily tired. Loo (2002) suggests that such children do not respond to Western dietary regimens. The role of acupuncture in treating obesity is to help to strengthen the Spleen and Kidneys and to encourage the clearing of Phlegm and Dampness.

A Cochrane review (Ernst 1997) of the use of acupuncture and acupressure looked at four randomised controlled trials using the Kleijnen et al (1991) scale, and included trials using active and sham acupuncture. The overall conclusion was that there was no evidence to support the use of acupuncture in weight control. These results need to be evaluated in the light of previous discussion on the credibility of systematic reviews of acupuncture where sham acupuncture has been used. Sun Fengmin (1994) used acupuncture in simple obesity, of the type excess Heat in Stomach and Intestines, to see if there was a relationship between the effect of acupuncture on weight reduction and calorific intake. 661 cases were reviewed and compared with a control group of 56. Of the treatment group, 219 had an adiposity of 20–30% and 307 of 30–50%. Auricular acupuncture was combined with body acupuncture. The auricular stud was stimulated three times a day by the patient. After one course of treatment lasting 1 month, 21.6% of patients were cured, i.e. body weight was standard or within normal limits (i.e. body fat <20% in men and <33% in women), 24.4% had markedly improved and 45.2% had improved.

Other interventions

For overweight due to purely emotional causes, the homeopathic remedies of Nat. mur, Calcarea and Phytolacca berry are indicated. Patients may be supported by the Bach flower remedies, which could include remedies such as Chestnut bud to break the cycle of weight loss and gain, Impatiens to help patients stick to the regime long term and not expect immediate results, Gentian to provide encouragement after breaking the diet and Walnut to help adapt to the new eating pattern. Again, any of the therapies which have been shown to be effective in controlling stress and anxiety would be useful adjunct treatments for patients wanting to lose weight.

CONCLUSION

From descriptions of CAM therapies and treatments throughout this book and elsewhere, it is clear that CAM has much to offer patients who might suffer from poor or altered body image. The healing and validating touch of massage, the building of confidence through hypnosis, the role of the Bach flower remedies in dealing with a range of emotional reactions, the use of t'ai chi and yoga to calm and relax, all can help adolescents to be aware of and relate well to their bodies.

REFERENCES

Coman G 1992 Hypnosis in the treatment of bulimia: a review of the literature. Australian Journal of Clinical and Experimental Hypnosis 20(2): 89–104

Coman G, Evans B 1995 Clinical update on eating disorders and obesity: implications for treatment with hypnosis. Australian Journal of Clinical and Experimental Hypnosis 23(1): 1–13

Crago M, Shisslak C, Estes L 1996 Eating disturbances among American minority groups: a review. International Journal of Eating Disorders 19: 239–248

Ernst E 1997 Acupuncture and acupressure for weight reduction? A systematic review. Wiener Klinische Wochenschrift 109(2): 60–62

Field T 2000 Touch therapy. Churchill Livingstone, Edinburgh

Fieldhouse P 1996 Food and nutrition: customs and culture, 2nd edn. Stanley Thornes, Cheltenham

Fornari V, Dancyer I, Schneider M 2001 Parental medical neglect in the treatment of adolescents with anorexia nervosa. International Journal of Eating Disorders 29(3): 358–362

Frasquilho F, Oakley D 1997 Hypnotisability, dissociation and three factors of eating behaviour. Contemporary Hypnosis 14(2): 105–111

Golden N, Sacker I 1984 An overview of the aetiology, diagnosis and management of anorexia nervosa. Clinical Pediatrics 23: 209–214

Groth-Marnat G, Schumaker J 1989 Locus of control as a predictor of severity of weight control strategies in bulimics. Psychology and Human Development 2(2): 61–66

Groth-Marnat G, Schumaker J 1990 Hypnotisability, attitudes towards eating and concern with body size in a female college population. American Journal of Clinical Hypnosis 32: 194–200

Gupta M, Gupta A, Schork N 1995 Perceived touch deprivation and body image: some observations among eating disordered and non clinical subjects. Journal of Psychosomatic Research 39: 459–464

Hill J, Peters J 1998 Environmental contributions to the obesity epidemic. Science 280: 1371–1373

Johnson C, Larson R 1982 Bulimia: an analysis of moods and behaviour. Psychosomatic Medicine 44: 341–351

Kleijnen J, Ter Riet G, Knipschild P 1991 Acupuncture and asthma: a review of controlled trials. Thorax 46(11): 799–802

Kohn M, Golden N 2001 Eating disorders in children and adolescents: epidemiology, diagnosis and treatment. Paediatric Drugs 3(2): 91–99

Kreipe R 1995 Eating disorders among children and adolescents. Pediatric Review 16: 370–379

Loo M 2002 Pediatric acupuncture. Churchill Livingstone, Edinburgh

Robarts J, Sloboda A 1994 Perspectives on music therapy with people suffering from anorexia nervosa. British Journal of Music Therapy 8(1): 7–14

Schaumberg L, Patsdaughter C, Selder F 1995 Hypnosis as a clinical intervention for weight reduction and self-esteem improvement in young adult women. International Journal of Psychiatric Nursing Research 1(3): 99–107

Smeijsters H 1996 Music therapy with anorexia nervosa: an integrative theoretical and methodological perspective. British Journal of Music Therapy 10(2): 3–12

Strober M, Freeman R, Morrell W 1997 The long term course of severe anorexia nervosa: survival, analysis of recovery, relapse and outcome predictors over 10–15 years in a prospective study. International Journal of Eating Disorders 22: 339–360

Sun F, Liu Z, Liu Z 1994 Effect of acupuncture on calorific intake of patients with simple obesity. International Journal of Clinical Acupuncture 5(4): 379–387

White A, Nicolaas G, Forster K et al 1993 Health survey for England 1991. HMSO, London

15 Problems with elimination

CHAPTER CONTENTS

- **Urinary tract infections   192**
  Homeopathy   192
  Herbalism and aromatherapy   192
  TCM   193
- **Irritable bowel syndrome   193**
  Aromatherapy   193

Homeopathy   194
TCM   194
Hypnosis   195
- **References   195**

URINARY TRACT INFECTIONS

As young people become more sexually active there is the increased risk of urinary tract infections, and cystitis is one such condition which responds well to CAM.

Homeopathy

Apis. mel, Cantharis, Lycopodium and Pulsatilla are all recommended homeopathic remedies for cystitis and bladder complaints, depending on the individual symptoms.

Herbalism and aromatherapy

Recently, cranberry juice has been advocated in the treatment of cystitis. It has been shown to reduce the frequency of urinary tract infections by being effective in inhibiting both bacterial adherence to mucosa and the growth of yeast.

One study by Avorn et al (1994) was set in a home for the elderly and was a well-designed randomised, double blind, placebo controlled trial. Over a 6-month period the experimental group were given a daily dose of 300 mL of cranberry juice and the control group a flavoured placebo drink. Urine samples were taken for baseline measurements and continued to be taken by a nurse during the trial. Although the differences between the groups did not achieve statistical significance, there was a substantial reduction in bacteriuria and pyuria in the experimental group, i.e. an incidence of 15% compared with an incidence of 28.1% in the control group. Similarly, there was a reduction in the prescription of antibiotics in 16 instances in the control group and in 8 in the cranberry juice group. Further research was conducted by Kontiokari (2001) over a 6-month period.

Using three groups of women who had urinary tract infections, comparison was made between groups taking cranberry juice, lactobacillus GG drink and a non-intervention group. Results indicated that in the cranberry juice group the re-infection rate was 16% and in the other groups 39% and 36% respectively.

Since cystitis is most commonly caused by *E. coli*, essential oils to which the organism is sensitive would be of value.

TCM

In TCM terms, bacterial infections are caused by external Damp/Heat, external Dampness entering the body by the lower channels and settling in the Bladder. When this happens it gives rise to painful urination, back pain and restlessness. Chronic recurrent cystitis is caused by Spleen-Qi deficiency, which may be constitutional, or Kidney-Yin deficiency, which leads to Bladder-Yin deficiency resulting in Bladder Heat accumulation. Treatment in all cases is to disperse Dampness, tonify Spleen and disperse Heat.

IRRITABLE BOWEL SYNDROME

More problematic than constipation is the frequent loose stools due to irritable bowel syndrome (IBS). IBS is a chronic, recurring disorder which may continue for many years. It is the most common functional gastro-intestinal disorder seen in both primary and secondary care. Its symptoms include abdominal pain, loose frequent stools, and the passing of mucus and constipation. Luscome (2000), in his review of the research on the quality of life of people suffering from IBS, noted that they had significantly lower scores on both the physical and mental health scales on the Short Form–36 (SF–36) compared with controls. It is noted that IBS negatively affects general health, vitality, social functioning, bodily pain, diet, sexual function and sleep, and leads to lost time from work. Lydiard (2001) examined the high levels of psychiatric disorders found in patients presenting with IBS, including general anxiety disorder, panic attacks, social phobia and major depression. Arun et al (1993) reported that IBS patients perceived life events as more stressful than did patients in a control group.

Aromatherapy

A number of therapies have been shown to be of value in treating IBS. It has been noted earlier that neroli is a good essential oil for combating stress and anxiety, and it would therefore be of value in the treatment of diarrhoea caused by stressful circumstances, such as exams or interviews. It can be used either in the bath, as a massage or inhaled before the stressful event. Other antispasmodic oils which could prove useful include chamomile, cypress, lavender and peppermint.

A number of studies have been conducted on the use of peppermint oil for IBS. In 1979 Rees et al (1979), using 18 patients who took one or two capsules daily in a double blind crossover trial, reported more symptom-free days and fewer severe symptoms for those taking the oil. The researchers concluded that the action of the oil was carminative, with potent antispasmodic properties. The botanical source of the oil was not stated. This antispasmodic effect was investigated by Taylor et al (1983) using guinea pig ileum, which was subjected to a range of stimulants in the presence of increasing amounts of peppermint oil. The oil was found to inhibit muscle contraction by interfering with the mobility of calcium ions. This was disputed by Lis-Balchin (1999), who deduced that the mode of action was post-synaptic.

A further study by Dew et al (1984) used 29 patients in a double blind crossover trial using peppermint oil or placebo. Over a 2-week period, patients recorded the severity of abdominal symptoms, stool frequency and side effects. Patients taking peppermint oil all reported feeling significantly better and had reduced abdominal symptoms compared with the placebo group. The botanical source of the oil was not stated. However, Nash et al (1986) achieved different results in their study when they compared peppermint oil with placebo in a dose of two capsules three times a day and found that there was no difference between the two groups. The researchers concluded that this may have been due to the fact that the dose was not patient controlled. The most recent study by Micklefield et al (2000) examined the type of capsule used and noted that enteric coated capsules had a better effect, since the oil in the non-enteric coated capsules was diminished in effectiveness by gastric juices.

Homeopathy

A homeopath might suggest Argent. nit for diarrhoea due to excitement or worry over a specific event, and Arsen. alb for attacks of food poisoning. A number of these remedies are also useful for irritable bowel syndrome.

TCM

In Traditional Chinese Medicine, three patterns of disharmony can be differentiated: excess pattern, with stagnation of Qi in the Liver and Intestines; deficiency pattern, with deficiency of Spleen-Qi; or mixed deficiency and excess pattern, with Liver invading the Spleen and deficiency of Lung-Qi with stagnation of Qi in the Large Intestine. Treatment using acupuncture is aimed at choosing points which will correct the imbalance (Lewis 1992).

Two studies of the use of Chinese herbal remedies in the treatment of IBS have been undertaken. Bensoussan et al (1998), using a double blind randomised placebo controlled trial, assigned patients to one of three groups, taking individualised Chinese formulations, a standard Chinese formulation or placebo. The trial was conducted over 16 weeks and outcomes were evaluated by a gastroenterologist and a traditional Chinese herbalist. Compared with the placebo group, both the active herbal groups had significant improvement in their symptoms and reported that they experienced a significantly reduced degree of interference with life activities caused by IBS symptoms. Individualised herbal formulations were no more effective than the standard preparation. However, at follow-up 14 weeks later, only the individualised formulation group of patients maintained their improvement. Similar results were obtained by Stevinson (1999).

Hypnosis

A number of studies have demonstrated the efficacy of hypnosis in the treatment of irritable bowel syndrome. Two cases have been described in which hypnotic suggestions included symptom relief, coping with the unavailability of a lavatory and the suggestion that the client would be able to 'hold on' appropriately and feel in control of the situation (Walker 1988). In another trial involving 30 subjects, half of whom received hypnosis, the outcome for the hypnosis group was superior to that for the control group (Whorwell et al 1987). Similar results were observed in a group of 33 patients with IBS, of whom 20 were significantly improved. 11 of these lost almost all their symptoms and this improvement was maintained at a 3-month follow-up (Harvey et al 1989). Suggestions used included visualisation of the stool passing along the intestine with the sphincters contracting smoothly and securely.

REFERENCES

Arun P, Kanwal K, Vyas J et al 1993 Life events and irritable bowel syndrome. Indian Journal of Clinical Psychology 20(2): 108–112

Avorn J, Monane M, Gurwitz J et al 1994 Reduction of bacteria and pyuria after ingestion of cranberry juice. Journal of American Medical Association 271(10): 751–754

Bensoussan A, Talley N, Hing M et al 1998 Treatment of irritable bowel syndrome with Chinese herbal medicine: a randomised controlled trial. Journal of American Medical Association 280(18): 1585–1589

Dew M, Evans B, Rhodes J 1984 Peppermint oil for the irritable bowel syndrome: a multicentre trial. British Journal of Clinical Practice 38(11–12): 394–398

Harvey R, Hinton R, Gunary R et al 1989 Individual and group hypnotherapy in the treatment of refractory irritable bowel syndrome. Lancet 1: 424–425

Kontiokari T 2001 Randomised trial of cranberry lingonberry juice and lactobacillus GG drink for the prevention of urinary tract infections in women. British Medical Journal 322(7310): 1571–1573

Lewis P 1992 Irritable bowel syndrome: emotional factors and acupuncture treatment. Journal of Chinese Medicine 40: 9–12

Lis-Balchin M, Hart S 1999 Studies on the mode of action of peppermint oil Mentha x piperita L in guinea pig ileum in vitro. Medical Science Research 27: 307–309

Luscome F 2000 Health related quality of life and associated psychological factors in irritable bowel syndrome: a review. Quality of Life Research March 9(2): 161–176

Lydiard B 2001 Irritable bowel syndrome, anxiety and depression: what are the links? Journal of Clinical Psychiatry 62(suppl 8): 38–45

Micklefield G, Greving I, May B 2000 Effects of peppermint oil and caraway oil on gastro duodenal motility. Phytotherapy Research 14: 20–23

Nash P, Gould S, Bernardo D 1986 Peppermint oil does not relieve the pain of irritable bowel syndrome. British Journal of Clinical Practice 40(7): 292–293

Rees W, Evans B, Rhodes J 1979 Treating irritable bowel syndrome with peppermint oil. British Medical Journal 2(6194): 835–836

Stevinson C 1999 Chinese herbal medicine effective for irritable bowel syndrome. Focus on Alternative and Complementary Therapies 2: 68

Taylor B, Luscombe D, Duthie H 1983 Inhibitory effect of peppermint oil on gastrointestinal smooth muscle. Gut 24: A992

Walker L 1988 Hypnosis in the treatment of irritable bowel syndrome. In: Heap M (ed) Hypnosis: current clinical experimental and forensic practices. Croom Helm, London

Whorwell P, Prior A, Colgan S 1987 Hypnotherapy in severe irritable bowel syndrome: further experience. Gut 28: 423–425

16 Problems related to working and playing

CHAPTER CONTENTS

- **Addictive behaviours 196**
- **Health promotion 196**
- **Models of addiction 197**
  Smoking 197
  Alcohol abuse 198
- **Interventions used for smoking 198**
  Acupuncture 198
  Hypnosis 199
  Herbalism 200
  Aromatherapy 200
  Other interventions 201

- **Interventions used for alcohol abuse 201**
  Bach flower remedies 201
  Herbalism 201
  TCM 201
- **Drug abuse 201**
  Ayurvedic medicine 201
  TCM 202
  Yoga 203
  Herbalism 203
  Anthroposophical medicine 203
- **Conclusion 204**
- **References 204**

ADDICTIVE BEHAVIOURS

Adolescence is a time of great change and stress, when young people are searching for acceptance and identity, and it is perhaps not surprising that sometimes their natural desire to experiment, and their tendency to be influenced by their peers, can lead them into adopting a range of unhealthy and dangerous behaviours, such as smoking, over-indulgence in alcohol and experimentation with drugs.

Bandura (1977) has highlighted the relationship between learning by imitation and the concept of self-efficacy, which he identifies as a personality trait related to confidence in one's own ability to achieve desired goals. Heather and Robertson (1997) noted that people with low self-esteem were more likely than those with high self-esteem to imitate undesirable behaviours.

With this in mind, it is clear that CAM may be useful in addressing such behaviour in two main areas. First, CAM can offer help with the underlying problems, often related to self-esteem, that lead to the injurious behaviour. Secondly, CAM can give support in dealing with the behaviour itself, whether in helping young people to cope with withdrawal symptoms or in providing longer-term support during rehabilitation.

HEALTH PROMOTION

The paediatric nurse's role in health promotion is of particular importance in this area of injurious behaviour, and this role sits well with the holistic philosophy of complementary therapies. Whitehead (1999) discussed the relationship between complementary therapies and health promotion, drawing upon a number of sources to support his argument (Labonte 1993, Benson & Latter 1998, Caelli 1998). He identified the key areas that are common to the philosophies of CAM and health promotion, i.e. holism, collaboration, partnership with client, self-determination and the attainment of positive health.

McDonald (1998), noting that nurses have a major role in health promotion since they constitute a large healthcare work force, highlights the need for additional education for health promotion and for nurses to have an 'understanding of other services … to which nurses could refer patients'. Some of these services could include complementary therapies. Implicit within the nurse's role is the duty to maintain current knowledge and to be aware of best evidence, in order to be in a position to enable the client to make an informed choice about his or her own health needs.

Watson (1985) described the role of the nurse as that of a catalyst, assisting the client to grow and change, and there are a number of models of change that enable the nurse to assess the client. One of these is the readiness-to-change model by Prochaska and DiClemente (1984), which consists of five stages:

- Precontemplation
- Contemplation
- Preparing to change
- Making the change
- Maintenance of the change.

All clients go through all the stages, frequently more than once, and relapse on the part of the client is normal (Prochaska et al 1992). Where complementary therapies are of particular value is that they can be utilised within all the stages of the cycle, and different therapies can be used at different stages.

MODELS OF ADDICTION

Smoking

Chassen et al (1996) noted that there is a marked increase in the incidence of smoking in mid-adolescence, and confirmed that the majority of adult smokers started smoking in early adolescence. Central to the development and, particularly, the continuation of smoking as an activity is the development of a physical dependence on the key ingredient, nicotine. It has been claimed that, over a period of years, tobacco manufacturers have steadily increased the levels of nicotine in their products to increase and maintain their addictiveness (Porter 1997). Support for this theory is offered by Davison and Duffy (1982) and Hatziandreu et al (1990). Behavioural factors involved in cigarette smoking include the escape/avoidance response (Pomerlau 1979). Murray et al (1988) noted that among young adults, boredom was a key reason for smoking, whilst young women smoked for pleasure and the reduction of negative affect. The role of stress in smoking has been confirmed by Murray et al (1983) and Colby et al (1994), while McNeill (1991) noted that young smokers reported that they smoked for its calming effect. A number of social theories of smoking have been forward, including learned behaviour, the concept of smoking as a social marker during the day, and smoking as a form of social interaction (Murray et al 1988).

Looking at these theories related to smoking, it is clear that some of the models, more than others, suggest that complementary therapies can have a role to play in treatment. Smoking based on tension reduction or on addiction may be more responsive to treatment by complementary therapies. Interventions that help to reduce withdrawal symptoms such as irritability, difficulties in concentration, anxiety, restlessness and depressed mood may be helpful (Stolerman & Jarvis 1995). Complementary therapies also have a role in the long term as supportive therapies in the maintenance phase. Wynd (1992) reviewed the literature on the use of relaxation and guided imagery to reduce stress following smoking cessation. He noted that the best predictor of good outcome during smoking relapse crises was the ability to cope with stress, and he supported the use of imagery as a coping tool.

Alcohol abuse

As with cigarette smoking, there are a number of models for alcohol abuse, including the addiction model, the disease model and the learning model. In common with cigarette smoking, a key factor in treatment is reduction of tension (Sayette & Hufford 1997). The effects of excessive alcohol consumption cannot be overestimated and it is the key factor in many accidents, particularly road accidents (Department of Transport 1996), but also other incidents including falls, fires, drowning etc. (Eckhardt et al 1981, Plueckham 1982). Theories related to alcohol abuse include genetic predisposition, disease and addiction. As with smoking cessation, some of these theories, more than others, suggest that alcohol abuse may be responsive to complementary therapies.

INTERVENTIONS USED FOR SMOKING

Acupuncture

One therapy for the treatment of addiction in general that has been researched extensively is acupuncture. When any drug that has a psychotropic effect is consumed, a feeling of euphoria and abnormal exhilaration results. In TCM terms this results in a change in the Shen (or consciousness), and continual abuse leads to troubled sleep and insomnia. Earlier reference has been made to calming the Shen to promote sleep. Depending on the particular addiction, further specific effects are noted; for example, in tobacco addiction, there is a further disharmony in Lung-Yin (Given 1998).

If we look on smoking as a stress reduction mechanism, a good substitute would be an intervention that addresses the stress and substitutes the 'feel good' factor. We have already noted that acupuncture works in reducing stress levels and relieving depression. Lewith and Kenyon (1984), in their review on pain, have suggested that acupuncture also works by stimulating the release of endorphins and encephalin, both of which are natural opiates.

A number of studies have been conducted into the use of acupuncture in giving up smoking. In their review, Vincent and Richardson (1987) concluded that acupuncture was as successful as other treatments for smoking cessation. Silagy (1994) re-evaluated the research on acupuncture and smoking and noted that the outcome measurements cited were equal to those of nicotine replacement therapy and that the site of needle insertion was not important. Lewith (1995) confirmed that acupuncture could, in a non-specific way, trigger the release of endorphins and thus aid withdrawal in a number of addictions. The most recent assessment of acupuncture is the Cochrane initiative (see list of websites), which concluded that, whilst acupuncture appeared promising as a clinical intervention, there was insufficient evidence at present to recommend it as an effective form of therapy for smoking cessation. However, this review is flawed by the inclusion of studies that used 'sham' acupuncture (discussed in Chapter 2) in the research design, thus confounding the results. In addition, nowhere in the trials reviewed was there any indication of how the subjects were selected or how they were assessed on the readiness-to-change model. The review concluded that the use of acupuncture was 'promising' and the known physical effects of acupuncture would, following assessment by the practitioner, appear to be able to offer some clients some help.

Hypnosis

One difficulty in assessing the effectiveness of hypnosis is the absence of recent clinical trials. The latest trial quoted by the Cochrane library suggests that there appears to be little advantage in using hypnosis over other interventions (Abbot et al 2003). This finding contradicts another extensive review of 600 studies of hypnosis by Viswesvaran and Schmidt (1992), which demonstrated hypnosis to be the most effective intervention in achieving smoking cessation. However, in their literature review in 1995, Spanos et al evaluated previous work and indicated that the effectiveness of hypnosis was unclear. They pointed out that studies either suffered from not having a control group, or were anecdotal and had unspecified or inadequate follow-up assessment. In their discussion, Spanos et al suggested that one variable that seemed to differentiate between successful and unsuccessful outcomes was the amount of effort, or as they termed it 'sacrifice', needed from the subjects. Giving blood samples to the investigator to determine nicotine levels and having to pay for the treatment were specific indicators for success. Other indicators were subjects choosing to undergo hypnosis, rather than being assigned randomly to the other treatment groups, and undergoing treatment which was congruent with expectations. These results were compared with those of clinical psychologists, who claimed least success with smoking cessation, possibly because the treatment was free. Perry et al (1979) showed significant correlation between indices of motivation and smoking cessation. Assessment on the readiness-to-change model is particularly important since hypnosis will not work if the client is 'sent' for treatment. For optimal results, clients have to be committed to making the necessary changes, and to addressing and developing them between sessions and after therapy has been concluded. It can be seen from this that hypnosis is not a single intervention leading to measurable results, but an ongoing intervention involving self-hypnosis, which the clients can utilise as they need.

Whilst hypnosis is not a potent means of changing behaviour, it is uniquely effective in helping individuals to achieve what they already want to do. In addition, it is particularly indicated when there is an underlying, perhaps not acknowledged, pay off with their present behaviour. Clients may smoke or may have taken up smoking in response to stress, peer pressure or as an act of adolescent rebellion when the use of smoking to upset significant adults is more important than any future health considerations. Using uncovering techniques, hypnosis can address these specific problems as well as directly addressing the act of smoking itself. Howie (1996) lists five areas of approach in the treatment of addictions:

- Amplification and reinforcement of resolve
- Reduction of perceived need, reason and desire to engage in addictive behaviours
- Alleviation of fears associated with abstinence from the addictive substance
- Enhancement of relaxation response
- Ego strengthening.

He also suggests that in the use of hypnosis in the treatment of addictive behaviour, it is necessary to employ a variety of approaches and techniques, tailored to the client's particular needs and goals.

Herbalism

Other therapies that have been indicated as useful in smoking cessation include the use of the herb lobelia (*Lobelia inflata*), also known as Indian tobacco. One of its constituents, lobeline, has peripheral and central effects similar to those of nicotine, but less potent. Traditionally, the herb has been used for respiratory conditions and has antispasmodic and expectorant properties (Barnes et al 2002). However, a review of the research into the effects of this herb by the Cochrane library (Stead & Hughes 2003) indicated that there is no evidence to support its role in smoking cessation.

Aromatherapy

One study using aromatherapy to aid smoking cessation indicated that the use of black pepper (*Piper nigrum*) could mitigate the effects of withdrawal symptoms from nicotine. The theory supporting this study relies on the fact that sensory cues suppress certain withdrawal symptoms, including the craving for cigarettes. By replicating the respiratory tract cues associated with cigarette smoke, it is possible to reduce craving for cigarettes and decrease cigarette smoke intake (Rose & Behm 1994). In this study it was hypothesised that the airway irritant effects of black pepper would suppress craving for cigarettes. Having abstained from smoking for 8 hours, the subjects were randomly assigned to one of three groups, none of which involved the administration of nicotine. The subjects were assessed over 3 hours, during which they were able to 'smoke' either the black pepper, menthol or a dummy cigarette. The black pepper group reported not only a reduced craving for nicotine and reduced somatic symptoms related to anxiety, but also positive mood changes. It was suggested that the active constituents of pepper might have activated the sensory cues of cigarette smoke.

Other interventions

Ayurvedic medicine would counsel against smoking and would advocate the use of transcendental meditation as an aid to quitting.

INTERVENTIONS USED FOR ALCOHOL ABUSE

Bach flower remedies

Patients who choose to use Bach flower remedies in the treatment of alcohol dependence might take Elm (for those who feel that responsibilities will overwhelm them), Gentian (to overcome relapses) and Centaury (to release them from their dependence on alcohol).

Herbalism

Examples of herbs that help in the healing process are the group called the hepatic herbs, including dandelion root (*Taraxacum officinale*), artichoke (*Cynara scolymus*), centaury (*Centaurium erythraea*), hart's tongue (*Phyllitis scolpendrium*) and bittersweet (*Solanum dulcamara*) (Mills 1994).

TCM

In TCM, alcoholism is seen as a problem of too much Heat in the body damaging the Liver. Herbs would be given to take the Heat out of the Liver and the Blood. Psychological factors relating to alcoholism are recognised and patients encouraged to seek professional help.

DRUG ABUSE

Ayurvedic medicine

Sharma et al (1994) describe the implementation of a programme to prevent alcohol and drug abuse amongst juveniles at risk. They acknowledge that alcohol and drug abuse have multiple and interacting causes but highlight specifically the role of the person's ability to cope with stress and anxiety. They identify risk factors as including depression, anxiety, emotional distress and antisocial behaviour. In their paper they describe the role and value of transcendental meditation (TM) in treating substance abuse, as a system of personal development rather than as a specific treatment. During the practice of TM the subject is in a stage of restful alertness, but it is its biochemical effects that make TM particularly valuable for use in treating drug abuse. TM has been shown to normalise biochemical functioning and rebalance the neurotransmitters directly involved in psychological functioning. In their review of the efficacy of TM in the treatment of opiate dependency, Gelderloos et al (1991) examine the results of 24 studies. All the studies showed positive effects for the use of TM but Gelderloos et al acknowledge the possibility of self-selection or responder bias in the results. They also confirm Sharma's assertion that TM is not in itself a treatment but is a technique for personal development and that any changes in substance usage would be considered as 'side effects' of the practice of TM. The use of TM has been implicated in the reduction of psychological distress, including depression (Brooks & Scarano 1985), in the enhancement of self-esteem (Alexander et al 1990), and in the improvement of resistance to stress (Brooks & Scarano 1985, Mills 1987). Gelderloos et al (1991) suggest that TM provides a natural way for abusers to achieve the same effects as they do from drugs, i.e. relief from stress, increased self-esteem, feelings of wellbeing and a meaning in life.

TCM

In TCM, the manifestation of opiate dependency is determined by the drug involved, e.g. cocaine dependency manifests itself as Lung-Qi deficiency and heroin dependency as Phlegm-Heat. Given (1998) reviews the variety of presenting symptoms and therapeutic approaches that might be used. Research into the value of acupuncture in the treatment of opiate dependency has yielded variable results. Some of the variations can be attributed to aspects of the condition under investigation. Wells et al (1995) noted problems of recruitment and retention of subjects whilst Moon and Latessa (1994), who were researching the use of acupuncture for addiction within the American probation service, noted that a number of their subjects were lost to the study in ways not normally associated with experimental research (i.e. they had to be retrieved from jail having been 'busted' for possession on a regular basis). 21% of the experimental group were arrested, 15% because of a new conviction; 31% of the comparison group were similarly accounted for. In their review of other intervention studies, Moon and Latessa (1994) note a number of principles for successful intervention, which include targeting high risk groups (Andrews et al 1990).

Wells et al (1995) investigated the use of acupuncture in decreasing withdrawal symptoms and to increase the stability of methadone patients on treatment. In this study, real and sham auricular acupuncture (1–3 mm away from the active point) were used. Results indicated that acupuncture appeared to have little effect on reported withdrawal and other physical symptoms, with the sham acupuncture group finding the treatment more helpful than the true acupuncture group. Since the researchers were using auricular acupuncture, they suggested that energy might migrate from the non-specific (sham) acupuncture points to where it is most useful.

Similar results were noted by Bullock et al (1999) in the use of acupuncture in the treatment of cocaine addiction. They too used sham acupuncture and noted no difference between sham and real acupuncture groups. They also acknowledged the specific subject problems of this type of research. However, they did acknowledge that their attempt to adhere to the standards of contemporary research design might not have been appropriate and that randomised placebo controlled study should not have been used. They suggested that perhaps the treatment should be used in its optimal form and then analysed into its component parts for examination.

In his excellent article about the Lincoln clinic in the Bronx, Blow (1994) describes how alcohol and opiate addictions have been treated successfully since 1974 in this clinic, which is a model for other detoxification clinics. Acknowledging the limitations of assessing the effectiveness of acupuncture using classical research methods, the clinic has used a survey analysis instead. From this they note that 90% of acute withdrawal symptoms are relieved and 60% of patients remain drug and alcohol-free after a period of several months. They also note that other supportive measures such as counselling are needed.

Yoga

The beneficial effects of yoga on stress levels have been noted by Panjawani et al (1995) and were discussed earlier. Shaffer et al (1997) compared yoga with dynamic psychotherapy in enhancing methadone maintenance treatment. This study suffered some of the compliance problems experienced by Moon and Latessa (1994). Although there was no difference between the two groups, the authors did suggest that yoga offered an additional treatment intervention. At a personal level, a number of subjects considered that the yoga was pivotal in their recovery by increasing their sense of wellbeing, whilst the breathing exercises helped another subject to control anxiety.

Herbalism

Rasmussen (1998), a herbalist with a particular expertise in treating drug dependency, points out that reliance on orthodox drugs to aid detoxification suffers from a number of disadvantages. Key amongst them is the fact that the drugs used are frequently the same as those to which the client is addicted. He goes on to review the range of herbal remedies that have been used alongside methadone to reduce the effects of opiate withdrawal in the detoxification unit he runs in New Zealand. Initially the client is stabilised on methadone which is then decreased on a daily basis, while herbal remedies are given at the same time. These remedies include corydalis (*Corydalis ambigua*), which is traditionally used as an analgesic and tranquilliser and contains papaveraceae-type alkaloids, Californian poppy (*Eschscholtzia californica*) and cramp bark (*Viburnum opulus*), which is of particular value in reducing the muscle cramps and aches that can occur midway during withdrawal. Other remedies include those already discussed in relation to stress, anxiety and depression.

Anthroposophical medicine

In their book about Anthroposophical medicine, Evans and Rodger (2000) describe the work of two Anthroposophical clinics, one in Germany and one in Holland, which have been set up as drug rehabilitation centres. They make the point that, in the experience of the Anthroposophical therapists at the centre, few addicts choose to try to 'kick the habit' before the age of 21. They attribute this to the belief in Anthroposophical medicine that the forces of the ego become freed from their unconscious activity at about this age. Treatment follows the developmental stages of childhood which have been described in earlier chapters, in order to restore the addict's damaged constitutional elements, the etheric and astral bodies and the ego, which are the product of successful maturation. Initially, the therapists concentrate on restoring the client's physical health and on withdrawal from the drug. This is achieved through a combination of whole food, diet and work. During the second phase, treatment concentrates on artistic activity and group discussions. This phase corresponds to the childhood developmental stage of age 7–14 years. It is described as an environment of cultural nutrition similar to school and aims to provide clients with the emotional and cultural input which they have so often lacked. During this time, clients will be treated with Anthroposophical medication and other therapies to augment the treatment. In the next stage, emphasis is placed on the development of responsibility and independence. This relates to the developmental stage from 14 to 21 years and an individualised programme is followed by each resident. Using this approach, the clinics claim a success rate of 52%, although it is not clear how success is defined. Certainly the holistic and developmental approach has much to recommend it.

CONCLUSION

At a macro level the evidence for the usefulness of complementary therapies in health promotion in the area of addictive behaviours is equivocal, due, in part, to the multivariate nature of the methodological faults and the limitations of meta-analysis (addressed in Ch. 1). Specifically, the use of Western research methodology with Eastern medical systems is problematic (Given 1998, Cole & Shanley 1998, Birch 1997, 1998). Hammerschlag's (1998) early caution about clinical trials of acupuncture could be applied to all therapies that have been evaluated using this methodology. Research within the health promotion arena is flawed by its failure to acknowledge the relationship between motivation and behaviour change, specifically, it fails to take into account that the process of behaviour change is not linear, and that relapse is the norm and does not necessarily indicate failure. As Cole and Shanley (1998) suggested, the limitation of controlled trials is that they fail to acknowledge the complexity of human nature. However, following detailed assessment of the client, therapy and stage of change, complementary therapies would appear to have a role to play in health promotion in this area, either as direct or supportive interventions.

REFERENCES

Abbot N, Stead L, White A et al 2003 Hypnotherapy for smoking cessation (Cochrane Review). The Cochrane Library Issue 1 www.cochrane.org/reabstr/ ab001008.htm

Alexander C, Davies J, Dixon C et al 1990 Growth of higher stages of consciousness: the vedic psychology of human development. In: Alexander C, Langer E (eds) Higher stages of human development. Perspectives on adult growth. Oxford University Press, Oxford

Andrews D, Zinger I, Hoge R et al 1990 Does correctional treatment work? A clinically relevant and psychologically informed meta analysis. Criminology 28: 369–404

Bandura A 1977 Self efficacy: toward a unifying theory of behaviour change. Psychological Review 84: 191–215

Barnes J, Anderson L, Phillipson J 2002 Herbal medicines: a guide for health care professionals, 2nd edn. Pharmaceutical Press, London

Benson A, Latter S 1998 Implementing health promoting nursing: the integration of interpersonal skills and health promotion. Journal of Advanced Nursing 27: 100–107

Birch S 1997 Issues to consider in determining an adequate treatment in a clinical trial of acupuncture. Complementary Therapies in Medicine 5: 8–12

Birch S 1998 Diversity and acupuncture: acupuncture is not a coherent or historically stable tradition. In: Vickers A (ed) Examining complementary medicine. Stanley Thornes, Cheltenham

Blow D 1994 The acupuncture treatment of alcohol and chemical dependency. Journal of Chinese Medicine May: 5–8

Brooks J, Scarano T 1985 Transcendental Meditation in the treatment of post Vietnam adjustment. Journal of Counselling Development 64: 212–215

Bullock M, Kiresuk T, Pheley A 1999 Auricular acupuncture in the treatment of cocaine abuse. Journal of Substance Abuse Treatment 16(1): 31–38

Caelli K 1998 Shared understandings: negotiating the meanings of health via concept mapping. Nurse Education Today 18: 317–321

Chassen C, Presson C, Rose J et al 1996 The natural history of cigarettes from adolescence to adulthood: demographic predictors of continuity and change. Health Psychology 15: 478–484

Colby J, Linsky A, Straus M 1994 Social stress and state-to-state differences in smoking and smoking related mortality in the United States. Social Science and Medicine 38: 373–381

Cole A, Shanley E 1998 Complementary therapies as a means of developing the scope of professional nursing practice. Journal of Advanced Nursing 27: 1171–1176

Davison G, Duffy M 1982 Smoking habits of long term survivors of surgery for lung cancer. Thorax 37: 331–333

Department of Transport 1996 Road accidents, Great Britain, the casualty report. Department of Transport, London

Eckhardt M, Harford T, Kaelber C et al 1981 Health hazards associated with alcohol consumption. Journal of American Medical Association 246: 648–666

Evans M, Rodger I 2000 Healing for body, soul and spirit: an introduction to anthroposophical medicine. Floris Books, Edinburgh

Gelderloos P, Walton K, Orme-Johnson D 1991 Effectiveness of Transcendental Meditation program in preventing and treating substance misuse: a review. International Journal of Addictions 26(3): 293–325

Given S 1998 Understanding addiction the Chinese way. International Journal of Alternative and Complementary Medicine 16(2): 26–30

Hammerschlag R 1998 Methodological and ethical issues in clinical trials of acupuncture. Journal of Alternative and Complementary Medicine 4(2): 159–171

Hatziandreu D, Pierce J, Lefkopoulou M 1990 Quitting smoking in the United States in 1986. Journal of the National Cancer Institute 82: 1402–1406

Heather N, Robertson I 1997 Problem drinking. Oxford University Press, Oxford

Howie D 1996 Contemporary developments in hypnotherapy applied to addictive behaviour, part 1. Journal of Substance Misuse 1: 9–12

Labonte R 1993 Health promotion and empowerment: practice frameworks. Centre for Health Promotion, University of Toronto, USA

Lewith G 1995 The treatment of tobacco addiction. Complementary Therapies in Medicine 3(3): 142–145

Lewith G, Kenyon J 1984 Physiological and psychological explanations for the mechanism of acupuncture as a treatment for chronic pain. Social Science and Medicine 19(12): 1367–1378

McDonald E 1998 The role of project 2000 educated nurses in health promotion within the hospital setting. Nurse Education Today 18: 213–220

McNeill A 1991 The development of dependence on smoking in children. British Journal of Addiction 86: 589–592

Mills P 1987 Cardiovascular and adrenergic reactivity and beta-adrenergic receptor sensitivity in practitioners of the Transcendental Meditation program and Type A behavior. Doctoral dissertation. Department of Neuroscience, Maharishi International University, Fairfield, Iowa

Mills S 1994 A complete guide to modern herbalism. Thorsons, London

Moon M, Latessa E 1994 Drug treatment in adult probation: an evaluation of an outpatient and acupuncture program. Evaluation and Program Planning 17(2): 217–226

Murray M, Swan A, Mattar N 1983 The task of nursing and risk of smoking. Journal of Advanced Nursing 8: 131–138

Murray M, Jarrett L, Swan A 1988 Smoking among young adults. Goer, Aldershot

Panjawani U, Gupta H, Singh S et al 1995 Effect of sahaja yoga practice on stress management in patients with epilepsy. Indian Journal of Physiological Pharmacology 39(2): 111–116

Perry C, Gelfand R, Markovich P 1979 The relevance of hypnotic susceptibility to clinical context. Journal of Abnormal Psychology 88: 592–603

Plueckhan V 1982 Alcohol consumption and death by drowning in adults: a 24 year epidemiological analysis. Journal of Studies on Alcohol 43: 445–452

Pomerlau D 1979 Behavioural factors in the establishment, maintenance and cessation of smoking. In: Smoking and health: a report of the Surgeon General. US Department of Health, Education and Welfare, Washington DC p 161–162

Porter R 1997 The greatest benefit to mankind: a medical history of humanity. Norton, New York

Prochaska J, DiClemente C 1984 The transtheoretical approach: crossing traditional foundations of change. Don Jones/Irwin Harnewood, Ill

Prochaska J, DiClemente C, Norcross J 1992 In search of how people change. American Psychologist 47: 1102–1114

Rasmussen P 1998 A role for phytotherapy in the treatment of benzodiazepine and opiate withdrawal. Modern Phytotherapist 4(1): 11–19

Rose J, Behm F 1994 Inhalation of vapour from black pepper extract reduces smoking withdrawal symptoms. Drug and Alcohol Dependence 34: 225–229

Sayette M, Hufford M 1997 Alcohol abuse/alcoholism. In: Baum A, Newman S, Weinman J (eds) Cambridge handbook of psychology, health and medicine. Cambridge University Press, Cambridge

Shaffer H, LaSalvia T, Stein J 1997 Comparing hatha yoga with dynamic group psychotherapy for enhancing methadone maintenance treatment. A randomised

clinical trial. Alternative Therapies 3(4): 57–66

Sharma H, Dillbeck M, Dillbeck S 1994 Implementation of the transcendental meditation program and Maharishi Ayurveda to prevent alcohol and drug abuse among juveniles at risk. Alcoholism Treatment Quarterly II (3/4): 429–457

Sharma H, Clark C 1998 Contemporary Ayurveda. Churchill Livingstone, Edinburgh

Silagy C, Mant D, Fowler G 1994 Meta analysis of efficacy of nicotine replacement therapy in smoking cessation. Lancet 343(8890): 139–142

Spanos N, Mondoux T, Burgess C 1995 Comparison of multi-component hypnotic and non hypnotic treatments for smoking. Contemporary Hypnosis 12(1): 12–19

Stead L, Hughes J 2003 Lobeline for smoking cessation (Cochrane Review). The Cochrane Library Issue 1 www.cochrane.org/reabstr/ab000124.htm

Stolerman I, Jarvis M 1995 The scientific case that nicotine is addictive. Psychopharmacology 117: 2–10

Vincent C, Richardson P 1987 Acupuncture for some common disorders: a review of the evaluative research. Journal of the Royal College of General Practitioners 37: 77–81

Visweswaran C, Schmidt F 1992 A meta-analytic comparison of the effectiveness of smoking cessation methods. Journal of Applied Psychology 77(4): 554–561

Watson J 1985 Nursing: the philosophy and science of caring. Colorado Associated University Press, Colorado

Wells E, Jackson R, Diaz R 1995 Acupuncture as an adjunct to methadone treatment services. American Journal of Addictions 4(3): 198–214

Whitehead D 1999 The relationship between health promotion and complementary therapies. Complementary Therapies in Nursing and Midwifery 5(6): 171–175

Wynd C 1992 Relaxation imagery used for stress reduction in the prevention of smoking relapse. Journal of Advanced Nursing 17: 294–302

Recommended reading

Bott V 1996 Spiritual science and the art of healing: Rudolf Steiner's anthropo sophical medicine. Healing Arts Press, Vermont

Bremness L 1995 Herbs. Dorling Kindersley, London

Culpeper N 1653 Complete herbal: a book of natural remedies for ancient ills. Wordsworth Editions, Hertfordshire

Davis P 1996 Aromatherapy: an A–Z. CW Daniel, Saffron Walden

Dimond B. 1996 The legal aspects of child health care. Mosby, London

Dimond B 1998 The legal aspects of complementary therapy practice: a guide for health care professionals. Churchill Livingstone, Edinburgh

Dougans I 1996 Complete reflexology: therapeutic foot massage for health and well-being. Element Books, Shaftesbury, Dorset

Evans M, Rodger I 2000 Healing for body, soul and spirit: an introduction to anthroposophical medicine. Floris Books, Edinburgh

Field T 2000 Touch therapy. Churchill Livingstone, Edinburgh

Gemmell D 1997 Everyday homeopathy. Beaconsfield Publishers, Beaconsfield, UK

Gibson D 1996 Studies of homeopathic remedies. Beaconsfield Publishers, Beaconsfield, UK

Heap M, Aravind K 2002 Hartland's medical and dental hypnosis. Churchill Livingstone, Edinburgh

Heap M, Dryden W (eds) 1993 Hypnotherapy: a handbook. Open University Press, Milton Keynes

Howard J 1991 The Bach flower remedies step by step. CW Daniel, Saffron Walden

Howard J 1994 Growing up with the Bach flower remedies. CW Daniel, Saffron Walden

Jonas M, Levin L 1999 (eds) Essentials of complementary and alternative medicine. Lippincott, Williams & Wilkins, London

Kaptchuk T 2000 Chinese medicine: the web that has no weaver. Rider, London

Lett A 2000 Reflex zone therapy for health professionals. Churchill Livingstone, Edinburgh

Lockie A 1990 The family guide to homeopathy. Penguin Books, Middlesex, England

Lockie A, Geddes N 1996 The complete guide to homeopathy, the principles and practice of treatment. Dorling Kindersley, London

Loo M 2002 Pediatric acupuncture. Churchill Livingstone, Edinburgh

Maciocia G 2000 The practice of Chinese medicine. Churchill Livingstone, Edinburgh

Mackereth P, Tiran D 2002 (eds) Clinical reflexology: a guide for health professionals. Churchill Livingstone, Edinburgh

MacNamara S 1995 Traditional Chinese medicine. Hamish Hamilton, London

Mantle F 1999 Complementary therapies: is there an evidence base? Nursing Times Clinical Monographs No 15. NT Books, Emap Healthcare, London

Micozzi M 1996 Fundamentals of complementary and alternative medicine. Churchill Livingstone, Edinburgh

Mills S 1989 The complete guide to modern herbalism. Thorsons, London

Mills S 1991 The essential herbal medicine. ARKANA, Penguin Books, London

Mills S, Bone K 2000 Principles and practice of phytotherapy: modern herbal medicine. Churchill Livingstone, Edinburgh

Morrison J 1994 The book of Ayurveda: a guide to personal well being. Gaia Books, London

Olness K, Kohen D 1996 Hypnosis and hypnotherapy with children. Guildford Press, London

Rankin-Box D 2001 The nurse's handbook of complementary therapies: a guide for nurses and the caring professions. Baillière Tindall, London

Richardson J 2002 The importance of information resources in complementary therapies. Complementary Therapies in Nursing and Midwifely 8(3): 125–129

Spencer J, Jacobs J 1999 (eds) Complementary/alternative medicine: an evidence based approach. Mosby, London

Sumner J 2000 The natural history of medicinal plants. Timber Press, Oregon

Swayne J 1998 homeopathic method: implications for clinical practice and medical science. Churchill Livingstone, Edinburgh

Vickers A 1993 Complementary medicine and disability: alternatives for people with disabling conditions. Chapman & Hall, London

Vickers A 1996 Massage and aromatherapy: a guide for health professionals. Chapman & Hall, London

Vincent C, Furnham A 1997 (eds) Complementary medicine: a research perspective. Wiley, London

Appendix 1

CAM USAGE CLIENT ASSESSMENT TOOL

Do you take any vitamin or herbal supplements?
Have you considered using acupuncture, homeopathy or any other complementary therapy?
How do you use this therapy?
Does it work for you?
Where did you learn about it?
Does the use of alternative therapies fit into your social, cultural or spiritual beliefs?
Do your family, doctor or friends know you use complementary therapies?
Are you able to discuss this with them?
What do you know about the therapies you use?
Do you need any more information about it/them?
Do you integrate conventional and alternative therapies?
Why are you interested in complementary therapies?
What have you heard about their effects on your particular illness/problem?
Did anyone recommend this treatment for you?

Assessment

Limited use
Use with conventional medicine
Abandons conventional medicine
Well-researched information
Information from reliable and unreliable sources
Little knowledge/poor sources

(Adapted with kind permission from the Ullrich–Hodge Alternative Therapy Assessment Model, 1999)

REFERENCE

Ullrich S, Hodge P 1999 The Ullrich–Hodge
Alternative Therapy Assessment Model:
teaching students to evaluate patients for use,
motivation and risks. Nurse Educator 24(6):
19–23

Appendix 2

USEFUL ADDRESSES

Anthroposophical medicine

Anthroposophical Nurses Association in Great Britain
Secretary
Flat 4, 18 Alexandra Grove
London N4 2LF

Ayurveda

The Ayurvedic Company of Great Britain Ltd.
81 Wimpole Street
London W1G 9RF
www.ayurvedagb.com

TCM

The British Acupuncture Council
63 Jeddo Road
London W12 9HQ
www.acupuncture.org.uk

The College of Traditional Acupuncture (UK)
Tao House
Queensway, Royal Leamington Spa
Warwickshire CV31-3L2
01926 422121

International College of Oriental Medicine UK
Green Hedges House
Green Hedges Avenue, East Grinstead
West Sussex RH19 1DZ
01342 313106

Traditional Chinese Medicine/Acupuncture
Centre for Community Care and Primary Health
University of Westminster
309 Regent Street
London W1R-8Al
0207911 5082

Northern College of Acupuncture
124 Acomb Road
York YO2 4EY
01914 785120

The College of Integrated Chinese Medicine
19 Castle Street
Reading RG1 7SB
0118 950 8880

The London College of Traditional Acupuncture
HR House
447 High Road
Finchley
London N12 0AF
020 8371 0820

Aromatherapy

Aromatherapy Associations Council (AOC)
3 Layers Close
Braybrooke
Market Harborough
Leicester LE16 8LN
01858 434242

International Federation of Aromatherapists (IFA)
Department of Continuing Education
Royal Masonic Hospital
Ravenscourt Park
London W6 0TN
0208 846 8066

International Society for Professional Aromatherapists (ISPA)
41 Leicester Road
Hinkley
Leicestershire LE10 1LW
01455 637 987

Bach flower remedies

The Edward Bach Foundation
Mount Vernon
Sotwell
Oxon OX10 0PX
01491 834678
www.bachcentre.com

Herbal Medicine

National Institute of Medical Herbalists
56 Long Street
Exeter
Devon EX4 6AH
01392 426022
http://www.btinternet.com/~nimh/

Homeopathy

Faculty of Homeopathy
Academic Department
The Glasgow Homeopathic Hospital
1053 Great Western Road
Glasgow G42 0XQ
0141 2111616
www.trusthomeopathy.org/faculty

Faculty of Homeopathy
15 Clerkenwell Close
London EC1R 0AA
0207 7566 7810
www.trusthomeopathy.org/faculty

Hypnosis

British Society of Experimental and Clinical Hypnosis
Hon Sec. Ann Williamson
Hollybank House
Lees Road
Mossley
Lancs OL5 OPL

British Society of Medical and Dental Hypnosis
National Office
17 Keppel View Road
Kimberworth
Rotherham
South Yorkshire S61 2AR

Massage

British Massage Therapy Council
Green Bank House
65a Adelphi Street
Preston PR1 7BH
01772 881063

Clare Maxwell-Hudson's Massage Training Centre
PO Box 457
London NW2 4BR
0208 4506494

Reflexology

Association of Reflexologists
27 Old Gloucester Street
London WC1 3XX
0207 237 6523

British School Reflex Zone Therapy of the Feet
23 Marsh Hall
Talisman Way
Wembley Park
London HA9 8JJ
0208 904 4825

British Reflexology Association
Monks Orchard
Whitbourne
Worcester WR6 5RB
01886 212707

Shiatsu

British Shiatsu Council
121 Sheen Road
Richmond
Surrey TW9 1YJ
0208 852 1080

Shiatsu Society
Barber House
Storeys Bar Road
Fengate
Peterborough PE1 5YS
01733 758 341
www.shiatsu.org.uk

Music therapy

British Society for Music Therapy
Roehampton Institute
Digby Stuart College
Roehampton Lane
London SW15 5PU

Useful peer reviewed journals

Complementary Therapies in Nursing and Midwifery
Churchill Livingstone, Edinburgh

Complementary Therapies in Medicine
Churchill Livingstone, Edinburgh

Focus on Alternative and Complementary Therapies (FACT)
Pharmaceutical Press, Oxon

Appendix 3

USEFUL WEB SITES

A number of websites have been identified as of use for information about and evaluation of CAM.

OMNI (Organised Medical Network Information) gateway provides free access to internet sites covering health and medicine
http://omni.ac.uk

General web sites include:

The Cochrane Library
http://www.cochrane.org

The Research Council for Complementary Medicine
http://www.rcm.org.uk

The Prince of Wales Foundation for Integrated Medicine
http://www.fimed.org

The National Centre for Complementary and Alternative Medicine (NCCAM)
http://nccam.nih.gov/nccam/databases.html

Complementary Therapies in Nursing and Midwifery
http://www.harcourt-international.com/journals/ctnm

AMED (Alternative and Allied Medicine Database)
(available in NHS libraries)

Cinahl (Cumulative Index to Nursing and Allied Health Literature)
(Available in NHS libraries)

FACT from Exeter
http://www.ex.ac.uk/FACT/

HerbMed
http://www.herbmed.org

Foundation for Traditional Chinese Medicine
http://www.rscom.com/tcm

Index

A

abdominal massage *see* massage
academic performance, PMS 168
accumulation, Ayurvedic disease
    stage 18
acne 177–180
  academic functioning 178
  acupuncture 180
  Anthroposophical medicine 179
  antimicrobials 178, 179
  aromatherapy 178
  Ayurvedic medicine 179
  Bach flower remedies 180
  body image 177–178
  conventional treatment 178
  diet 179–180
  forgotten disease 178
  herbalism 179
  homeopathy 180
  PMS exacerbation 169
  scarring 178
  stress association 177
  TCM 179–180
Aconite 54
  acute respiratory distress 66
  emergency department 118
  epilepsy treatment 124
  headaches 87
  sleep disorders, children 72
  wounds 143
Acts of Parliament 41–43
acupressure *see* massage
acupuncture
  acne 180
  analgesia 83
  asthma treatment 64–65
  Cochrane initiative 199
  colds and allergic rhinitis 58
  depression 155–156
  diabetes 104
  disease prophylaxis 52
  dysmenorrhoea 173
  eczema treatment 137
  efficacy investigation problems
    35–36, 36–37
  electro-needling 122–123
  endorphins 83, 199
  epilepsy 122–123
  hyperactivity 128
  hypoglycaemic effects 105
  insomnia treatment 73
  meridians 13
  migraine 89

  mobility problems 119
  multiple sclerosis 119
  nausea and vomiting
    chemotherapy 100
    postoperative 98–100
  neurotransmitters released 83
  nightmares treatment 73
  obesity 189–190
  pain in children 82–83
  PMS 169
  points, massage *see* massage,
    acupressure
  psoriasis 181–182
  Qi flow enhancement 13
  serotonin levels 73
  sham/placebo 36, 58, 199, 202
  small children adaptation 15
  smoking 198–199
  upper respiratory tract conditions
    58
acute respiratory distress 66–67
addictions (adolescents)
  behaviour 196
  health promotion 196–197
  interventions used 198–204
  models of 197–198
  see also alcohol abuse; drug
    abuse; smoking
addresses, organizations 210–213
  (Appendix)
adolescents
  body image *see* body image
  CAM usage, reasons for 148
  development 147–148
  health care needs 148–149
  lazy misdiagnosis 130
  nurses role 148–149, 196–197
  rebellion 148
  stereotype 151
  see also specific topics
adulteration, risks 10
agar, constipation 112
Agaricus muscarius, psoriasis 182
agnus castus
  acne 179
  dysmenorrhoea 174
  PMS 170
Agrimony, eczema 140
agrimony, hypoglycaemic effects 104
alcohol
  herbal sedatives, therapeutic
    enhancement 163
  restriction 162
alcohol abuse 201
  Bach flower remedies 201

  herbalism 201
  models for 198
  TCM 201
Alexander technique, mobility
    difficulties 120
allantoin 141
allergens
  chamomile 64
  compositae family 64
  desensitisation 56
  elimination 56–57
  in the home 56
  house dust mites *see* house dust
    mite allergens
  TCM herbs for 58
allergic asthma *see* asthma
allergic rhinitis (children) 55–57
  acupuncture 58
  Anthroposophical medicine 56
  antihistamine reduction 56
  aromatherapy 56–57
  herbalism 56
  homeopathy 55–56
  population statistics 55
  symptoms 55
allergies, diagnostic tests 95–96
almond, antibacterial properties 51
aloe vera
  gel 142
  psoriasis 181
  wounds 142
altered body image 134, 144
Alumia, eczema treatment 137
Amalaki 18
  acne 179
American Cancer Society, diet
    review 96–97
American Psychological Association,
    agnus castus 170
Amerlaki, acne 179
amrit kalash 53
anaesthesia
  herbal effect 28
  hypnosis 81, 139, 144
  postoperative vomiting *see* nausea
    and vomiting
  reflexology effect 27
  sweet orange oil, recovery
    characteristics 75
  see also pain (children)
angelica
  antibacterial properties 51
  headaches 89
animal bites 143
animal magnetism 19

anorexia nervosa 185–187
  aetiology 185
  Bach flower remedies 187
  cross over disorder 188
  epidemiology 186
  family factors 185
  homeopathy 187
  hypnosis 187
  massage 186–187
  music therapy 187
  symptoms 186
  t'ai chi and yoga 187
Anthroposophical medicine 15–17
  acne 179
  allergic rhinitis treatment 56
  asthma treatment 64
  astral body 16
    massage effect 25
    pain theory 84, 143
    sleep withdrawal 76
    social sense development 48
  body reshaping 48, 54
  burns 143
  Camphill communities 120
  colds 54–55
  cosmic influences 16
  depression 156
  developmental stages
    adolescence 148
    children 16–17, 48
  drug abuse 203–204
  eczema 136–137
  efficacy evaluation 38
  ego 16
    connection 48
    drug addicts 203–204
    inflammation 84–85, 143
    sleep withdrawal 48
  elements, human relationship 16
  enuresis 116
  eurythmy 121
  four body system 16
  history 15–16
  illness and soul development 17
  liver see liver
  massage 25
  migraine remedy 89
  music 29
  organization 210 (Appendix)
  pain in children 84–85
  past lives and past deeds 120
  philosophy 15–16
  predestination concept 120
  psoriasis 182
  range of interventions 16
  seven year cycles 16–17, 48
  skin 136–137
  sleep disorders
    adolescents 166
    children 76
  three main systems 16
  trained practitioners 17
    survey on use and
      evaluation 38
  treatment 16
  wounds 143

antibiotics
  advent 4–5
  nicotinamide gel 178
  reduction with cranberry juice,
    cystitis 192
  resistant pathogens 140, 141
  upper respiratory tract conditions,
    inappropriate use 49–50
anticoagulation therapy, St John's
    wort contraindication 152
antifungal properties, essential oils
    52
antimicrobial properties
  aromatherapy essential oils 51–52
  herbal preparations
    acne 179
    respiratory infections 51
    wound infections 140–141,
      142
Antimonium crudum, acne 180
antimony, eczema treatment 137
antiseptic oils 52
antiviral properties, herbs 50–51
anxiety see stress and anxiety
apigenin, sedative properties 75
Apis. mel, cystitis 192
Apis, pain relief 84
apple diet 179
apple juice, diarrhoea 113
Argentum nit
  anorexia nervosa 187
  IBS 194
  motion sickness 102
Arnica, wounds 143
aromatherapy/essential oil(s) 24–25
  acne 178
  administration 24, 25
  allergic rhinitis 56–57
  antimicrobial properties 51–52
  blood pressure changes 154
  breathing problems (children)
    51–52
  burns discrepancy 140
  cerebral palsy 119
  citrus fragrance effect 153–154
  constipation 112
  constituents 24
  depression 153–154
  diarrhoea 114
  dysmenorrhoea 174
  eczema 135–136
  epilepsy 121–122
  evidence for efficacy 25
  history 24
  IBS 193–194
  massage efficacy 25
  mood profiling 154
  organizations 211 (Appendix)
  pain in children 85
  patented inhalations 51
  PMS 168
  safety see safety issues
  sleep disorders
    adolescents 165–166
    children 74–76
  smoking 200

wounds 140
  see also specific types
arrow, acute respiratory distress 66
Arsen. alb
  IBS 194
  safety 71
  sleep disorders, children 71
artichoke, alcohol dependence 201
artificial somnambulism 19
asanas see yoga
asthma 58–66
  Anthroposophical medicine 64
  Ayurvedic medicine 61–62
  emotions/mood 58, 59, 64
  exercise-induced 65
  herbalism 63–64
  homeopathy see homeopathy
  hypnosis see hypnosis
  incidence 58
  massage 60
  pranayama 62
  psychological factors 58–59
  reflexology 65–66
  TCM 64–65
  TM 62
  yoga 62
astral body see Anthroposophical
    medicine
attention deficit disorder (ADD)
    124
  see also hyperactivity
attention deficit hyperactivity
    disorder (ADHD) 124–125
  see also hyperactivity
auricular stud 190
Avena Sativa, sleep aid 76, 166
ayur 17
Ayurvedic medicine 17–19
  acne 179
  affective disorders 156–157
  asthma treatment 61–62
  Ayurveda concept 17–18
  breathing problems 53
  constipation 110
  depression 156–157
  diabetes 103
  diet see diet
  disease process stages 18
  disease prophylaxis 53
  doshas 17–18
    anxiety and depression
      156–157
    balancing see diet(s)
    daily predominance 74
    dominance and illness tendency
      18
    illness propensity 61
    kapha definition 18
    obstruction 61
    pain involvement 83
    pitta definition 18
    pranayama type dictation 62
    sleep patterns 74
    vata definition 18
    see also kapha; pitta; vata
  dreams 74

drug abuse 201–202
dysmenorrhoea 174
epilepsy 123–124
evidence for efficacy 19
exam stress 157, 158
five elements 17
headaches 89
hyperactivity 126–128
    additive elimination 127
    oily food 127
    pancha karma 128
    pita type and vata type 127
    pranayama breathing 128
massage see massage
menses and purification 171
mobility problems 120
organization 210 (Appendix)
pain classification 83–84
pain in children 83–84
philosophy 17–18
PMS 171
primordial energy 17
psoriasis 182
sleep disorders
    adolescents 165
    children 74
smoking 201
three vital energies 17–18
treatment 18–19
vital energy 5, 6
wounds 142
yoga see yoga

B

babies
    massage effect 105
    sleep pattern 70
    unsettled 71
    weight gain 105–106
Bach, Dr Edward 22–23
Bach flower remedies 22–24
    acne 180
    alcohol abuse 201
    anorexia nervosa 187
    depression 153
    dispensing 23
    distillation methods 23
    eczema 139–140
    emergency department 118
    emotional rebalancing 22, 23
    energy imprinting on water 23
    enuresis 116
    epilepsy treatment 124
    evidence for efficacy 24
    history 22–23
    obesity 190
    patient empowerment 22–23
    personality plasticity 23
    philosophy 22–23
    PMS 168
    prescription 23
    Rescue Remedy see Rescue
        Remedy

safety 10
sleep disorders in adolescents 165
backward bend asana 165
Baihui point 73
Balder 152
Balsamicum ointment, eczema
    treatment 137
barbiturates 164
bay, antibacterial properties 51
bed wetting see enuresis
Beech, PMS 168
bee products see honey; propolis
Belladonna
    dysmenorrhoea 174
    enuresis 115
    headaches 87
    pain relief 84
    sleep aid 76, 166
benzoate preservatives 125
benzodiazepine
    brahmighritham vs 123
    valerian vs 164
benzoyl peroxide 178
bergamot, depression 153
bergamot oil, PMS 168
beta-glucuronidase injections,
    hyperactivity 126
bibhitaki 18
Bidor, migraine remedy 89
biomedical system, philosophy 5, 6
bitter orange oil see neroli oil
bittersweet, alcohol dependence 201
black pepper, smoking cessation
    200
Blackthorne, asthma treatment 64
blood, TCM terms 13
    stagnant, in pain 82
blood pressure, changes with
    essential oils 154
boat asana 62
body image (adolescents)
    acne 177–178
    anorexia nervosa 185
    sexuality 167, 190
body image (children)
    eczema 134
    wounds/burns 144
Boschma, holism definition 7
Bourbon geranium oil, fungistatic
    activity 56
bow asana 62
brahmighritham, epilepsy control
    123
breathing exercises see pranayama
breathing problems (children)
    49–69
    see also asthma; upper respiratory
        tract conditions
breath of fire asana 62
bronchitis, yoga positions 62
bronchodilators, hypnosis, reduction
    59
Bryonia
    colds 54
    constipation 112
    headaches 87–88

bulimia nervosa 188
    hypnosis 188
burdock, hypoglycaemic effects 104
burn(s) (children)
    Anthroposophical medicine 143
    aromatherapy discrepancy 140
    debridement 144
    herbalism 141
    patients
        hypnosis 82, 143–144
        massage 144
        music therapy 144
    see also wound(s)

C

calamus root
    anticonvulsive properties 123
    Cree tribe usage 123
    kapha stimulation 61
Calc. phos, dysmenorrhoea 174
calcium, dysmenorrhoea 172
calendula
    burns 143
    eczema treatment 137
Californian poppy, drug dependency
    203
CAM
    effectiveness see clinical
        effectiveness
    history 4
    integration, evidence base
        39–40
    nurses see nurse(s)/nursing
    philosophy 5–8
        individual responsibility 7
    therapies/interventions
        classification 3, 12–29
        groups 3
        range practiced, UK estimate 3
    usage 4–5
        client assessment tool 209
            (Appendix)
        emergency department see
            emergency department
        ethnic groups 4
        NHS vs private sector 7–8, 40
        parental reasons for 8, 148
Camphill communities 120
camphor, antibacterial properties
    51
Cancer Act, unsubstantiated claims
    41–42
cancer diets 96–97
Candida, cinnamon effect 52
Candida albicans 52, 174
Cantharis, cystitis 192
cascara, constipation 112
castor-oil enemas 96
Causticum, enuresis 115
Centaury, alcohol dependence 201
cerasee, hypoglycaemic effects 104
cerebral palsy 119
CFS see chronic fatigue syndrome

chamomile/chamomile oil
  asthma treatment 63
  constipation 112
  depression 153
  diarrhoea 114
  dysmenorrhoea 174
  eczema 135–136
    vs hydrocortisone ointment
      138
  history of therapeutic use 63–64
  IBS 193
  insomnia 75
  oil distilling 75
  pain relief 85
  PMS 168
  postoperative nausea and
    vomiting 98
  Roman and German 75
  sedative activity and extracts 75
  sedative properties 75, 163
  stress and anxiety 158
  unsettled babies 71
Chamomilla
  diarrhoea 113
  unsettled babies 71
channels 13
Chemical Hazard Information and
    Packaging (CHIP) regulations
    12
chemotherapy, nausea and vomiting
    see nausea and vomiting
Cherry Plum 23
  PMS 168
Chestnut bud, obesity 190
child abuse, enuresis 114
children 8–10
  body image 134, 144
  CAM usage, parental reasons 8
  concerns 8–9
  development theories 47–48
  naturopathy risk 8–9
  oncology patients 8
  t'ai chi, TCM concept 15
  see also specific topics
Children Act (1989), appropriate
    treatment 42
children's oil 75
China remedy, diarrhoea 113
Chinese herbs, safety 10
chocolate, hyperactive children 126,
    127
chronic fatigue syndrome (CFS)
    129–131
  adolescents 'lazy' misdiagnosis
    130
  gender differences 130
  herbalism 130
  massage 131
  nutritional supplements 130
  prevalence 130
  symptoms 129
  TCM 131
chronic non-specific diarrhoea
    (CNSD) 112–113
  apple juice 113
chrysanthemum, headaches 89

chrysarobin 181
Cinnabaris, sinusitis remedy 57
cinnamon bark
    anti-allergy preparation 58
    antimicrobial properties 51, 52,
      61
citral oil, fungistatic activity 56
citronellol oil, fungistatic activity 56
citrus fragrance, depression 153
citrus oil
  depression 153
  hypersensitivity 12
Clematis 23
clindamycin gel, acne 178
clinical effectiveness 33–40
  evaluation criteria 34
  evidence-based practice 33–34
    definition 34
    emergence, reasons for 33
  evidential strength categories
    34–35
  human complexity 35
  integrating CAM 39–40
  legal issues see legal and
    professional issues
  miscellaneous approaches 37–39
  peer-reviewed journals 213
    (Appendix)
  proving mechanism 37–38
  publication bias 37
  randomised controlled trials
    35–36
  statistical significance 34
  systematic reviews 36–37
clinical supervision 40–41
clove, antibacterial properties 51
cobra asana 62, 165
coca cola, hyperactive children
    125–126, 127
cocaine dependency 202
Cocculus, motion sickness 102
Cochrane library 199, 200
Code of Professional Conduct
    (2002) 41
coenzyme Q, CFS treatment 130
Coffea cruda
  motion sickness 102
  sleep aid 164–165
Coffea tosta, sleep aid 76, 166
coffee
  enemas 96
  excessive ingestion 164–165,
    166
  restriction 162, 172
cold (TCM external force) 14
colds (children) 53–55
  acupuncture 58
  Anthroposophical medicine
    54–55
  herbalism 53–54
  homeopathy 54
combudoron, burns 143
comfrey
  protein containment 141
  toxicity 142
  wounds 141–142

communication problems
    (adolescents) see depression;
    stress and anxiety
compositae family, allergies 64
Conception vessel 13
Conners Teacher Rating Scale,
    hyperactivity 128–129
consent, legal and professional issues
    42
constipation (children) 109–112
  aromatherapy 112
  Ayurvedic medicine 110
  common occurrence periods 110
  conventional treatment 110
  herbalism 112
  homeopathy 112
  hypnosis 112
  incidence 109–110
  massage 111–112
  TCM 110–111
contraceptive pill, St John's wort 152
Control of Substances Hazardous to
    Health (COSHH) 12, 43
coriander
  antimicrobial properties 52
  hypoglycaemic effects 104
corpse asana 157, 165
cortisol levels, measurement 60,
    154, 158
corydalis
  drug dependency 203
  headaches 89
cosmic influences 16
  herbalism 27
cow's milk, hyperactivity 125
Crab apple
  acne 180
  anorexia nervosa 187
  depression 153
  eczema 139
  PMS 168
cramp bark, drug dependency 203
cranberry juice, cystitis 192
croton oil test 138
Culpeper, St John's wort 141, 152
cuttle fish 152
cypress oil, IBS 193
cystic fibrosis
  reflexology 65–66
  tea tree prophylaxis 52
cystitis 192–193
  cranberry juice 192
  Herbalism and aromatherapy 192
  homeopathy 192
  TCM 192–193

D

dairy products, hyperactivity 125
damp (TCM external force) 14
dandelion
  alcohol dependence 201
  diuretic 28
  hypoglycaemic effects 104

dark, fear of 71, 77
Data Protection Act 43
deadly nightshade, poisoning 84
Dead sea, psoriasis 183
deep sleep *see* non-rapid eye
    movement (NREM) sleep
Defensive Qi 64
deposition, Ayurvedic disease stage
    18
depression (adolescents) 151–157
    acupuncture 155–156
    Anthroposophical medicine 156
    aromatherapy 153–154
    Ayurvedic medicine 156–157
    Bach flower remedies 153
    classic symptoms 151
    conventional antidepressant
        similarity 152, 156
    cultural differences 154
    diet 157
    fluoxetine 151
    herbalism 151–152
    homeopathy 152–153
    hops contraindication 163
    hypersomnia in 162
    IBS and 193
    measuring 154
    mothers 105–106, 158
    pain perception 79
    paroxetine 151
    safety issues 152, 153, 163
    scales 154
    TCM 155–156
    women 156
    see also stress and anxiety
dermatology *see* burn(s); eczema;
    wound(s)
development
    adolescence 147–148
    childhood 47–48
development theories, children
    47–48
diabetes mellitus (children) 102–105
    Ayurvedic medicine 103
    CAM, long term use 102–103
        types uses 103
    herbalism 104
    incidence 102
    insulin dose reduction 104
    symptoms 102
    TCM 103–104
    type 1 102
    type 2 102
diarrhoea (0–11yrs) 112–114
    apple juice trigger 113
    aromatherapy 114
    causes 112–113
    fruit and milk induced 113
    green stools 113
    homeopathy 113
    psychological origin 114
    TCM 113
    toddlers occurrence 112
    watery stools 113
    see also chronic non-specific
        diarrhoea (CNSD)

diet(s)
    1 week apple diet 179
    acne 179–180
    additive exclusion 125–126, 127
    Ayurvedic dosha balancing
        asthma 61
        depression 157
        hyperactivity 127
        insomnia 74
        PMS 171
    CFS supplementation 130
    dangerous 96–97
    diarrhoea tendency 113
    dysmenorrhoea 172
    eating and drinking problems
        adolescents 185–191
        children 94–108
    food allergies, diagnostic tests
        95–96
    Gerson 96
    hyperactivity 125–126, 127
    legal considerations 42
    macrobiotic 97
    migraine precipitation 86
    obesity 189
    obesity and diabetes 102
        Chinese population 103
    PMS and nutrition 171, 172
    protein 157
    restrictive 96–97
    TCM 64, 97, 113
    vegetarian 127, 179
    zinc deficiency *see* zinc deficiency
Diplococcus pneumoniae
    respiratory infections 51
    rhinitis 56
dithranol 181, 182
doctor(s), Anthroposophical
    approach to illness 16–17
dog's mercury, eczema treatment
    137
doshas *see* Ayurvedic medicine
Douglas fir, stress and depression
    154
dreams
    Ayurvedic theory 74
    dominant dosha reflection 74
    spirit world 76
drug abuse (adolescents) 201–204
    Anthroposophical medicine
        203–204
    Ayurvedic medicine 201–202
    herbalism 203
    TCM 202–203
    yoga 203
dysmenorrhoea 172–174
    abdominal massage 174
    acupuncture 173–174
    approaches to treatment 172–173
    aromatherapy 174
    Ayurvedic medicine 174
    diet 172
    foot massage 173
    fruit and eggs 172
    herbalism 174
    homeopathy 174

over-the-counter analgesics 173
TCM 173–174

E

E. coli see Escherichia coli
earth
    developmental stages 48
    five element theory 14
earth apple 64
eating and drinking problems
    adolescents 185–191
        see also anorexia nervosa;
            bulimia nervosa; obesity
    children 94–108
        see also diabetes; nausea and
            vomiting
eating disorder inventory (EDI) 186
echinacea
    antibacterial properties 50
    CFS treatment 130
    immunostimulant properties 50
    immunosuppressed patients
        50–51
    origin 50
    respiratory tract infections 50–51
Echinacea augustifolia see echinacea
eczema (children) 135–140
    Anthroposophical medicine
        136–137
    aromatherapy 135–136
    Bach flower remedies 139–140
    CAM vs hydrocortisone 136, 138
    conventional treatments 135
    herbalism 138
    homeopathy 137
    hypnosis 139
    incidence 135
    itching 137
    itch/scratch/itch cycle 139
    liver synergy 136
    massage 138
    parental stress 135
    psychological factors 135, 136,
        139
    reflexology 139
    symptoms 135
    TCM 137–138
    UK diagnostic criteria 135
effectiveness *see* clinical effectiveness
ego
    strengthening
        asthma sufferers 59
        insomnia 77
    see also Anthroposophical
        medicine
elderflower
    antiviral properties 54
    colds 53–54
elimination problems
    adolescents *see* cystitis; irritable
        bowel syndrome
    children *see* constipation;
        diarrhoea; enuresis

Elm
　　alcohol dependence 201
　　anorexia nervosa 187
emergency department
　　hypnosis application 82, 143
　　integration 118
　　ventilated patient 66–67
emotions/mood
　　anxiety see stress and anxiety
　　asthma 58, 59, 64
　　Bach flower remedies 22, 23
　　constipation 111
　　depression see depression
　　eczema 135, 136, 139
　　lungs association 61
　　music 29
　　outburst control 129
　　pain perception 80
　　PMS 168
　　problems, acupuncture for 73
　　profiling 154
　　TCM philosophy 155
endorphins
　　acupuncture 83, 199
　　massage 80
enemas
　　constipation 110
　　safety issues 96
energy imprinting, water
　　Bach flower remedies 23
　　homeopathy 21
enuresis (children) 114–116
　　Anthroposophical medicine 116
　　bladder signals 114
　　dreaming 115
　　effects of 114
　　herbalism 115
　　homeopathy 115
　　hypnosis 115
　　incidence 114
　　nocturnal behaviour 114
　　presentation 114
　　　remedy identification 115
　　reflexology 115–116
　　TCM 116
EPD injections, hyperactivity 126
ephedra see ma-huang
epilepsy (children)
　　aromatherapy 121–122
　　auto-hypnosis 121–122
　　ayurvedic medicine 123–124
　　electro-acupuncture 122–123
　　grand mal and petit mal 121
　　ground ivy contraindications 56
　　herbalism 123
　　homeopathy 124
　　patients' essential oil preference 122
　　precipitation 121
　　prevalence 121
　　Sahaja yoga 123–124
　　seizures 121, 122, 123
　　smell memory 121
　　TCM 122–123
Epstein–Barr, CSF implication 129
Equistium, enuresis 115
Erikson's developmental stages 47–48
Erysidoron 179

Escherichia coli
　　cystitis 192
　　respiratory infections 50, 51, 52
　　wounds 141, 142
Essence 13
essential oils see aromatherapy/ essential oil(s)
etheric body 16
　　maternal connection 48
ethnic groups, usage 4
eucalyptus oil, house dust mite allergens 57
euphorbia, asthma treatment 63
eurythmy, Anthroposophical medicine 121
evidence-based practice see clinical effectiveness
Ewin, Dabney 82, 143

F

family issues
　　acne 177
　　anorexia 185
　　circumstances and hyperactivity 126, 127
　　depressed mothers and baby growth 105–106
　　development
　　　adolescent 148
　　　childhood 48
　　enuresis and child abuse 114
　　obesity 189
　　reasons for CAM usage 8, 148
　　sleep disorders effect 71
Ferrum phos, colds 54
feverfew
　　headaches 86–87, 89
　　migraine 86–87
fire
　　developmental stages 48
　　five element theory 13–14
fish posture 62
five element theory see Traditional Chinese Medicine
flint, sinusitis remedy 57
fluoxetine 151
fruitarian diet, legal considerations 42

G

Gallae halepenses, psoriasis 182
garlic, antibacterial properties 61
gate control theory 82
Gelsemium
　　colds 54
　　motion sickness 102
　　sleep disorders, children 72
Gencydo
　　allergic rhinitis 56
　　asthma treatment 64
genital herpes 174

Gentian
　　acne 180
　　alcohol dependence 201
　　eczema 139–140
　　obesity 190
geraniol, fungistatic activity 56
geranium oil
　　antibacterial properties 51
　　fungistatic activity 56
　　PMS 168
German commission E monographs 50
　　chamomile 75
　　feverfew 87
　　marshmallow 53
Gerson diet 96
ghee, wounds 142
Gillick competent children 42
ginger
　　anti-allergy preparation 58
　　baths 127
　　headaches 89
　　hypoglycaemic effects 104
　　motion sickness 101–102
　　postoperative nausea and vomiting 98
ginseng
　　CFS treatment 130
　　gypsum combination, hypoglycaemic effects 103–104
glove anaesthesia 81, 139
golden rod, allergic rhinitis 56
golden seal, allergic rhinitis 56
Gorse, depression 153
Governor vessel 13
grape vine, eczema treatment 136–137
Graphites
　　constipation 112
　　eczema treatment 137
ground ivy
　　allergic rhinitis 56
　　epilepsy contraindications 56
guava, hypoglycaemic effects 104
guided visualisation
　　nausea and vomiting, chemotherapy 100–101
　　unconscious patients 66
gynaecological infections, adolescents 174
gypsum
　　ginseng combination, hypoglycaemic effects 103–104
　　sleep disorders, children 72

H

Haemophilus influenzae, respiratory infections 49, 51
Hahnemann, Samuel 20–21, 137
hair analysis, allergy testing 95
half wheel asana 62

Hamilton rating scale for depression
  acupuncture 156
  citrus fragrance effect 154
Ham-Ying (1993), holism definition 7
haritaki 18
hart's tongue, alcohol dependence 201
hay fever *see* allergic rhinitis
headache and migraine (children) 85–93
  accompanying symptoms 86
  acupuncture 89
  Anthroposophical medicine 89
  contributing factors 86
  coping style 86
  diet precipitation 86
  herbalism *see* herbalism
  hot and cold presentation 87
  hypnosis 90–91
  incidence 85
  reflexology 91
  TCM 88–89
  tension 85
headstand asana 62
heart
  conditions and contraindications 152, 163
  TCM sleep association 72, 155
    acupuncture points 72–73
Heart 6 73
Heart 7 72–73
heat (TCM external force) 14
Hepar. sulphuris calcareum, sinusitis remedy 57
Hepatodoron, eczema treatment 136–137
herb(s), shape and colour, therapeutic property reflection concept 141
herbalism 27–28
  acne 179
  alcohol abuse 201
  allergic rhinitis 56
  antimicrobials 51, 140–141, 142
  antivirals 50–51
  asthma treatment 63–64
  breathing problems 50–51
  burns 141
  CFS 130
  colds 53–54
  constipation 112
  depression 151–152
  diabetes 104
  diagnosis 28
  drug abuse 203
  dysmenorrhoea 174
  eczema 138
  enuresis 115
  epilepsy 123
  headaches and migraine 86–87
    back of head 88
    blurred vision 88
    emotional stress 87
    heat/cold exposure 87
    night 87–88
    right sided 88

history 27
  nausea and vomiting
    motion sickness 102
    postoperative 98
  nervous restoratives 163
  organization 211 (Appendix)
  PMS 170
  psoriasis 181
  remedies and classification 28
  safety 28
  sleep disorders in adolescents 163–164
  smoking 200
  stress and anxiety 158
  superstition 27
  synergism 28
  vital energy 5–6
  wound 140–142
  see also specific herbs
Herpes genitalis 174
Herpes virus, CSF implication 129
Herscu, epilepsy treatment 124
holism
  definition 6
    variations 7
  nursing and 7–8
  philosophy 6–8
holistic
  nursing 7
  term misuse 6
Holly, PMS 168
homeopathic interview 21
homeopathic pathogenic trial (HPT) 37
homeopathy 20–22
  acne 180
  allergic rhinitis 55–56
  anorexia nervosa 187
  asthma treatment 62–63
    constitutional type 62
  colds 54
  constipation 112
  cystitis 192
  depression 152–153
  diarrhoea 113
  dilution 21
  dosage 21
  dysmenorrhoea 174
  eczema treatment 137
  energy imprinting on water 21
  enuresis 115
  epilepsy 124
  evidence for efficacy 22
    proving mechanism 37–38
  healing process concept 22
  history 20–21
  hypoglycaemic effects 105
  IBS 194
  like treating like 20
  motion sickness 102
  obesity 190
  organizations 212 (Appendix)
  pain in children 84
  patient interview prior to 21
  philosophy 20–21
  PMS 169
  potencies 21, 22

prescription 21–22
  psoriasis 182
  remedy dispensing 22
  remedy imprinting 21
  safety 10
  sinusitis 57
  sleep disorders, children 71–72
  substances used 21
    extraction and preparation 21
  vital energy 5–6
  wounds 143
honey
  acne 180
  allergic rhinitis 56
  antimicrobial properties 140–141
    source and potency 141
  contaminants 141
  key ingredients 141
  monofloral 141
  Rescue Remedy 23
  standards for medicinal use 141
  wound care 140–141
    history 140
hop pillow 72
hops, sedative effect 76, 163, 166
horsetail, enuresis 115
Hospital Anxiety and Depression Score (HADS), acupuncture 156
house dust mite allergens
  aromatherapy preparation 55–56
  eucalyptus oil 57
  homeopathic preparation 55–56, 63
House of Commons Select Committee on Health, adolescent health needs 148–149
House of Lords Select Committee on Science and Technology 3
Human Rights Act 33
hyacinth, stress and depression 154
hyperactivity 124–129
  aromatherapy 129
  Ayurvedic medicine *see* Ayurvedic medicine
  Conners Teacher Rating Scale 128–129
  conventional treatment 125
  dairy foods 125
  EPD injections 126
  family circumstance 126, 127
  food additives 125–126
    exclusion diet 126
  herbalism 129
  hypnosis 129
  massage 127, 129
  pitta type and vata type 127
  Ritalin 125, 127
  structured lifestyle and daily routine 126, 127
  supplements 125
  symptoms 124
  vata provoking 126–127
  vegetarianism 127
  zinc deficiency 125–126
hypericum *see* St John's wort

hypnosis 19–20
  age-related susceptibility 20
  anaesthesia 81, 139, 144
  anorexia nervosa 187
  asthma therapy 59–60
    acute attacks 60
    underlying emotional aspects
      59
  bulimia nervosa 188
  burns 82, 143–144
  confidence gaining 20
  constipation 112
  eczema 139
  emergency room application 82,
    143
  enuresis 115
  epilepsy, smell memory 121–122
  explaining 20
  glove anaesthesia 81, 139
  headache and migraine 90–91
  history 19
  IBS 195
  imagery 82
  key aim 20
  nausea and vomiting
    chemotherapy 101
    postoperative 98
  obesity 189
  organizations 212 (Appendix)
  pain in children 81–82
    application techniques 81–82
  parental reassurance 20
  positive side effects 82
  safe place technique 76–77, 163
  safety 11
    acute asthma attack 60
  sleep disorders
    adolescents 163
    children 76–77
  smoking 199–200
  surgery and 19
  trance concept 19
  trance equivalent state 82, 143

I

Ignatia
  depression 152
  motion sickness 102
illness, soul development 17
immunisation
  Anthroposophical avoidance 17
  TCM concept 15
immunity
  atopic vs non-atopic individual
    55
  echinacea effect 50–51
  rasayanas effect 53
immunosuppressed patients,
  echinacea use 50–51
Impatiens
  obesity 190
  PMS 168
imported herbs, safety 10

Indian cluster bean, hypoglycaemic
  effects 104
Indian herbs, safety 10
Indian tobacco see lobelia
infection(s), respiratory,
  aromatherapy for 51–52
inflammation 84–85
insomnia see sleep disorders
Internet prescriptions 9
iris, migraines 88
Irish Medical Board, ban on St
  John's wort 152
irritable bowel syndrome (IBS)
  193–195
  aromatherapy 193–194
  homeopathy 194
  hypnosis 195
  TCM 194
isocones 72, 73, 166
isoprenaline, tylophora vs asthmatics
  61

J

Jing 13, 128
journals, peer-reviewed 213
  (Appendix)

K

Kali. brom
  acne 180
  sleep disorders, young children 72
Kamillosan cream, eczema treatment
  136
kapha
  asthma 61
  definition 18
  excess, in pain 83
  headache 89
  pranayama type in asthma 62
  see also ayurvedic medicine,
    doshas
karela, hypoglycaemic effects 104
Kidney 6 (in TCM) 73
kidneys, TCM function 64
kinesiology, allergy testing 95
Klebsiella pneumoniae
  respiratory infections 51
  wounds 142
Kleine–Levin syndrome 162
Knightia excela 141
Kutaj, acne 179
Kutaj bark, acne 179
kut root, epilepsy control 123

L

lactobacilli, Anthroposophical
  lifestyle 54–55

Larch, acne 180
laurel, antibacterial properties 52
lavender oil
  anticonvulsive properties 122
  burns 140
  constipation 112
  depression 153
  diarrhoea 114
  dysmenorrhoea 174
  IBS 193
  pain relief 85, 90
  sedative properties 74–75,
    165–166
laxatives, constipation 110, 112
Ledum, puncture wounds 143
legal and professional issues 41–43
  accountability 41
  advertising when unqualified
    41–42
  consent 42
  enemas for children 110
  nutrition 42
  orthodox treatment rejection 42
  regulating bodies 43
  unsubstantiated claims 41–42
lemon balm
  asthma treatment 63
  melancholy 63
  sedative properties 76, 163
lemongrass, antifungal properties
    52
lemon oil, depression 153
leopard's bane, burns 143
leukaemia, echinacea use 51
licorice
  anti-allergy preparation 58
  antimicrobial properties 61
  hypoglycaemic effects 104
  kapha stimulation 61
  wounds 142
lime blossoms, sedative effects 165
lime flowers
  asthma treatment 63
  cardiac patients contraindication
    163
  cardiovascular conditions 64
  sedative effect 163
linseed, constipation 112
liver
  aloe vera tonic 142
  Anthroposophical medicine
    organ of life theory 156
    skin correlation 136–137
  bile stimulation diet 96
  toxicity, comfrey 142
Liver-Qi
  deficiency 111
  definition 13
    see also Traditional Chinese
      Medicine
  stagnation 169
lobelia
  asthma treatment 63–64
  safety 63
  smoking cessation 200
lotus asana 157

lovage, antibacterial properties 51
lucid sleep 19
Lung-Qi 13
    see also Traditional Chinese
        Medicine
lungs
    emotion association 61
    skin correlation 137
    therapeutic vomiting for
        congestion 61
    vulnerability stage 48
lychee, hypoglycaemic effects 104
Lycopodium
    cystitis 192
    depression 152
    migraines 88

M

macrobiotic diet, legal
        considerations 42
macrobiotic diets 97
magnesium
    dysmenorrhoea 172
    intramuscular, CFS treatment 130
Maharishi Ayurveda (MAV) 17
ma-huang
    anti-allergy preparation 58
    asthma treatment 63, 65
    safety 63
MAK 4/MAK 5 53
Malvae comp. tea 166
mandarin oil, eczema 135–136
manifestation, ayurvedic disease
        stage 18
Manuka honey 141
MAOI 152, 163
marigold, eczema treatment 137
marjoram
    antibacterial properties 51
    headache/migraine relief 90
marjoram oil, dysmenorrhoea 174
Marquis de Chastenet de Puységur
        19
marshmallow plant, colds 53
massage 25–26
    abdominal 25, 111–112, 174
    acupressure
        childhood sleep disorders
            72–73
        isocones 72, 73, 166
        meridians 13
        motion sickness 101
        obesity 190
        over the counter kits 72
        postoperative nausea and
            vomiting 98–100
        Qi flow enhancement 13, 25
    adolescents 158
    anorexia nervosa 186–187
    anxiety reduction *see* stress and
        anxiety
    asthma treatment 60
    astral body effect 25

Ayurvedic medicine 120, 127, 174
    children 25
    babies 105
    burns patients 144
    cerebral palsy 119
    CFS 131
    constipation 111–112
        benefits 111
    dysmenorrhoea 173, 174
    eczema 136
    endorphin levels 80
    epilepsy 121
    foot for dysmenorrhoea 173
    headaches 90
    hyperactivity 127, 129
    hypoglycaemic effects 105
    intensive care units 66
    mobility problems 120
    neonates and weight gain
        105–106
    nursing 26
    organizations 212–213
        (Appendix)
    pain in children 80–81
    PMS 168–169
    Rolfing 26
    serotonin levels 80
    stress reduction *see* stress and
        anxiety
    systems 26
    techniques 26
    Tui Na *see* Tui Na (TCM child
        massage)
ME *see* chronic fatigue syndrome
medical competence 11
Melaleuca alternifolia 52
mentals, homeopathy 21
meridians *see* Traditional Chinese
        Medicine
Mesmer, Anton 19
metal
    developmental stages 47
    five element theory 14
methicillin resistant staphylococcus
        aureus (MRSA) 140
methotrexate, psoriasis 181
methylphenidate hydrochloride 125
migraine *see* headache and migraine
Mimulus, anorexia nervosa 187
MIND charity, depression and
        culture 154
Minor Blue Dragon, anti-allergy
        preparation 58
misdiagnosis danger 11
mistletoe, hypoglycaemic effects
        104
mobility and movement 118–133
    abnormal 121–129
    chronic fatigue syndrome *see*
        chronic fatigue syndrome
    epilepsy *see* epilepsy
    hyperactivity *see* hyperactivity
    limited 118–121
    special needs 119
modalities, homeopathy 21
models of change 197

monoamine oxidase inhibitor
        (MAOI) 152, 163
monocytes, echinacea effect 50
monoterpenes 24
mood profiling, aromatherapy 154
motion sickness *see* nausea and
        vomiting
movement problems *see* mobility
        and movement
MRSA 140
muguet, depression 154
multiple sclerosis, acupuncture for
        119
music therapy 28–29
    anorexia nervosa 187
    burns patients 144
    feeling expression 29
    history 28–29
    nausea and vomiting,
        chemotherapy 100–101
    organization 213 (Appendix)
    pain in children 85
    physical changes 29
    ventilated patient 66–67
Mustard
    acne 180
    depression 153
    PMS 168
Mycobacterium tuberculosis,
        respiratory infections 49
myrrh, wound care, history 140

N

narcolepsy 162
Nat. mur
    anorexia nervosa 187
    colds 54
    depression 152
    PMS 169
National Heart and Lung Institute,
        propolis research 51
natural killer (NK) cells, echinacea
        effect 50
natural therapies, side effects
        misconception 10
naturopathy, paediatric risk 11
nausea and vomiting (children)
        98–102
    chemotherapy 100–101
        acupuncture and acupressure
            (TCM) 100
        guided imagery 100–101
        hypnosis 101
    motion sickness 102
        acupressure 101
        herbalism 102
        TCM 101
    postoperative 98–100
        acupuncture and acupressure
            98–100
        herbalism 98
        hypnosis 98
        TCM 98–100

neonates *see* babies
neroli oil
  anxiety reduction 66
  depression 153
  diarrhoea 114
  IBS 193
  sedative effects 75, 165
nervous restoratives 163
nettle
  burns 143
  hypoglycaemic effects 104
New Zealand honey 141
Nicotiana, asthma treatment 64
nicotinamide, acne 178
nightmares (children)
  occurrence 71
  treatment 72, 73, 77
non-rapid eye movement (NREM)
    sleep
  definition 70
    children vs adults 71
  serotonin effect 73, 81
nosods 55
nurse(s)/nursing
  abdominal massage 111–112
  adolescent health needs 148–149,
    196–197
  Anthroposophical approach to
    illness 16–17
  antibiotics, education 49–50
  aromatherapy oil on burns
    140
  assessment of evidential strength
    39
  CAM synergy 7
  chronic pain
    objectives 80
    problems 80
  clinical supervision 40–41
  codes of practice 41
  confusion issues 11, 140
  diabetic patients, considerations
    105
  evidential strength 39
    effective remedy 33
  holism and 7–8
  informed decisions 42
  integration 40
    development 43
  legal and professional issues *see*
    legal and professional issues
  massage 26
  models of change 197
  professional skills development
    40–41
  role 9–10
Nursing and Midwifery Council,
    professional issues 41
Nursing Times, massage
    recommendation 26
nut grass, epilepsy control 123
nutmeg oil, stress reduction 154
nutrition *see* diet
Nutritive Qi 64
Nux vomica
  constipation 112

sleep disorders
  adolescents 164
  children 72

O

oatmeal, psoriasis 181
oats 76, 166
  acne 180
obesity 188–190
  aetiology 188–189
  Bach flower remedies 190
  China occurrence 103
  definition 189
  food factors 189
  homeopathy 190
  hypnosis 189
  TCM 189–190
  type 2 diabetes 102
occupational dermatitis 12
opiate dependency 202, 203
Optivite 172
orange oil
  depression 153
  eczema 135–136
oregano, antimicrobial properties
    52
orthodox medicine
  advent 4–5
  adverse herbal interactions 11
  co-morbidity 5
  delay in seeking, safety issues 11
  integrating CAM 39–40
  rejection, legal issues 42
osmanthus, stress and depression
    154
over-the-counter (OTC) remedies
    3–4
  acupressure kits 72
  herbal 28
  homeopathic 21–22
  Irish Medical Board ban on St
    John's wort 152
  menstrual pain medication 173
  stress and anxiety 158
  tee tree oil 52
oyster shells, sinusitis remedy 57

P

paediatrics *see* children
pain (adolescents), period *see*
    dysmenorrhoea
pain (children) 79–93
  acupuncture 82–83
  analgesia
    inadequacy 79
    natural 80–81, 83
  Anthroposophical medicine
    84–85
  anxiety perception 79
  aromatherapy 85

Ayurvedic medicine 83–84
  types 83–84
clinical guideline for 80
depression perception 79
dimmer switch 82
emotions/mood 80
headache *see* headache and
    migraine
homeopathy 84
hypnosis 81–82
inflammation 84–85
massage 80–81
music therapy 85
myths 79–80
perception 79
  altering 81
  factors affecting 80, 81
  procedures identified, causing 80
  psychological factors 81
  TCM 82–83
  toleration vs adult 80
  transfer 82
  treatment *see specific therapies*
palm tree asana 62, 157
PAMs 11
Panax ginseng 130
pancha karma 18
  depression 157
  dysmennorhoea 174
  hyperactivity 128
pansy, eczema treatment 137
paroxetine 151
passiflora
  sedative effects 165
  stress and anxiety 158
passion flower, sedative properties
    76, 163
past lives and past deeds,
    Anthroposophical medicine
    120
pau pau, hypoglycaemic effects 104
peony, anti-allergy preparation 58
peppermint
  diarrhoea 114
  headache/migraine relief 90
  postoperative nausea and
    vomiting 98
peppermint oil, IBS 194
Pericardium 6
  anti-emetic properties 98–99, 100
  motion sickness 101
Pericardium 7 73
period pain *see* dysmenorrhoea
personality plasticity, Bach flower
    remedies 23
Peru balsam tree, eczema treatment
    137
phagocytosis enhancement
  echinacea 50
  propolis 51
phenols 12
Phlegm 111
Phos. ac, diarrhoea 113
Piaget's developmental stages 47, 48
pimento, antibacterial properties
    51

pitta
  definition 18
  dreams 74
  excess, in pain 83
  headache 89
  pranayama type in asthma 62
  see also Ayurvedic medicine,
    doshas
plough asana 62, 157
PMS see premenstrual syndrome
    (PMS)
prana, definition 6
pranayama
  asthma 62
  hyperactivity 128
Pre-Heaven Essense 15
premenstrual syndrome (PMS)
    168–176
  academic performance 168
  acupuncture 170
  aromatherapy 168
  Ayurvedic medicine 171
  Bach flower remedies 168
  dietary recommendations 171, 172
  herbalism 170
  homeopathy 169
  massage 168–169
  menstruation stages 169
  Optivite supplement 172
  reflexology 171–172
  sub-categories and symptoms 168
  TCM 169–170
Press Complaints Council 9
pressure sores 142
primordial energy, ayurvedic
    medicine 17
Prince of Wales Foundation for
    Integrated Health 40
probiotics 55
professions allied to medicine
    (PAMs) 11
Profile of Mood States 169
propolis
  gynaecological infections 174
  respiratory tract infections 51
  thrush 174
  topical use 141
  wounds 141
protein, mood effect 157
Proteus mirabilis, respiratory
    infections 50
Proteus vulgaris, respiratory
    infections 53
proving (homeopathy)
  arrow 66
  evidence for efficacy 37–38
  Psorinium 137
provocation, ayurvedic disease stage
    18
Pseudomonas aeruginosa
  respiratory infections 51, 52, 53
  rhinitis 56
  wounds 142
psoriasis (adolescents) 181–183
  acupuncture 181–182
  Anthroposophical medicine 182

Ayurvedic medicine 182
  conventional treatment 181
  Dead sea bathing 183
  herbalism 181
  homeopathy 182
  other interventions 183
  psychological interventions 182
  rice bran broth bathing 182
  stress association 177, 183
  TCM 181–182
  ultraviolet light 181
Psorinium, eczema treatment 137
psyllium seed, constipation 112
Pulsatilla
  allergic rhinitis 56
  anorexia nervosa 187
  cystitis 192
  dysmenorrhoea 174
  PMS 169
  sinusitis remedy 57
pulse reading, TCM diagnosis 14,
    155
pyrasidol-type antidepressants 156
pyridoxine, 157

Q
Qi (vital energy)
  deficiency 57, 82
  definition 13
  depression 155
  diarrhoea 113
  headaches 88
  nutrition and 97
  stagnant, in pain 82
  see also Liver-Qi; Traditional
    Chinese Medicine
Qigong
  asthma relief 65
  breathing, disease prophylaxis 53
  change of body image 144
  children 15
  definition 14
  enuresis 116
  history 13
  mobility problems 119–120
Quackwatch web site 126
Quartz 179
  psoriasis 182

R
randomised controlled trials
    35–36
  see also clinical effectiveness
rapid eye movement (REM) sleep
    70–71
  serotonin effect 73
rasayanas 53
Recognition and Assessment of
    Acute Pain in Children 80
Red Chestnut, sleep disorders 165

Red Cross Society, burns 140
reflexology 26–27
  advantages 27
  anaesthesia effect 27
  areas involved 26
  asthma 65–66
  body zones 26
  clinical competence 11
  diagnostic tool 26
  eczema 139
  enuresis 115–116
  headache 91
  healing crisis 115–116
  history 26
  hypoglycaemic effects 105
  meridians 13
  modern developments 27
  philosophy 26
  PMS 171–172
  reflex points 26, 27
  respiration problems 65–66
  sleep aid 74
  stress and anxiety 158
  zone therapy 65–66
rehmannia
  diabetes 103, 104
  TCM formulas 103
Rehmannia Eight Formula, diabetes
    103
Rehmannia Six Formula, diabetes
    103, 104
renal disease, ground ivy
    contraindications 56
Rescue Remedy
  acne 180
  components 23
  depression 153
Research Council for
    Complementary Medicine,
    clinical effectiveness studies
    39
respiratory disease, age-related
    vulnerability 49
  see also upper respiratory tract
    conditions
rhinitis, definition 55
rhubarb root, constipation 112
rice bran broth bathing, psoriasis
    182
Ritalin 125, 127
Rock Rose 23
Rock water, anorexia nervosa 187
Rolfing, massage technique 26
rosemary/rosemary oil
  antibacterial properties 52
  anticonvulsive properties 122
  depression 153
  PMS 168
  sedative properties 163
rose oil
  depression 153
  PMS 168
  sedative effect 165
  sexuality 168
rosewood, antifungal properties
    52

Royal College of Nursing
Complementary Therapy
Forum 7–8
Rubisan, psoriasis 182

S

safety issues 10–12
adverse effects
classification 11
confusion and conflicts 12
reporting system absence 12
Arsen. alb 71
calamus root 61
cardiac conditions 152, 163
comfrey 142
compositae family, anaphylactic
reactions 64
dangerous diets 96–97
deadly nightshade 84
depression 152, 153, 163
diabetic patients 105
enemas 96
essential oils 11–12, 24–25
epileptic seizure precipitation
121
Gerson diet 96
ground ivy 56
herbal sedatives 163, 164
hops 163
intervention appropriateness
11
lime flowers 163
lobelia 63
macrobiotic diet 97
ma-huang 63
paediatric concerns 8–9
passion flower 163
renal disease 56
St John's wort 152
sage
antibacterial properties 52
hypoglycaemic effects 104
Sahaja yoga, epilepsy 123–124
sandalwood oil, sedative properties
165
savory, antifungal properties 52
scarring, acne 178
Scleranthus, acne 180
Scope of Professional Practice (1992)
41
Sea Bands 99, 100, 101
seasonal affective disorder 157
selenium deficiency, CFS 130
self image 134
senna, constipation 112
Sepia, depression 152
serotonin
acupuncture 73, 83
baby stress levels, measuring
105
depression 156
pain in children, massage 81, 90
serotonin re-uptake inhibitor 152

sesame oil
dysmenorrhoea 174
mobility problems 120, 127
sesquiterpenes 24
sexuality expression (adolescents)
167–176
sham acupuncture 36, 58, 199, 202
Shen 13, 73, 155, 198
Shinpi-To 65
Shitatsu, organizations 213
(Appendix)
shooting pain 84
Short Form-36 (SF-36) 193
Siberian ginseng 130
Silica, constipation 112
Silicea
migraines 88
sinusitis remedy 57
silver, psychological shock 166
sinusitis 57
propolis role 51
Sishenchong point 73
skin, lungs correlation 137
skin conditions see acne; burn(s);
eczema; psoriasis; wound(s)
skin reactions 12
skullcap
antispasmodic properties 123
sedative properties 163
sleep
enhanced, fatigue symptoms 131
patterns 70–71
neonate 70
somatostatin release 81
sleep disorders (adolescents)
162–166
Anthroposophical medicine 166
aromatherapy 165–166
Ayurvedic medicine 165
Bach flower remedies 165
conditions to exclude 162
conventional medication 164
curtailing time spent in bed 162
exploring underlying problems
163
general approaches 162–163
getting off to sleep fear 163
herbalism 163–164
homeopathy 164–165
hypersomnia 162
hypnosis 163
isocones 166
orthodox sedative therapy 163
overactive mind 164
problems on the mind 165
sleep-maintenance insomnia 162
sleep-onset insomnia 162
stimulus control 162
TCM 166
yoga 165
sleep disorders (children) 70–78
acupressure 72–73
acupuncture 73
afraid of the dark 71, 77
Anthroposophical medicine 76
aromatherapy 74–76

Ayurvedic medicine 74
babies 71
diet 74
dyssomnias 71
early morning waking 72
effect on family 71
ego strengthening 77
foot massage 74
herbalism 75
homeopathy 71–72
hypnosis 76–77
nervous 76
night crying 73
nightmares see nightmares
night terrors 72, 77
over-stimulated/over-excited 72
pain interruption/perception 79
parasomnias 71
predisposing factors 71
reflexology 74
self-control 77
sleepwalking 72
talking in sleep 72
TCM 72–73
therapeutic interventions see
specific therapies
smoking 197–201
acupuncture 198–199
aromatherapy 200
Ayurvedic medicine 201
herbalism 200
hypnosis 199–200
reasons for 197
social theories 197–198
stress association 197–198
Smuts, Jan, Holism word history 6
soapwort, elderflower and, antiviral
properties 54
social economics 4
somatostatin, sleep release 81
special needs, movement limitation
119
Spillberger's anxiety score 158
Spleen-Qi 13, 64
deficiency 111
see also Traditional Chinese
Medicine
spread, Ayurvedic disease stage 18
Staphylococcus aureus
antibiotic resistant strains 140, 141
respiratory infections 49, 50, 51,
52, 53
wound infections 140, 141, 142
Star of Bethlehem 23
State Anxiety Scale 60
State Anxiety Scale for Children 60
State Trait Anxiety Inventory 169,
186
Steiner, Rudolph
philosophy 15–16
spirituality 76, 166
St John's Ambulance, burns 140
St John's wort
CFS treatment 130
colds 54
contraindications 152

Culpeper's description 141, 152
depression 151–152
elderflower and, antiviral
    properties 54
history of use 152
interactions with other drugs 152
Irish Medical Board ban 152
pain relief 84
PMS 170
sedative properties 163, 164
wounds 141, 152
Streptococcus faecalis, respiratory
    infections 51
Streptococcus pneumoniae,
    respiratory infections 49
Streptococcus pyogenes
    respiratory infections 51
    wounds 141
Streptococcus viridians, respiratory
    infections 51
stress and anxiety (adolescents)
    157–159
    acne 177
    Ayurvedic medicine 158–159
    herbalism 158
    IBS association 193
    massage 158
    measures 156, 158, 169
    psoriasis 183
    reflexology 158
    smoking association 197–198
    t'ai chi 159
    TCM 159
    yoga 158–159
    see also depression
stress and anxiety (children)
    epilepsy associated 123–124
    hypnosis management 81
    massage 60, 90
        babies 105
        CSF patients 131
        intensive care 66
    measures 60
    neroli oil, reduction 66
    pain perception 79
    school affairs, constipation 111
    sleep, children 71
    t'ai chi 129
sugar
    aloe vera 142
    white 126, 127
    wound care, history 140
suggestion susceptibility, hypnosis 19
Sulphur
    acne 179, 180
    constipation 112
    eczema treatment 137
    sleep disorders, children 72
sunbathing, psoriasis 183
Sunder vati, acne 179
sun method, Bach flower remedies
    23, 153, 168
Sunth, acne 179
superstition, herbalism 27
Supply of Goods and Services Act 43
Swedish massage 26

Sweet Chestnut, depression 153
sweet orange oil, anaesthesia
    recovery 75

T

Tabacum, motion sickness 102
t'ai chi
    anorexia nervosa 187
    anxiety
        adolescents 159
        children 129
    Form 159
    hyperactivity 128–129
    mobility problems 120
    respiratory conditions 65
tarragon, hypoglycaemic effects 104
tartrazine (E102) 125, 126
Tarunya Peetika, acne 179
TB, unsubstantiated claims 41
tee tree oil 52
    acne 178
    thrush 174
TENS intervention 131, 173–174
tetanus 143
thalidomide disaster 5
thrush 174
thyme
    antibacterial properties 51
    hypoglycaemic effects 104
thyme leaved gratiola, epilepsy
    control 123
tin, asthma treatment 61
tongue appearance, TCM diagnosis
    14
tonsillectomy, vomiting after,
    acupuncture 99
tonsillitis, propolis role 51
Traditional Chinese Medicine
    (TCM) 12–15
    accupuncture *see* acupuncture
    acne 179–180
    alcoholism 201
    asthma treatment 64–65
    bacterial infections 192
    CFS 131
    child characteristics 48
    cold (external force) 14
    constipation 110–111
    cystitis 192–193
    damp 14
    depression 155–156
    development
        adolescence 147
        childhood stages 15, 47, 48
    diabetes 103–104
    diagnostic process 14, 155
    diarrhoea 113
    diet 64, 97, 113
    disease prophylaxis 52–53
    drug abuse 202–203
    dysmenorrhoea 173–174
    eczema 137–138
    emotions 155

enuresis 116
epilepsy 122–123
evidence for efficacy 15
external forces, definition 14
five element theory 13–14
    abdominal massage 25
    behavioural influences 47
headache and migraine 88–89
heart *see* heart
heat 14
herbal prescription hierarchy
    14–15, 138
history 12–13, 15
hyperactivity 128–129
IBS 194
internal forces, definition 14
Jing 13, 128
liver *see* liver
massage treatment *see* massage,
    acupressure; Tui Na (TCM
    child massage)
menstruation stages 169
meridians 13
    acupuncture and acupressure
        usage 13, 25
    reflexology usage 26
mobility problems, limited
    movement 119–120
nausea and vomiting
    chemotherapy 100
    motion sickness 101
    postoperative 98–100
nutritional aspects 97
obesity 189–190
organizations 210–211
    (Appendix)
paediatrics use 15
pain in children 82–83
    causative factors 82
philosophy 13
PMS 169–170
psoriasis 181–182
Qi (vital energy), definition 13
Qigong treatment *see* Qigong
rice bran broth bathing 182
root of the tree (body) 173
seven emotions theory 155
Shen 13, 73, 155, 198
sleep disorders
    adolescents 166
    children 72–73
smoking 198–199
stress and anxiety 159
three treasures 13
tongue appearance diagnosis 14
treatment range 14
upper respiratory tract conditions
    57–58
vitalism concept 5–6
vulnerable organs 15, 48, 64
    pulse reading 14, 155
water stage 47–48
wood stage 48, 64, 111
Yin and Yang, definitions 13
    see also Yin and Yang
see also specific therapies

trance *see* hypnosis
transcendental meditation (TM)
    asthma 62
    drug abuse 201–202
trauma, hypnosis application 82
Trichomonas vaginalis 174
triphala 18
    constipation 110
    depression 157
tuberose, stress and depression
    154
Tui Na (TCM child massage) 15, 25
    diarrhoea 113
turmeric 61, 142
tylophora, isoprenaline vs,
    asthmatics 61

U

ulcers 141, 142
    see also wound(s)
Ullrich-Hodge Alternative Therapy
    Assessment Model 9–10
Ultimate Being, union 61–62
ultraviolet light, psoriasis 181
upper respiratory tract conditions
    (children) 53–58
    antibiotics, inappropriate use
        49–50
    aromatherapy patented
        inhalations 51
    superimposed infections 49
        leukaemia 51
    tea tree prophylaxis 52
    see also allergic rhinitis; colds;
        sinusitis
urinary tract infections *see* cystitis

V

valerian
    sleep aid 76, 163, 164, 166
    stress and anxiety 158
    vs benzodiazepine 164
vata
    definition 18
    dreams 74
    excess, in pain 83
    headache 89
    limited movement problems 120
    pranayama type in asthma 62
    see also Ayurvedic medicine,
        doshas

veda 17
vega test, allergies 95–96
vegetable juices, Gerson diet 96
vegetarian diet, hyperactivity
    treatment 127
ventilated patient 66–67
vervain, sedative properties 163
Vidanga, acne 179
viral infections
    CSFimplication 129
    echinacea for 50
visualisation techniques
    imagery for pain 82
    nausea and vomiting,
        chemotherapy 100–101
    night terrors 77
    ventilated patient 66
vital force 5–6
vitalism 5–6
vitamin B group 157

W

wakefulness, nocturnal, children 71
Walnut
    acne 180
    anorexia nervosa 187
    depression 153
    obesity 190
washing and dressing problems
    adolescents 177–184
        see also acne; psoriasis
    children 134–146
        see also burn(s); eczema;
            wound(s)
water hemlock, epilepsy treatment
    124
water stage (TCM) 47–48
websites 214 (Appendix)
wellbeing, philosophy 5
White Chestnut, sleep disorders 165
wild lettuce, sedative properties 163
Wild oat, acne 180
wild strawberry, eczema treatment
    136–137
Willow, acne 180
wind (TCM external force) 14
'winter disease, summer cure' theory
    15
Women's Precious Pills 173
wood stage (TCM) 48, 64, 111
wound(s) 140–143
    Anthroposophical medicine 143
    aromatherapy 140
    Ayurvedic medicine 142

    bee products for 140–141
    effective healing requirements
        144
    herbalism 140–142
    history of care 140
    homeopathy 143
    oil application discrepancy 140
    sepsis 140
    toxicity and comfrey 142
    ulcers 141, 142
    see also burn(s)

Y

Yellow Emperor's Inner Classic
    12–13
yellow jasmine *see* Gelsemium
Yin and Yang 13
    menstrual cycle 169
    nutrition and 97
    Yin deficiency
        constipation 111
        diabetes 103
    see also Traditional Chinese
        Medicine (TCM)
ylang ylang oil
    anticonvulsive properties 122
    depression 153
yoga 18
    anorexia nervosa 187
    asanas/positions 62, 157, 165
    asthma treatment 61, 62
    constipation aid 110
    depression 157
    drug abuse 203
    epilepsy 123–124
    glucose homeostasis 103
    headache treatment 89
    hyperactivity 128
    inducing sleep 74, 165
    respiratory conditions 61–62
    Sahaja 123–124
    stress and anxiety 158–159

Z

zinc deficiency
    CFS 130
    hyperactive children 125–126
    mental lethargy 157